NREMT STUDY GUIDE

LEARNIK

First edition, January 2025.

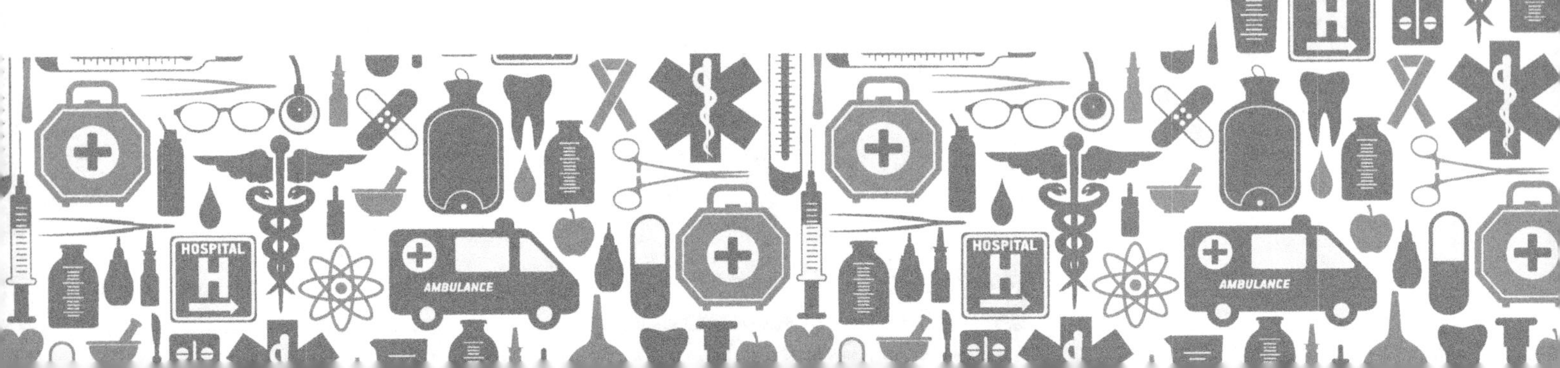

TABLE OF CONTENTS

TABLE OF CONTENTS

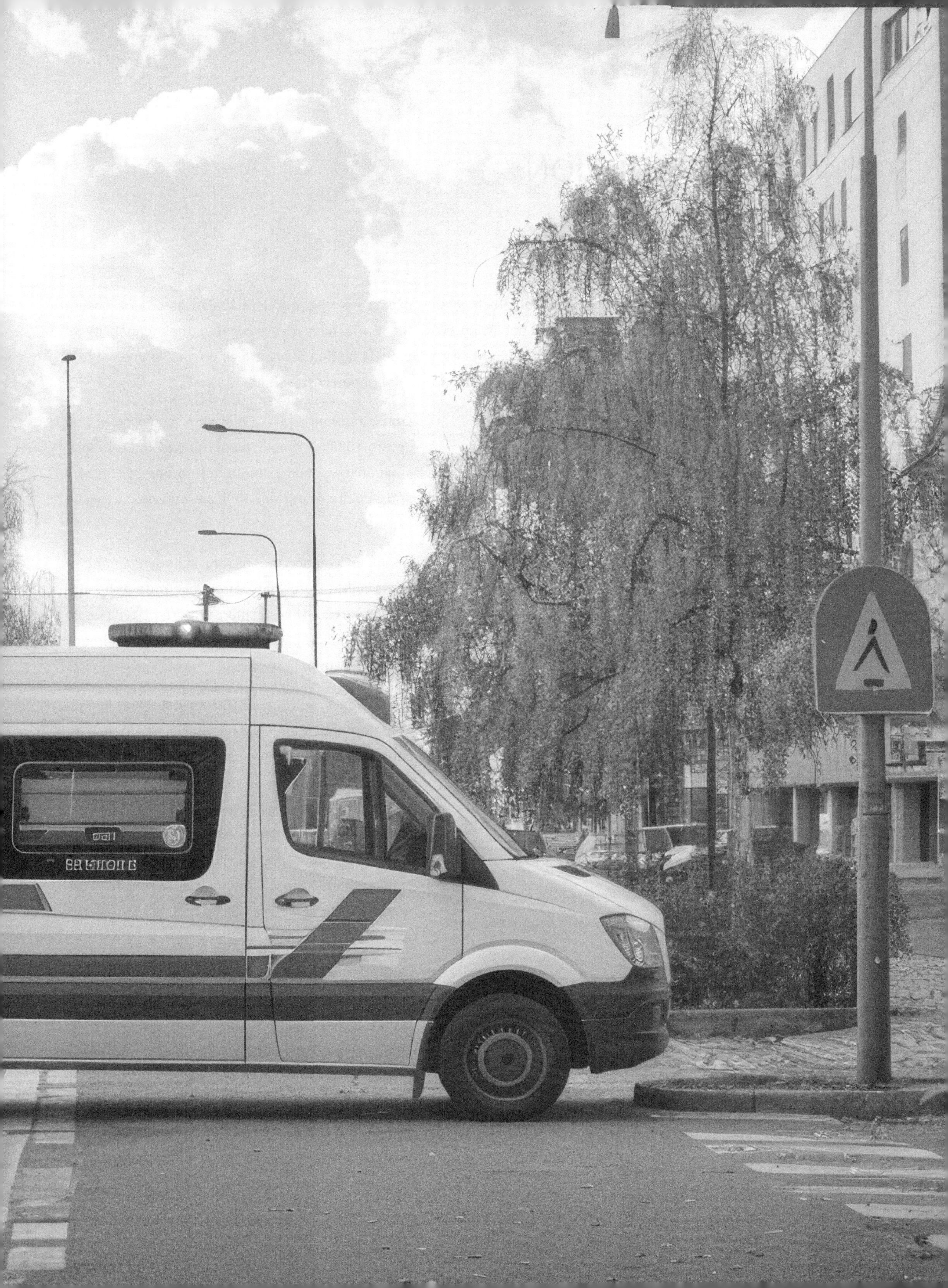

INTRODUCTION

Becoming an Emergency Medical Technician (EMT) is no small feat. It starts with achieving basic education requirements to equip aspirants with the skills needed for this high-pressure job. Anyone who dreams of becoming an EMT must first have a high school diploma or GED certificate. This education acts as a foundation, providing them with the essential skills that will later be fine-tuned through more specialized training programs.

Moreover, a government issued driver's license or identification will be required. Prospective EMTs must next secure CPR certification from reputable entities such as the American Red Cross or the American Heart Association. These courses teach essential life-saving skills, including one-person and two-person CPR, rescue breaths, and the use of an automated external defibrillator (AED).

Upon completion of CPR certification, individuals are required to register for an approved EMT course that provides comprehensive education on emergency medical procedures and state-sanctioned technology. This course imparts to learners both theoretical understanding and hands-on competency that are essential in actual emergency scenarios.

Certification is obtained after candidates pass two exams. The first is the NREMT cognitive exam—an all-encompassing computer-based test that tests knowledge in areas including, but not limited to: cardiology, trauma care, and respiration. The second is the psychomotor exam, a demonstration of mastery of essential emergency skills. These two exams are critical educational milestones to ensure the EMTs have demonstrated their capability to provide high-quality care when on site in emergency situations (Stevens, 2024).

Obtaining your EMT certification could grant you several fulfilling employment options. For example, you could work as a lifeguard to protect swimmers and acquire important first aid and water rescue expertise.

Health information technicians maintain patient records and ensure that data is accurate in healthcare settings. This position is perfect for people who appreciate handling paperwork and indirectly assisting with patient care.

In addition to performing fire rescues and mitigation, firefighters are fundamental in emergency response and critical medical care delivery. This job offers a combination of volunteer work and physical activities. Medical assistants assist healthcare providers with patient intake and examinations, combining patient care with administrative tasks, making them a great starting point for medical careers.

As a crucial conduit between the public and emergency services, emergency dispatchers are essential in channeling calls for assistance and organizing replies. This position requires one's ability to communicate and solve problems. Medical equipment service professionals provide a practical technical vocation in the healthcare sector by ensuring that medical equipment operates as intended.

In hospital emergency rooms, technicians help with patient monitoring and support medical staff. They also give indispensable treatment. This position is perfect for people who enjoy providing direct, high-pressure patient care.

Combining science and law enforcement, forensic science technicians examine crime scenes and gather evidence. They use biological, chemical, hematological, or serological tests to identify suspects. These tests help them gain a clearer understanding of how a crime took place.

Combat medics serve as first responders, educators, and critical care providers in combat environments. Those looking to contribute in high-pressure settings would be well-suited for this role. Paramedics respond to emergency calls, offering life-saving care and gaining experience in varied medical emergencies. First aid instructors teach essential care procedures, preparing others to handle emergencies effectively, a role perfect for those passionate about education and safety (Indeed Editorial Team, 2024).

Becoming an EMT can lead to many options for job progression. Becoming a Registered Nurse (RN) is one logical next step for EMTs. EMTs with a strong foundation in emergency care frequently do well in nursing programs and can pursue specializations in trauma, critical care, or emergency nursing.

Skilled EMTs can also pursue careers in teaching and training, where they can mentor aspiring EMTs or offer healthcare professionals ongoing education. By doing this, you can impart your knowledge and influence the emergency response workforce of the future.

Lastly, EMTs, such as public health officers or emergency preparedness coordinators, can transition into public health and safety roles. These positions focus on improving community health, developing emergency response plans, and managing public health initiatives, offering a broad impact on community wellbeing (LifeLine EMS, 2024).

One of the most essential skills for an EMT is performing effective patient assessments. This involves obtaining vital signs such as blood pressure and breathing rate from the patient; evaluating their medical history, including any pre-existing conditions or medications taken, and determining their level of consciousness. Secondary evaluations for specific body regions and mental state assessments must also be performed to ensure comprehensive care.

Cardiac knowledge is another demanding ability that EMTs should possess since they play a key role in basic life support techniques like CPR using AEDs. Defibrillation helps restore normal heart rhythm in patients who are experiencing cardiac arrest—a leading cause of death worldwide among adults.

Apart from the physical care procedures that EMTs provide at the scene while managing emergencies, emotional support is equally important: compassion should always be demonstrated toward individuals who are going through distressing situations due to ill health or injury concerns.

Listening is an essential skill for Emergency Medical Technicians. Patients should be carefully observed when they are speaking in order to accurately understand their mental and physical well-being. And this also plays a significant role during team collaboration with co-workers who may have other ideas on treating the patient.

An ability to think fast and rationalize decisions under stress is a must in the high-intensity job environment for EMTs, as it is essential to problem-solving. However, being able to promptly address patient needs through effective problem-solving can be particularly difficult due to the unpredictability and complexity of the situations. Communication skills are also a key component for EMTs. They must be able to communicate clearly and concisely with patients, their team, and other medical staff—especially in times of emergency. This involves providing easily comprehensible information: clear instructions on what needs to be done, accurate relay of patient conditions, and plain language descriptions of procedures to be undertaken (Stevens, 2023).

Every career has advantages and disadvantages, and you have to be able to recognize these before moving forward.

On the positive side, EMTs are first responders who frequently arrive at emergency scenes first. They play an invaluable role in keeping patients alive and stable until they can be transported to a hospital for further care. The position offers many chances for critical thinking and practical medical experience, which can be extremely satisfying for people with a strong desire to assist people in need.

Moreover, as EMTs transition to higher certification levels, such as EMT-increased or Paramedic, there is opportunity for job advancement through increased training. This progress improves abilities and creates opportunities for more specialized and higher-paying roles in the healthcare industry.

However, there are also some drawbacks to the work. EMTs frequently work long, erratic shifts in high-stress environments and must physically execute demanding duties like lifting patients. It can also be taxing to handle emotionally charged situations and answer calls that are not emergencies.

Furthermore, a large portion of the work involves paperwork and administrative duties, which increase workload and demand exacting attention to detail. Despite the difficulties, many people find it incredibly fulfilling to have the chance to positively impact people's lives. It's a profession that calls for fortitude, empathy, and a commitment to helping the community (Explore Medical Careers, n/a).

EMTs and paramedics are both essential, but they differ widely. EMTs take a training program that is at least 170 hours long. They learn basic skills for emergency situations such as CPR or oxygen delivery, as well as trauma management. EMTs skillfully evaluate patients to quickly detect any life-threatening conditions and provide appropriate basic emergency care.

Paramedics are trained much more extensively—between 1,200 and 1,800 hours, typically over six to 12 months. Their curriculum delves into advanced areas such as anatomy, physiology, cardiology, and even specialized medical procedures. Paramedics are able to carry out high-level interventions, such as administering various medications through different routes, including IV lines, or reading EKGs for diagnosis.

To become a Paramedic, one must first be certified as an EMT and typically have at least six months of experience in that role. Additional criteria for paramedic programs may include college-level coursework, health clearances, and background investigations.

Overall, paramedics and EMTs play important roles in emergency treatment; however, because paramedics have received more training and have a wider range of expertise, they can offer more advanced medical care (Mednet, n/a).

As you progress through this book, be sure to visit the Test Section at page 112 or page 170, where you'll find detailed instructions on how to access our valuable bonus materials via the Learnik e-learning platform, enhancing your study experience with additional resources

1 PREPARING FOR SUCCESS ON THE NREMT EXAM

PREPARING FOR SUCCESS ON THE NREMT EXAM

Meeting specific criteria is necessary to qualify for the National Registry of Emergency Medical Technicians (NREMT) exam. One of the primary requirements is that you must possess—or be able to obtain—a full and unrestricted Emergency Medical Service (EMS) license in your area of jurisdiction. Ineligibility may occur if your EMS license has been suspended, revoked, or voluntarily surrendered due to disciplinary actions; yet, participation in non-disciplinary rehabilitation programs for substance abuse does not affect eligibility for the exam.

To maintain your EMT certification, you have to go through all the primary certification conditions and also follow the guidelines, deadlines, and regulations that the NREMT establishes. These involve presenting an honest application and responding to any further information asked. Regarding recertification, you should submit your application before the expiration date.

Your eligibility will be reviewed if you have ever been convicted of a felony or a crime involving public health. You should pay all the applicable fees in full; if your payment is stopped or revoked, you will not be able to take the exam until it is settled. The NREMT also has the right to withhold or revoke certification if there are issues with exam security or integrity, even if you were not personally involved.

Lastly, you must submit accurate and valid information to prove you meet the NREMT's requirements. A secure website affiliated with the NREMT exam site is used for this process, and you must comply with the site's Terms of Use (NREMT, n/a).

Now, let us look at the steps to register for the NREMT exam to ensure you are properly prepared and verified before taking the test.

Step 1: If you do not already have a National Registry account, create one on the National Registry homepage.

Step 2: Fill out all required fields regarding your personal account information. Verify that the name matches your official ID or driver's license exactly; otherwise, you may not be allowed to enter the testing facility.

Step 3: Click on "Create a New Application" to apply for your exam. Check the Personal Information Summary and correct any errors by clicking on Manage Account Information. Choose the appropriate application level you wish to complete.

Step 4: Pay the fee. It is beneficial that you pay the application cost when completing the online form. While payment is not required at the time of registration, no Authorization to Test (ATT) Letter will be issued until payment is received and all required verifications are finished.

Step 5: Verify you have been approved to test. Once all application processes are completed and verified, a link to the Print/View Authorization To Test (ATT) Letter will appear, so make sure you check its status.

Step 6: Once the ATT link is available, click on it to view and print the letter. The ATT letter is valid for 90 days, so if it expires, a new application and fee will be required.

Step 7: Follow the instructions on the ATT letter to schedule your exam. You can schedule online via the Pearson VUE website or call 1-866-673-6896 for assistance (note that Pearson VUE charges an additional fee for phone scheduling) (NREMT, n/a).

Applying for the National Registry of Emergency Medical Technicians (NREMT) exam comes with specific fees. For those aiming to become an EMT, the application fee is $104 per attempt for the cognitive exam as of 2024. This fee applies each time you take the exam, so it's essential to thoroughly prepare to avoid multiple payments.

The NREMT has a refund policy in place for those who might need it. Refunds are available within 90 days of payment, minus an administrative fee. Refunds can be requested for several reasons such as an incomplete application, if the candidate decides not to pursue certification, or if a certified EMS provider opts out of recertifying (NREMT, n/a).

Additionally, as of October 1, 2015, all paper recertification applications submitted to the National Registry incur a $5.00 processing fee, which is added to the standard recertification cost for the respective level. However, online recertification remains the most efficient and cost-effective method, avoiding the additional processing fee and ensuring a smoother process overall (NREMT, n/a).

What happens if you fail the exam? The NREMT gives you three chances to pass the test before requiring you to enroll in a refresher course.

After an unsuccessful attempt, you will receive an email with feedback on your performance, indicating which areas were above passing, near passing, and below passing. This feedback should be prioritized to identify the subjects you need to focus on for your next attempt. You must wait 15 days from the date of your last examination before you can reschedule and retake the test (EMTprep, 2022).

To begin the retake process, visit the NREMT website and create an account if you do not already have one. Once logged in, you can start a new application. If no information has changed since your previous application, opt for the Express Application to transfer all previous details to your new application.

Next, you will need to submit the application fee again. Keep track of your application's progress through the Certification Application Status page to ensure no additional steps are required before you can schedule your exam. By following these steps and using the feedback provided, you can better prepare for your retake and improve your chances of passing on your next attempt (NREMT, n/a).

Nationally registered EMTs must renew their certification every two years to ensure they stay current with their skills and knowledge. There are two ways to recertify: passing the cognitive examination again or completing continuing education requirements. The EMT National Continued Competency Program (NCCP) mandates 40 hours of continuing education. This program is divided into three parts: the national component, the local/state component, and the individual component.

The National Registry accepts education from State EMS Offices, CAPCE accredited programs, and U.S. accredited academic institutions, all of which must be related to EMS patient care. International providers need to complete education from approved U.S. sources. Continuing education can be completed online through Distributive Education (DE) or via in-person courses. There are no longer limits on the amount of DE that can be used for recertification.

Certain types of courses and activities are not eligible for recertification, such as duplicate courses, clinical rotations, instructor courses, management/leadership courses, duty performance, preceptor hours, serving as a skilled examiner, and volunteer time. For more detailed information on what is accepted, refer to the Recertification Guide (NREMT, n/a).

Let us talk a bit about what will happen on exam day. The cognitive exam is taken on a computer. During this exam, you will be presented with mostly multiple-choice questions numbering between 70 and 120. Out of these, ten questions do not contribute to your final score; they are included as part of the new concept evaluation for upcoming tests. As the test taker, you are not informed which questions are unscored; therefore, it is advisable to approach every question as if it will impact your final result.

The test is a Computer Adaptive Test (CAT), which implies that it adapts the difficulty of the questions according to your responses. If you answer correctly, more challenging questions will follow suit—this technique is employed to evaluate if you are competent enough at the entry level standard for passing. The purpose is not to deceive you but to gauge your knowledge against a pre-set passing standard.

All facets of EMS care are considered in the examination which comprises airway, ventilation, oxygenation, trauma, cardiology, medical, and EMS operations. The majority (85%) of the questions center around adult patient care while the remaining 15% are dedicated to pediatric care (NREMT, n/a).

Sometimes, exams can be intimidating, especially when they determine your future as an EMT. But take a deep breath. To calm your nerves and instill a sense of confidence, here are some tips that should make your journey through the NREMT exam easier:

Tip 1: It is important to be well-versed in AHA Guidelines. Make sure you are aware of the current American Heart Association guidelines for CPR and Emergency Cardiovascular Care—these will be evaluated up to the Basic EMT training level.

Tip 2: Be aware of the exam structure. Realize that every question has one best choice despite several possible correct options. Concentrate on selecting the most suitable answer.

Tip 3: Recognize life-and-death moments. Look out for signs that point toward critical situations, such as changes in mental condition or unusual skin indications. In these cases, prioritize immediate actions.

Tip 4: Make sure to read the questions carefully. Watch closely to every word used in the questions and responses. Terms like "anterior," "posterior," "never," or "always," carry very different meanings and can significantly lead you astray.

Tip 5: Focus on airway management. Understand the importance of airways, respiration, and ventilation. Know when to ventilate versus when to oxygenate a patient.

Tip 6: Stick to national standards. The exam tests national EMS standards, not state or local protocols. Base your answers on national training guidelines.

Tip 7: Get familiar with the CAT format. The exam uses a computer adaptive test format. You cannot skip questions or change answers, so answer each question to the best of your ability.

Tip 8: Bring Required IDs. Ensure you have two forms of valid identification, including a government-issued photo ID and another with your name and signature (Beutler, 2019).

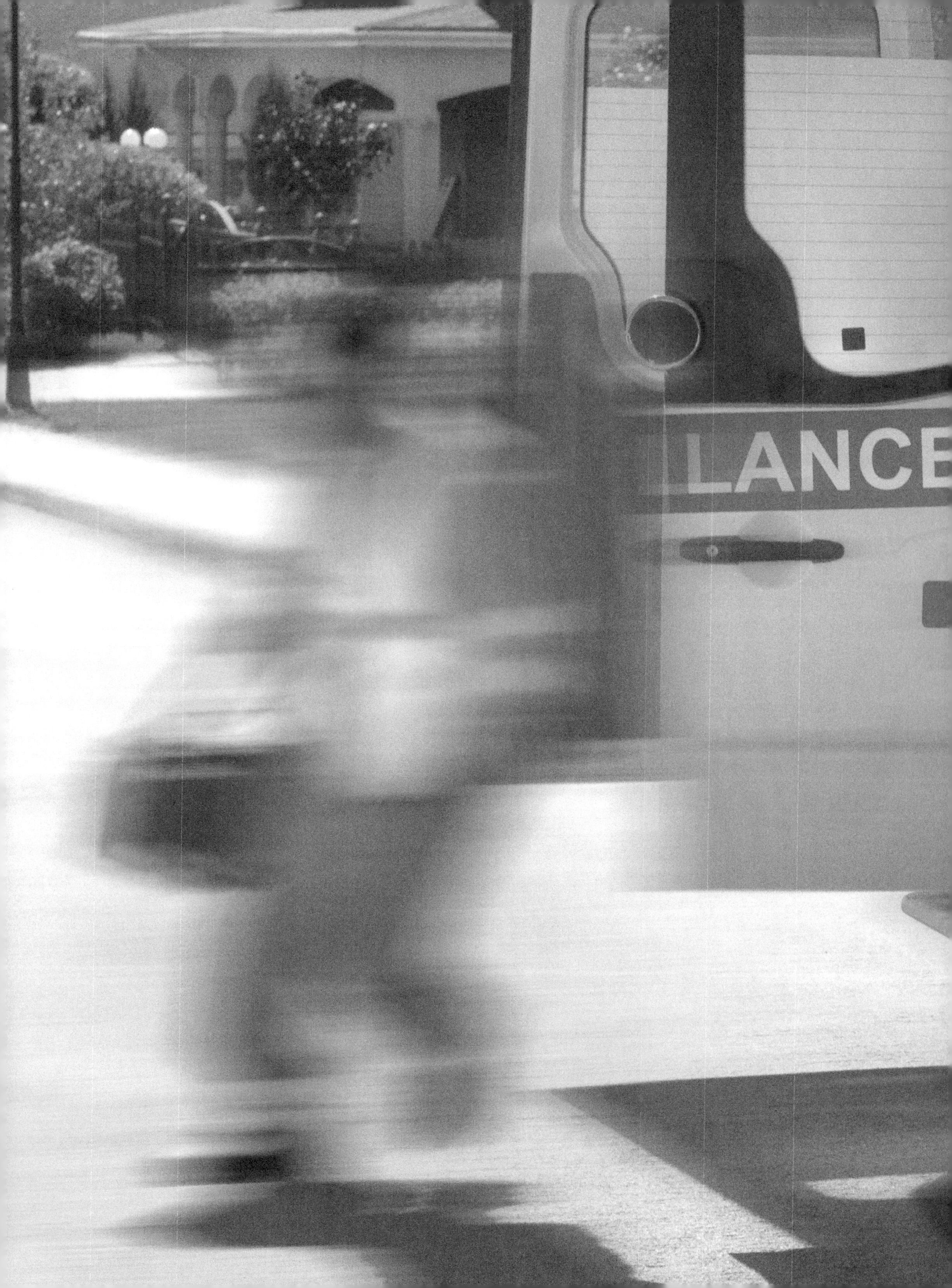

2 EMT ROLES AND RESPONSIBILITIES

EMT ROLES AND RESPONSIBILITIES

The history of EMTs reflects significant advancements driven by societal needs and medical practice. Until the mid-1960s, the U.S. had no formal emergency response services, with funeral home workers often serving as first responders. A 1965 report by the National Academy of Sciences highlighted the devastating impact of accidental injuries, prompting the transformation of military medics into civilian first responders.

The origins of EMTs can be traced back to battlefield medics during the Civil War when Major Jonathan Letterman established the U.S. Ambulance Corps. This model expanded in World War I, and post-war, when volunteers from fire departments and undertakers formed the first civilian emergency responders. The late 1950s and 1960s saw significant advancements with the American Heart Association training physicians, and subsequently EMTs, in CPR.

A pivotal moment came in 1966 with the publication of the white paper Accidental Death and Disability: The Neglected Disease of Modern Society. The report revealed that road accidents in 1965 claimed more American lives than the Korean War, prompting the development of an emergency response system modeled after Vietnam War medics. The first national standardized curriculum for EMTs was published in 1969, marking the formal beginning of modern EMT training (Vale, 2023).

Throughout the 1970s, the EMT profession gained recognition and legitimacy. The Highway Safety Act of 1966 mandated standardized training and improvements in emergency transport services. By 1973, the first recertification of a nationally registered EMT was processed, and guidelines for the national EMT-Paramedic curriculum were developed.

In the 1980s, emergency services became further standardized, and new roles like paramedics emerged to manage advanced medical tasks. The AIDS epidemic prompted the adoption of protective measures such as gloves and masks. The 1990s brought a focus on managed care and increased EMS visibility through popular TV shows. The National Registry continued refining curricula, conducting practice analysis studies, and enhancing communication systems with state EMS offices (NREMT, n/a).

Today, EMTs face new challenges, particularly post-COVID-19, including medical personnel shortages and emergency room capacity issues. Despite these challenges, the field continues to evolve, with developments in telehealth and expanded roles in mental health emergencies. The profession's history is a testament to the adaptability and innovation necessary in emergency medical services (Vale, 2023).

The field of public health is diverse, and it aims to promote community well-being through prevention, education, and responding to emergencies. Public health EMTs lead as first responders in medical emergencies. This responsibility not only entails primary care but also branches into other elements that concern the larger issue of community health and safety (Health.ny.gov, n/a).

EMTs usually show up at emergency sites before anybody else. Their capacity to quickly evaluate and stabilize a patient can be lifesaving, literally reducing morbidity and mortality rates. Their actions (such as managing airways or controlling bleeding) significantly impact critical situations where CPR may be performed.

An essential public health responsibility of EMTs is advocating for their patients. They not only offer medical care but also provide emotional support and reassurance to the patients and their families during times of stress. Communication is key to providing effective care: it helps the patients understand their condition and what is being done for them, reducing anxiety, and making them feel secure.

EMTs also address hospital overcrowding through proper decision-making on patient transport. Their evaluation on the scene helps to distinguish people who need immediate hospital care from those who can be taken care of in a less acute setting. Thus, resource optimization at the emergency department, whereby only those critically in need are taken to hospitals, is assured through this triage process.

Moreover, EMTs are integral to community health education. They engage in public outreach programs, teaching emergency preparedness, first aid, and basic life support. These educational efforts empower individuals with the knowledge and skills necessary to respond effectively to emergencies, enhancing community resilience.

EMTs' role in the continuum of care is necessary. When EMTs hand over patients to hospital staff, it ensures continuity of care and marks an important moment in the process. By providing detailed reports on the patient's condition and the care administered at the scene, EMTs facilitate a seamless transition that allows hospital staff to continue treatment without delay (Guardian EMT, 2023).

In addition to their emergency response duties, EMTs must maintain a prominent level of readiness. This involves regular training and adherence to protocols that ensure the safe handling of patients, including those with contagious infections or hazardous exposures. EMTs also play a role in safeguarding public health by following strict decontamination procedures and ensuring their equipment is in optimal condition (Health.ny.gov, n/a).

Medical, legal, and ethical issues are integral to an EMT's professional responsibilities. Understanding these areas ensures that EMTs provide appropriate and lawful care while maintaining high ethical standards.

Medical Issues: Organ donation requires signed legal documentation. EMTs should treat organ donors the same as other patients and communicate potential organ donations with medical direction. Medical identification tags are crucial during patient assessment as they provide information on medical conditions such as allergies, asthma, diabetes, or epilepsy. In cases of death, EMTs should always assume the patient is alive unless obvious signs like rigor mortis, dependent lividity, decapitation, decomposition, or obvious fatal injuries are present.

Legal Protection: EMTs are protected from lawsuits if they can document that they met the duty to act, practiced within their scope, and adhered to the standard of care. The "duty to act" requires on-duty EMTs to care for patients who need and consent to it. Off-duty EMTs may not be legally required to assist, but if they do, they must continue care until transferring it to another qualified provider.

Terms and Rules: The scope of practice defines what EMTs can legally do, and performing beyond this scope is illegal. The standard of care is the level of care an average provider in the community would offer. EMTs must follow medical directions, which include both offline protocols and online instructions from a doctor. Patient consent is essential; adults must give expressed consent, while implied consent is assumed for unresponsive patients or minors if a guardian is unavailable. Patient refusals must be documented, and EMTs should try to persuade patients to accept care, ensuring they are mentally competent.

Advanced directives like Do Not Resuscitate (DNR) orders should be followed if there is clear documentation. Confidentiality is protected under HIPAA, and EMTs should not disclose patient information unless necessary (EMT-Training, n/a). For instance, EMTs can share information with family members if the patient is unconscious and the EMT determines it is in the patient's best interest (Department of Health and Human Services, n/a). Insurance regulations, such as those under COBRA or EMTALA, ensure all patients receive emergency care regardless of their ability to pay. At crime scenes, EMTs must preserve evidence and communicate with law enforcement, documenting any unusual findings and avoiding actions that might destroy evidence.

Ethical Responsibilities: EMTs must treat all patients and colleagues with dignity and respect, maintain competency, document honestly, and advocate for the patient's best interests. Good Samaritan Laws protect off-duty EMTs from liability when providing care ethically.

Understanding these medical, legal, and ethical issues helps EMTs provide safe, lawful, and ethical care to their patients (EMT-Training, n/a).

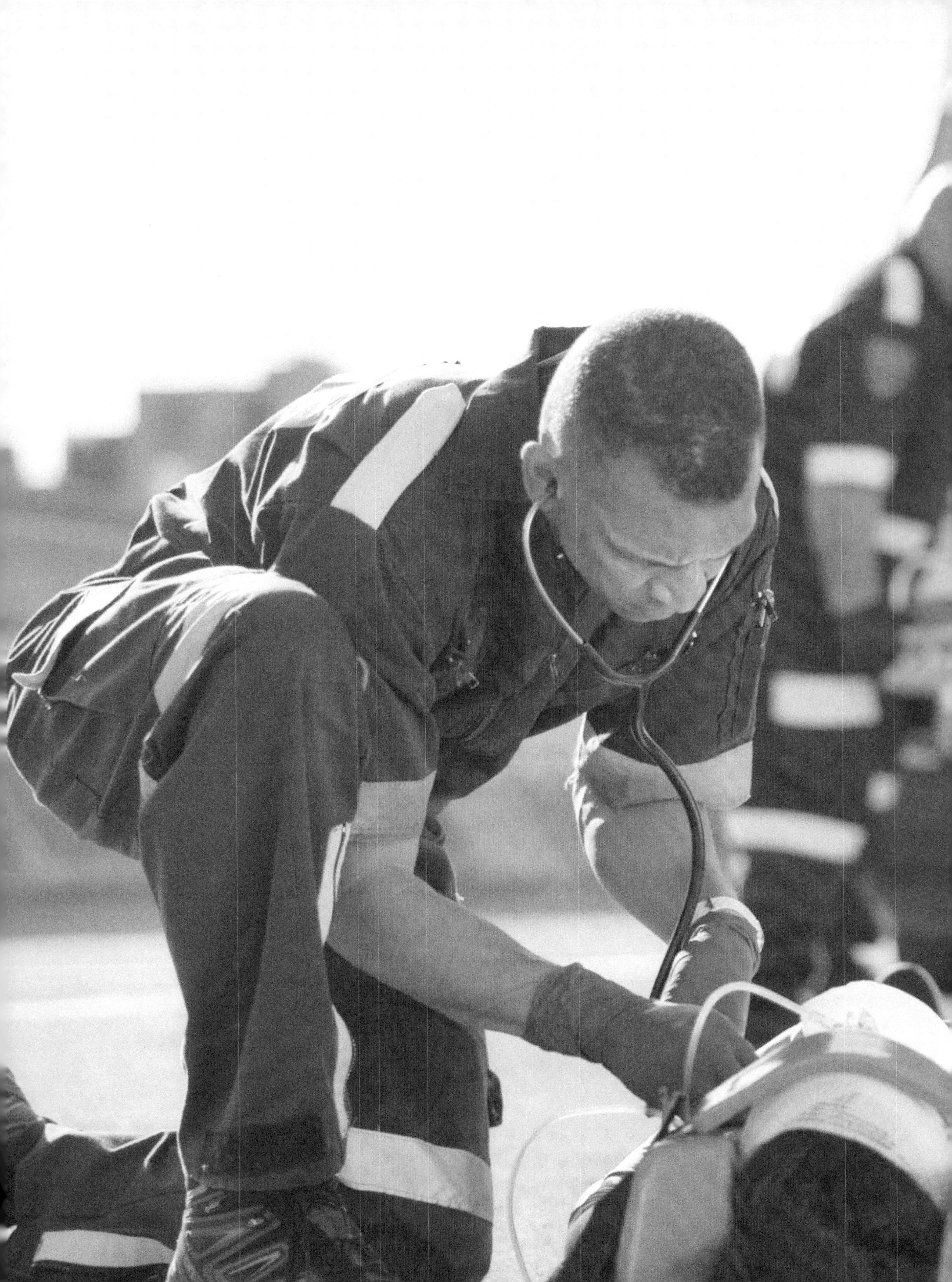

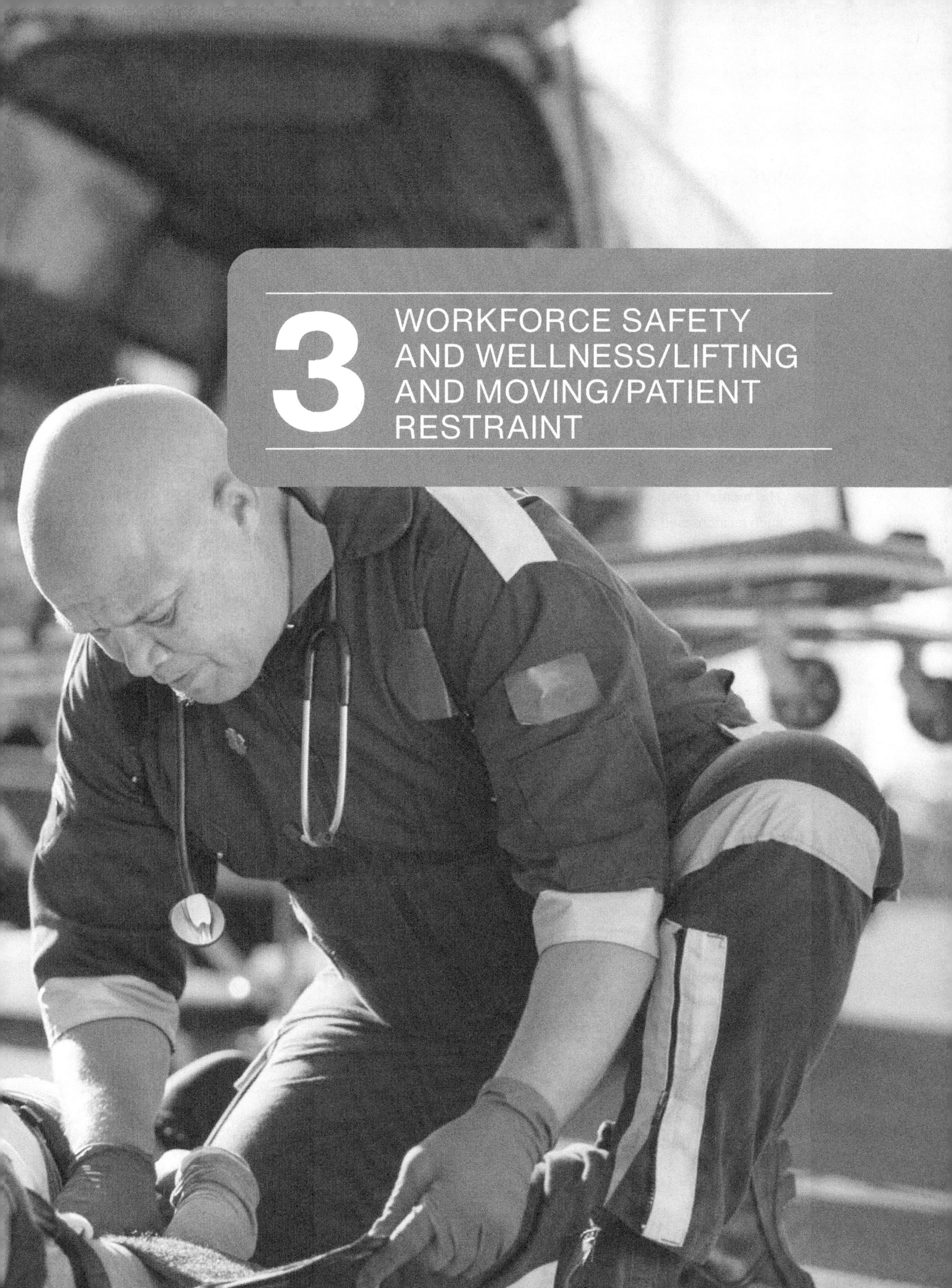

3 WORKFORCE SAFETY AND WELLNESS/LIFTING AND MOVING/PATIENT RESTRAINT

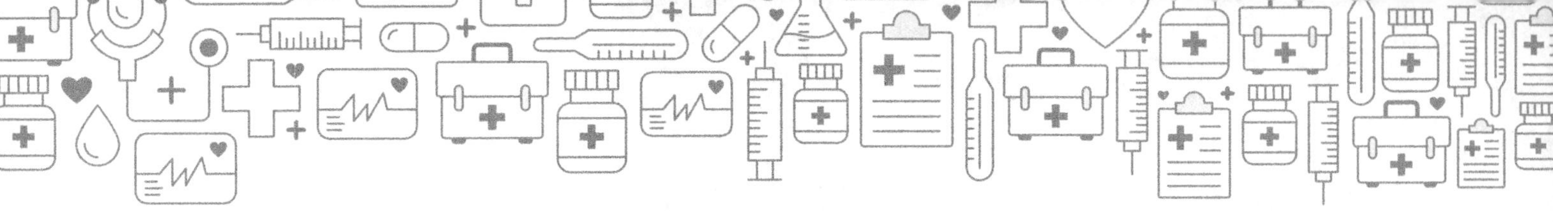

WORKFORCE SAFETY AND WELLNESS/LIFTING AND MOVING/PATIENT RESTRAINT

The demanding nature of this profession requires EMTs to prioritize their own safety and wellness to ensure they can effectively perform their duties. This involves understanding the importance of both physical and mental health, as well as recognizing and mitigating potential hazards on the job.

Regular exercise and proper nutrition are essential for maintaining physical health. Exercise not only keeps the body fit but also helps in managing stress by releasing endorphins. Incorporating activities like running, walking, or even physical hobbies can provide much-needed relief from stress. Additionally, eating a balanced diet rich in fruits, vegetables, and essential vitamins can bolster the immune system.

The mental health of EMS providers is often overlooked, yet it is a high priority. Signs of mental strain, such as increased anger, anxiety, or depression, need to be acknowledged and addressed promptly. Peer support and employee assistance programs can provide vital resources for those struggling with mental health issues. It is important for EMT providers to check in with themselves and their colleagues regularly to ensure everyone is coping well.

Adequate sleep is another basic component of health that is often compromised in this profession. Long shifts and irregular hours can lead to sleep deprivation, which negatively impacts both physical and mental health. EMT leaders should implement fatigue risk management programs and encourage practices like short naps during shifts to help mitigate these effects (Calams, 2020).

Prioritizing Safety on the Scene

Scene safety is critical for EMT providers because they frequently work in unpredictable and hazardous conditions. The priority while arriving at a situation is to secure personal safety, followed by the safety of colleagues, and finally the patient. This structure allows EMS providers to offer care without becoming victims themselves.

Scene safety is not a one-time evaluation; it requires constant reassessment. Conditions can change rapidly, and new hazards can emerge at any time. EMT providers must remain vigilant and be prepared to adapt to changing circumstances. This includes being aware of bystanders, potential threats from individuals or animals, and environmental hazards.

Preparation begins even before arriving at the scene. Information gathered by dispatch can provide valuable insights into potential dangers. For instance, knowing the scene involves a chemical spill or an area with high criminal activity could help providers take the required security measures.

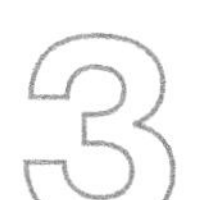

Upon arrival, keen observation is essential. Indicators such as fleeing individuals, agitated crowds, or unusual environmental signs like broken windows can signal danger. EMT providers should approach cautiously, with strategies in place for quick exits if needed. Maintaining awareness of the surroundings and the actions of those present can prevent many threats from escalating.

Providers need to be aware of the many risks they could face. Such as the presence of drugs or potentially dangerous products as well as knowing what safety precautions to take. It is frequently safer to avoid situations involving dangerous substances and to bring in specialized personnel instead. Understanding dangers and sticking to appropriate procedures will greatly mitigate them (Klein and Prasanna, 2023).

The importance of safety and wellness in the EMS profession cannot be overstated. EMS providers must prioritize their physical and mental health to effectively care for others. By recognizing the signs of stress and mental health issues, maintaining a healthy lifestyle, and constantly assessing scene safety, EMS providers can navigate the challenges of their profession more effectively.

To ensure overall safety, EMS providers must integrate physical safety measures with their mental health practices. This includes being prepared for the physical demands of lifting and moving patients. Proper training and adherence to protocols are essential in preventing injuries during these tasks.

When moving and positioning a patient, it is important to ensure that no injuries occur to yourself, your team, or the patient. You need training and practice because lifting and transferring patients might result in injury. Patients with head traumas, shock, spinal injuries, pregnancy, and obesity require specific lifting and moving strategies. Let us evaluate some tips for safe lifting and moving of patients.

TIP 1: PROPER BODY MECHANICS

Proper body mechanics are critical in lifting; the shoulder girdle should be aligned over the pelvis, and hands should be held close to the legs to minimize strain by keeping the force straight down the spinal column. Injuries can occur if you lift with a curved back or if the back is straight but significantly bent forward at the hips.

TIP 2: POWER LIFT TECHNIQUE

The power lift technique is recommended for safe lifting, where feet should be spread about 15 inches apart, with feet placed to balance the center of gravity. Bend at the knees to lower the upper body, then grasp the patient or stretcher with arms kept close to the sides of the body. Lift the patient by raising the upper body and straightening while keeping the weight as close to the body as possible. The power grip, with palms up and hands about ten inches apart, ensures maximum force from the hands.

TIP 3: WEIGHT AND DISTRIBUTION

Weight and distribution considerations include using a rolling device whenever possible and if not available, using a backboard with more weight on the head end. The diamond carry technique involves one EMT at the head and foot of the backboard and one on each side, while the one-handed carry allows rescuers to support the backboard with one hand each, facing forward. Patients must always be secured to prevent sliding. Wheeled ambulance stretchers, which weigh 40-145 pounds, are too heavy for stairs, necessitating a backboard or stair chair for conscious patients and a backboard for supine or immobilized patients. Coordination is valuable, so follow the team leader's directions and use preparatory commands and countdowns for synchronized lifting.

TIP 4: BODY MECHANICS FOR DRAGS AND TRANSFERS

Keep the back locked and straight and extend arms no more than 15 to 20 inches in front.

Kneel to minimize leaning distance when dragging a patient on the ground or across a bed.

To pull a patient from a different height:

» Bend knees until hips are below the plane's height.
» Extend arms 15 to 20 inches in front of the torso.

In hospitals, when transferring a patient from a stretcher to a bed:

» Ensure the stretcher is the same height or slightly higher than the bed.
» Drag the patient in increments while kneeling.

For logrolling a patient:

» Keep the back straight.
» Roll without stopping until the patient is on their side.

When rolling the wheeled ambulance stretcher:

» Push from the head end.
» Keep your arms close to the body.
» Slightly bend forward at the hips.

TIP 5: GENERAL CONSIDERATIONS FOR MOVING PATIENTS

Move in an orderly, planned, and unhurried manner to protect oneself and reduce the risk of worsening the patient's condition.

Plan ahead and select methods that involve the least amount of lifting and carrying.

Use emergency moves when there is a potential danger (e.g., fire or hazardous materials) preventing proper assessment and immediate care.

Techniques to prevent aggravation of spinal injuries include:

» Clothes drag
» Blanket drag
» Arm drag

Urgent moves may be necessary for patients with:

» Altered consciousness
» Inadequate ventilation
» Shock

The rapid extrication technique is used for patients needing urgent removal from a vehicle. It typically requires one minute or less and it should be avoided if no urgency exists.

TIP 6: NON-URGENT MOVES SPECIAL PATIENT CONSIDERATIONS

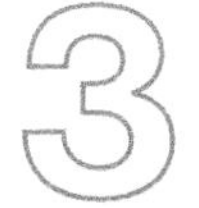

Use non-urgent moves when both the scene and patient are stable, requiring careful planning, sufficient personnel, obstacle removal, and proper equipment (Sharp School, n/a).

Methods include:

- Direct ground lift: Lifting a patient from the ground to a stretcher, involving two or more rescuers.
- Extremity lift: One rescuer lifts the patient's legs while another lifts under the arms.
- Direct carry: Transferring a patient from a bed to a stretcher by carrying them.
- Draw sheet method: Sliding a patient from one surface to another using a sheet.
- Scoop stretcher: Separating the stretcher into two halves, placing them on either side of the patient, and then fastening them together (EMT-Training, n/a).

TIP 7: SPECIAL PATIENT CONSIDERATIONS

When transferring geriatric patients, EMTs must deal with skeletal abnormalities such brittle bones and spinal curvatures, which can make immobilization and transportation difficult. Many patients are unable to rest supine on a backboard without risking more harm, therefore packaging and transportation must be carefully planned. Adopting a sympathetic and compassionate approach, speaking slowly, clarifying procedures, and anticipating needs might help reduce anxieties and elicit cooperation from these patients.

Bariatric patients face tremendous challenges as well. With around 35% of women and 31% of men over 19 in the United States being overweight or obese, there is a high demand for emergency treatment and transportation (Sharp School, n/a). This takes a physical toll on healthcare professionals and raises the risk of back problems. Although stretchers and equipment with greater weight capacities are available, securely carrying bigger patients remains a challenge.

TIP 8: MEDICAL RESTRAINTS

Medical restraints are used for combative patients. A minimum of five personnel are required for restraint, ensuring the patient is in a supine position to prevent positional asphyxia. It is essential to assess the patient's circulation after restraints are applied and document all information. Personnel considerations involve evaluating physical strength, available room for proper stance, and the need for additional lifting assistance to avoid rescuer injuries. The first key rule of lifting is to protect yourself so that you can remain effective in helping others (Sharp School, n/a).

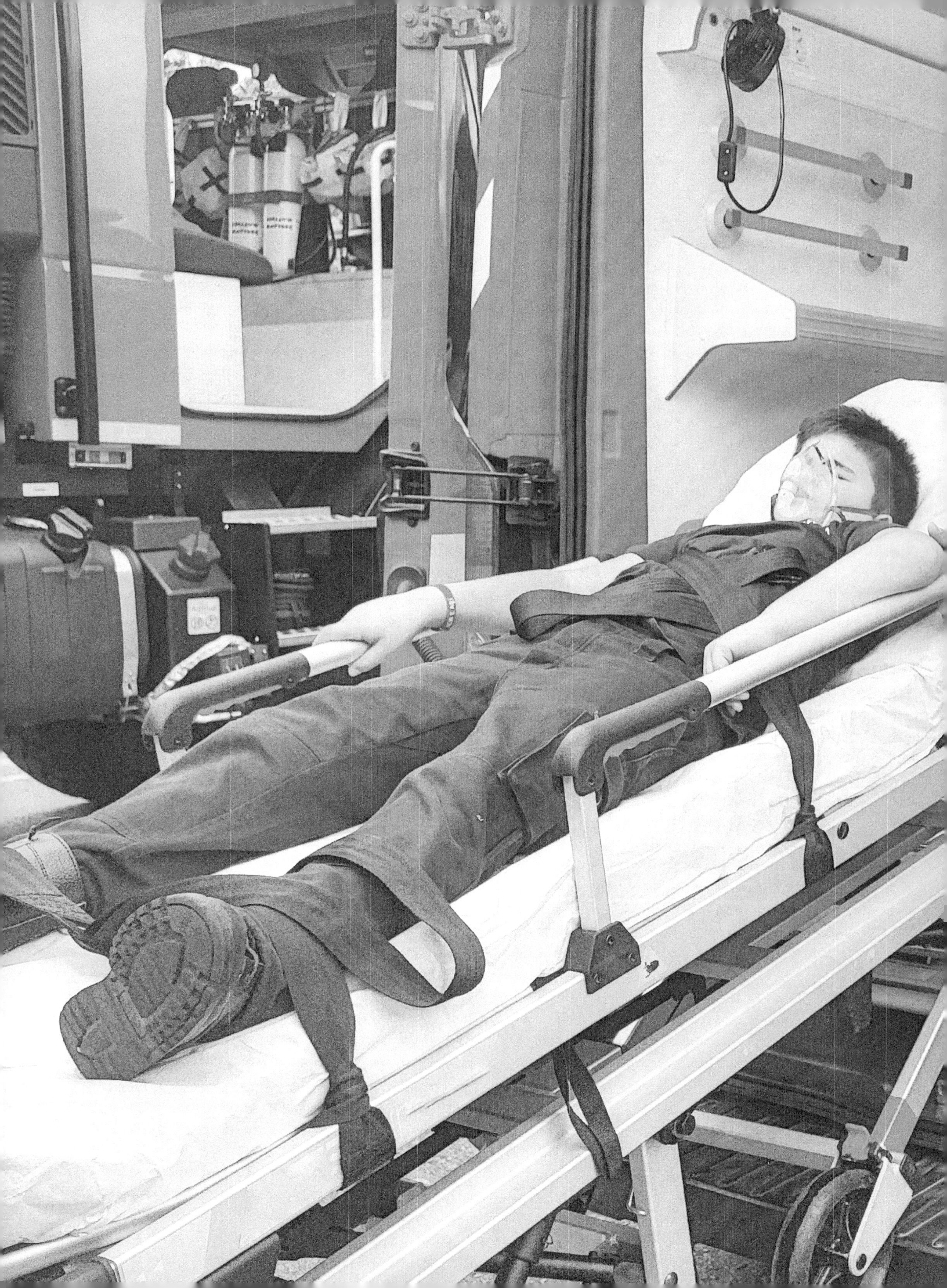

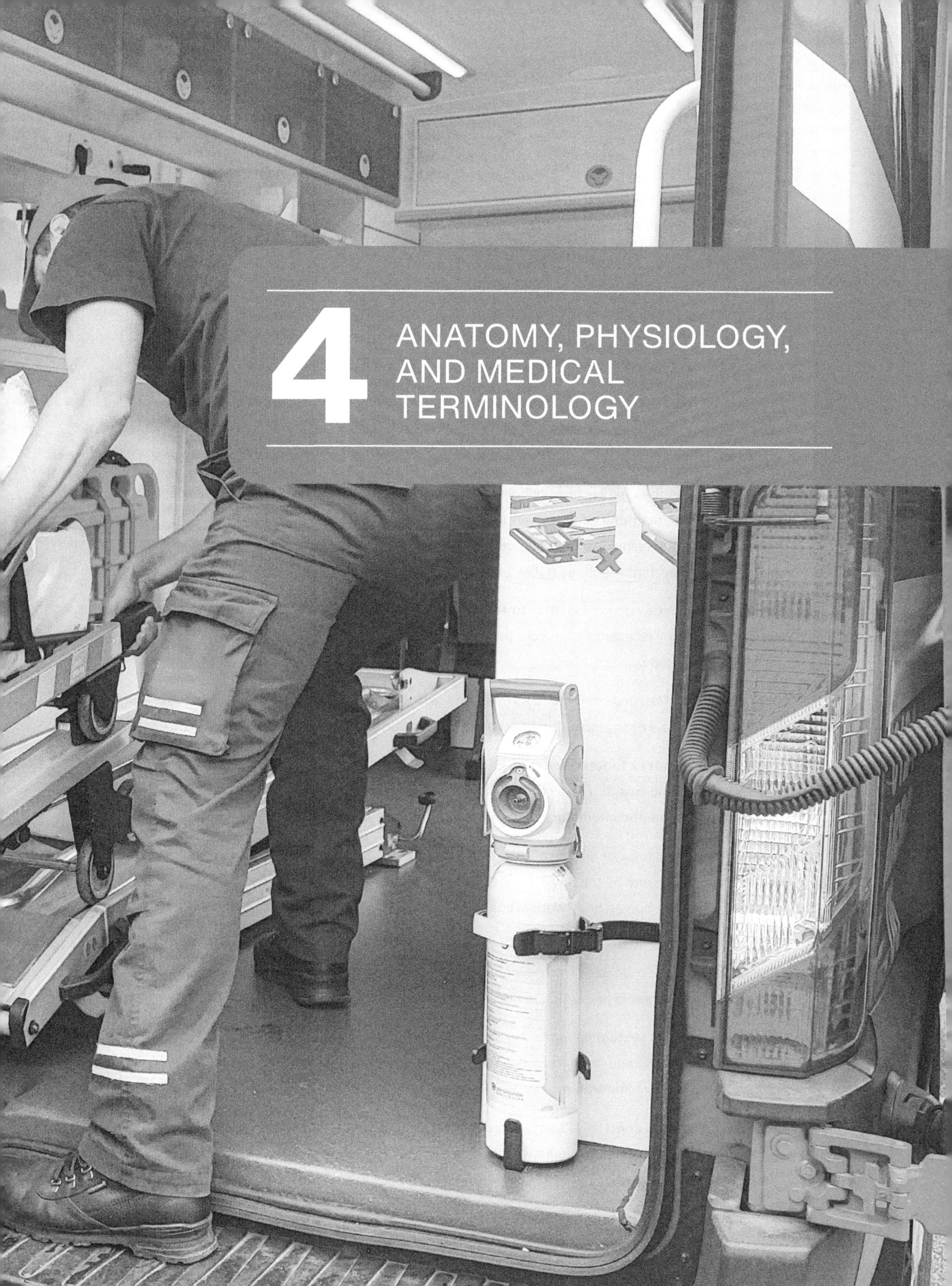

4 ANATOMY, PHYSIOLOGY, AND MEDICAL TERMINOLOGY

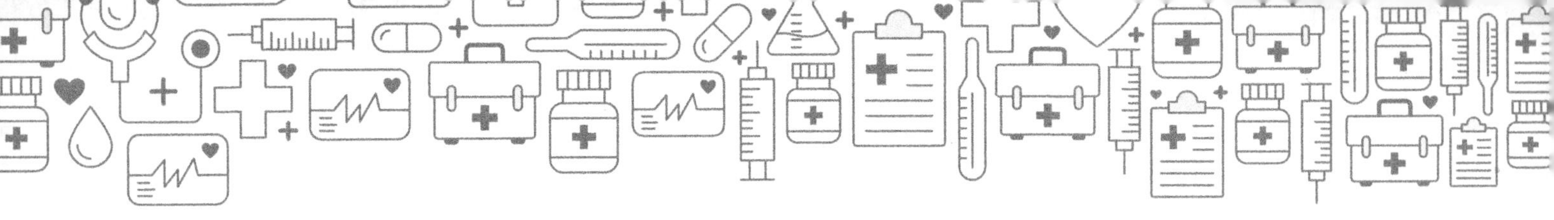

ANATOMY, PHYSIOLOGY, AND MEDICAL TERMINOLOGY

Basic Anatomy and Physiology

Anatomy is the study of the structure of the body and its parts, while physiology focuses on the functions and processes of those parts, such as how the heart pumps blood and how the lungs facilitate breathing. Understanding basic anatomy and physiology is fundamental for medical professionals, as it lays the foundation for diagnosing and treating illnesses and injuries (Betts et al., 2023).

At the most basic level, the body is composed of atoms, which are the smallest units of matter. These atoms combine to form molecules, the chemical building blocks of all body structures. Examples of molecules include water, proteins, and sugars, essential for various body functions.

The next level is the cellular level, where molecules combine to form cells. A cell is the smallest independently functioning unit of life. Even the smallest organisms, like bacteria, consist of single cells. In more complex organisms like humans, cells are the fundamental units that make up all living structures and conduct important functions (Libretexts, n/a).

Cells of similar types come together to form tissues. Tissues are groups of similar cells that perform a specific function. For example, muscle tissue enables movement, while nervous tissue transmits signals throughout the body.

Different types of tissues combine to form organs, which are anatomically distinct structures that perform specific functions. For example, the heart pumps blood, and the lungs facilitate breathing.

Organs work together to form systems. Each organ system performs major functions necessary for the body's survival and health. For instance, the digestive system breaks down food into nutrients that the body can use, while the circulatory system transports these nutrients throughout the body.

Finally, the highest level of organization is the organism itself. An organism, like a human being, is a living entity that can perform all the physiological functions necessary for life. All the cells, tissues, organs, and organ systems in a human body work in concert to maintain the life and health of the organism (Libretexts, n/a).

The human body is organized into several major systems, each with distinct functions that contribute to the body's overall health and functionality. Here is a brief overview of these major organ systems:

The integumentary system includes the skin, hair, nails, and glands. It serves as the body's first line of defense against environmental hazards. The skin protects internal structures, prevents dehydration, and helps regulate body temperature.

The skeletal system consists of bones, cartilage, ligaments, and joints. It provides structural support, protects vital organs, enables movement by serving as attachment points for muscles, and produces blood cells in the bone marrow (Betts et al., 2023).

The muscular system is made up of skeletal muscles, smooth muscles, and cardiac muscles. It enables movement, maintains posture, and produces heat. Skeletal muscles work with bones to create movement, while smooth muscles facilitate peristalsis, the wave-like contractions that move food through the intestines. Cardiac muscles are found in the heart and are responsible for pumping blood throughout the body by contracting rhythmically and continuously without conscious control (Lumen Learning, n/a).

The nervous system includes the brain, spinal cord, and peripheral nerves. It controls and coordinates body activities by transmitting electrical signals. It allows for quick responses to internal and external changes through the senses and motor functions (Betts et al., 2023). For example, if a doctor taps your knee with a reflex hammer, your spinal cord instantly sends a signal to your muscles to kick your leg. This quick reflex occurs without involving your brain and helps demonstrate the spinal cord's role in managing reflexes (Cleveland Clinic, 2021).

The endocrine system is composed of glands that produce hormones, such as the thyroid, adrenal glands, and pancreas. These hormones regulate metabolism, growth, reproduction, and other critical functions.

The cardiovascular system includes the heart and blood vessels. It circulates blood throughout the body, delivering oxygen and nutrients to tissues and removing waste products. The heart pumps blood, and the vessels carry it to various body parts.

The lymphatic system, which includes lymph nodes, lymph vessels, and the spleen, helps maintain fluid balance, absorbs fats from the digestive system, and provides defense against pathogens through immune responses.

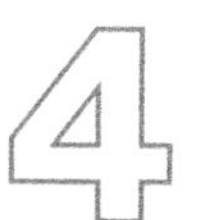

The respiratory system comprises the lungs, trachea, bronchi, and diaphragm. It is responsible for gas exchange, bringing oxygen into the body, and removing carbon dioxide. The diaphragm and other muscles facilitate breathing.

The digestive system includes the mouth, esophagus, stomach, intestines, liver, and pancreas. It breaks down food into nutrients the body can absorb and use for energy, growth, and repair.

The urinary system comprises the kidneys, ureters, bladder, and urethra. It removes waste products from the blood, regulates fluid and electrolyte balance, and maintains blood pressure.

The reproductive system differs in males and females and includes organs such as the ovaries, fallopian tubes, uterus, and vagina in females, and the testes, vas deferens, and penis in males. This system produces offspring and ensures the continuation of genetic material.

Each system works in concert with the others to maintain the body's overall health and function, highlighting the intricate and interdependent nature of human anatomy and physiology (Betts et al., 2023).

This complex coordination ensures the body can adapt to various internal and external changes, sustain life, and promote well-being. One of the key principles underlying this harmony is homeostasis.

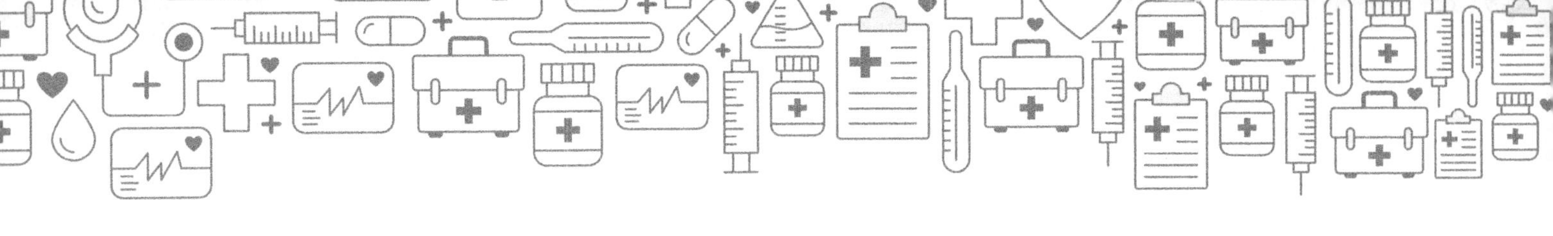

Homeostasis is the body's process of maintaining a stable internal environment despite changes in external conditions. This balance is necessary for the body's optimal functioning and survival.

Homeostasis relies on key components to regulate the body's internal environment effectively. The set point is the ideal value for a physiological parameter, such as the approximate 37°C (98.6°F) for body temperature, around which the normal range fluctuates. This ideal value serves as a target that the body strives to maintain.

Surrounding this set point is the normal range, which is the restricted range of values within which the body functions optimally and remains healthy. The normal range ensures that physiological conditions are kept within limits that support proper bodily function and overall health.

Homeostasis relies on feedback mechanisms, primarily negative, to maintain stability. This works to correct deviations from the set point, thereby maintaining homeostasis. This system involves three main components:

Sensor (Receptor): Detects changes in the physiological parameter and sends this information to the control center.

Control Center: Compares the detected value to the set point. If there is a significant deviation, it activates an effector.

Effector: Responds to signals from the control center to reverse the deviation and restore the parameter to its normal range.

For example, when body temperature rises above the set point, sensors in the skin and brain detect this change. The brain's temperature regulatory center then activates mechanisms like sweating and increased blood flow to the skin, which helps cool the body down.

While less common, positive feedback amplifies changes rather than reversing them, moving the system further from the set point. This mechanism is typically involved in processes that have a clear end point, such as childbirth or blood clotting. During childbirth, the release of oxytocin intensifies uterine contractions, pushing the baby further down the birth canal until delivery is complete (Betts et al., 2023).

Healthcare practitioners use specialized language known as medical terminology to ensure accuracy and prevent misconceptions. This language, which has its roots mostly in Greek and Latin, is organized so that each term expresses a particular aspect of the body and its state, facilitating efficient and clear communication between medical professionals (Biga et al., n/a).

For instance, during patient care, it allows for precise descriptions of symptoms and conditions, enabling accurate diagnoses and effective treatment plans. In medical records, standardized terminology ensures that patient histories and treatment details are documented comprehensively. Similarly, in prescriptions, clear language helps avoid errors in medication administration, while in medical billing, standardized codes ensure the accurate processing of insurance claims.

Additionally, medical terminology is essential in medical imaging, which helps describe findings from X-rays and scans and guide treatment decisions. In research and education, consistent terminology is needed for documenting and sharing scientific findings and for training future healthcare professionals (University of San Diego, n/a).

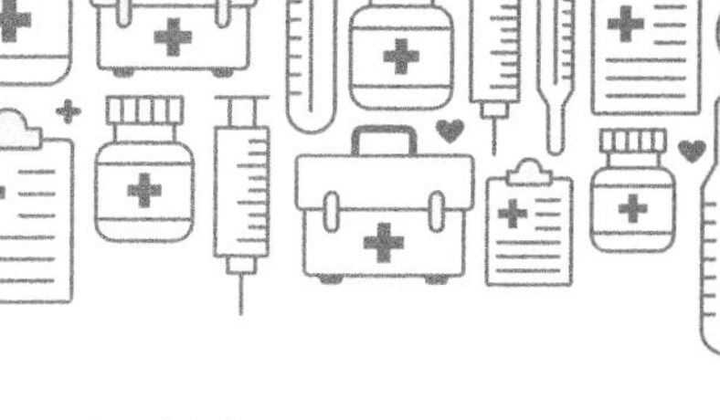

Understanding these planes is essential for interpreting medical images and describing anatomical movements accurately.

To better comprehend the significance and use of medical language, let us examine its foundational concepts, which include body planes, cavities, regional and directional terminologies, anatomical locations, and components.

Medical terms are composed of roots, prefixes, and suffixes. The root of a term often indicates the organ, tissue, or condition being referred to. For example, "cardio-" relates to the heart. Prefixes and suffixes modify these roots to provide additional details. For instance, the prefix "hyper-" means "over" or "excessive," and when combined with "tension" (pressure), it forms the term "hypertension," which describes high blood pressure (Biga et al., n/a).

Understanding medical terminology involves breaking down terms into their components to understand their meanings. For example, in everyday conversation, you might describe a common illness simply as a "cold" or "sore throat." However, in medical practice, this would be referred to with more specificity, such as "upper respiratory tract infection (URI) with acute pharyngitis." This demonstrates how medical terminology translates common symptoms into precise diagnoses.

Each medical term typically includes a root word, which provides the base meaning. Prefixes are added to the beginning of the root to modify its meaning, while suffixes are added to the end to further refine the term. For instance, "intravenous" combines the prefix "intra-" (within) with "venous" (relating to veins), describing something administered directly into a vein. Similarly, "myocardial infarction" breaks down into "myo-" (muscle), "-cardial" (of the heart), and "infarction" (tissue death), referring to what is commonly known as a heart attack (University of San Diego, n/a).

Directional terms are used to describe the locations of structures relative to other parts of the body. These include:

Anterior (ventral): Toward the front. For example, the toes are anterior to the foot.

Posterior (dorsal): Toward the back. The shoulder blades are posterior to the chest.

Superior (cranial): Toward the head. The head is superior to the neck.

Inferior (caudal): Toward the feet. The knees are inferior to the hips.

Medial: Toward the midline of the body. The nose is medial to the eyes.

Lateral: Away from the midline. The ears are lateral to the eyes.

Proximal: Closer to the point of attachment. The elbow is proximal to the wrist.

Distal: Further from the point of attachment. The fingers are distal to the elbow.

Superficial: Closer to the surface of the body. The skin is superficial to the muscles.

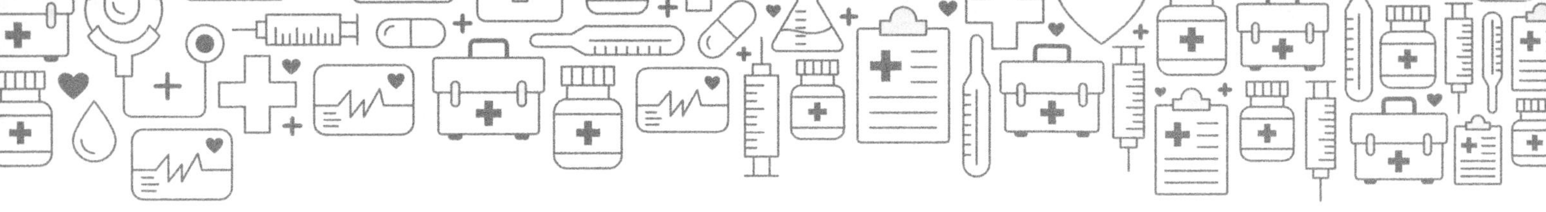

Deep: Further from the surface. The bones are deep to the muscles.

Body planes are imaginary lines that divide the body into sections. These planes help in describing locations and movements:

Sagittal Plane: Divides the body into right and left sides. If it runs down the midline, it is called the midsagittal plane; if off-center, it is called the parasagittal plane.

Frontal (Coronal) Plane: Divides the body into anterior (front) and posterior (back) sections.

Transverse Plane: Divides the body into superior (upper) and inferior (lower) parts.

The body contains several cavities that house and protect internal organs:

Cranial Cavity: Encloses the brain.

Thoracic Cavity: Houses the lungs and heart, protected by the rib cage.

Abdominopelvic Cavity: Divided into the abdominal cavity (digestive organs) and pelvic cavity (reproductive organs). This is the largest cavity and is not physically separated, but functionally distinct.

For detailed description and diagnosis, the abdominopelvic cavity is often divided into regions and quadrants:

Nine Regions: Used for detailed anatomical studies, including right and left hypochondriac regions, epigastric region, right and left lumbar regions, umbilical region, right and left iliac regions, and hypogastric region.

Four Quadrants: Commonly used in clinical settings for quick reference, dividing the abdomen into right upper quadrant (RUQ), left upper quadrant (LUQ), right lower quadrant (RLQ), and left lower quadrant (LLQ) (Biga et al., n/a).

We explored the structure and function of the human body, from the atomic level to complex organ systems. It outlines how atoms form molecules, which combine into cells, the smallest units of life. Cells form tissues, which build organs, and organs create systems essential for health. Key systems include integumentary, skeletal, muscular, nervous, endocrine, cardiovascular, lymphatic, respiratory, digestive, urinary, and reproductive systems. We also covered homeostasis, the body's internal balance mechanism, and emphasized the importance of medical terminology for accurate communication in healthcare.

4

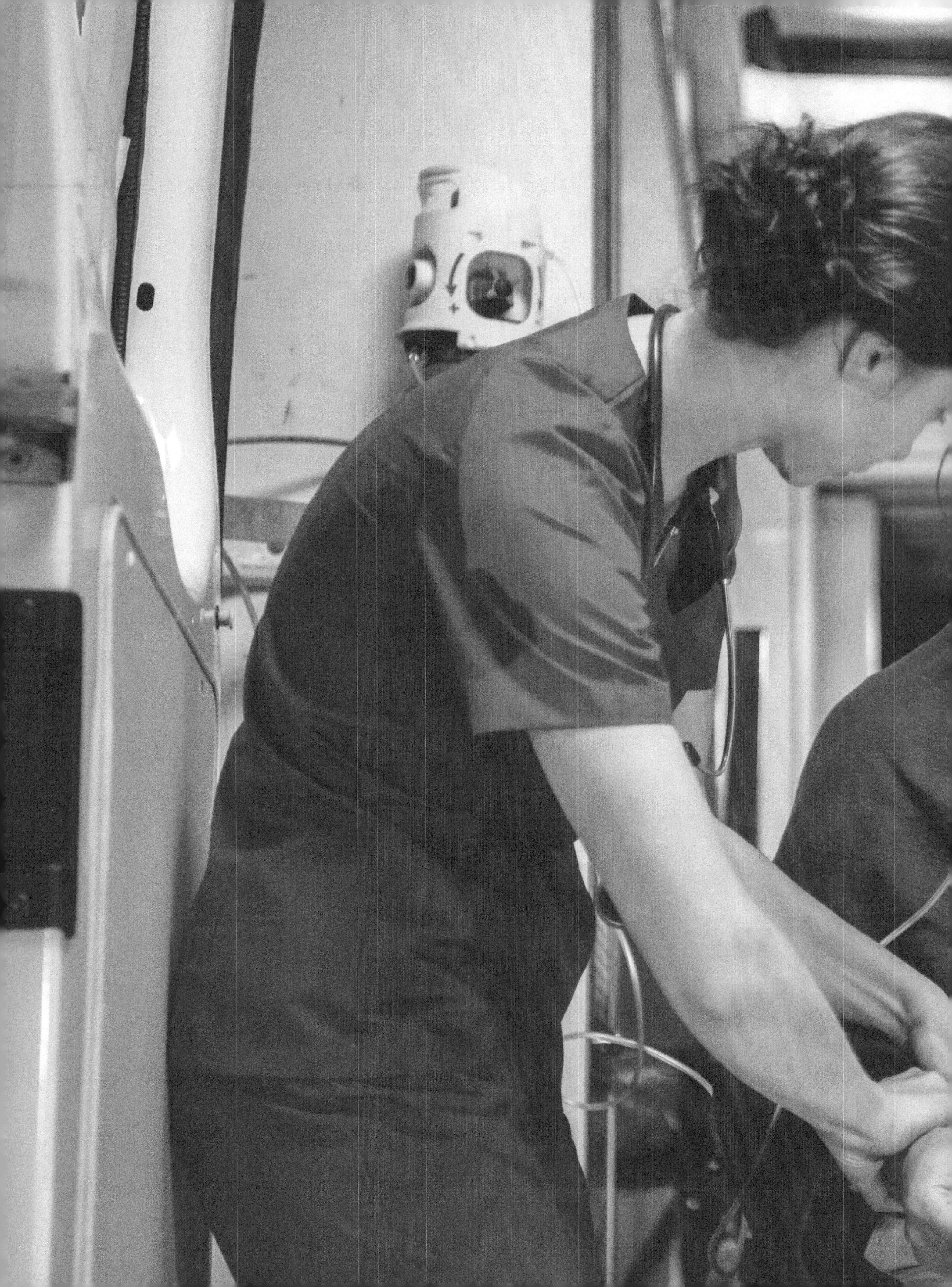

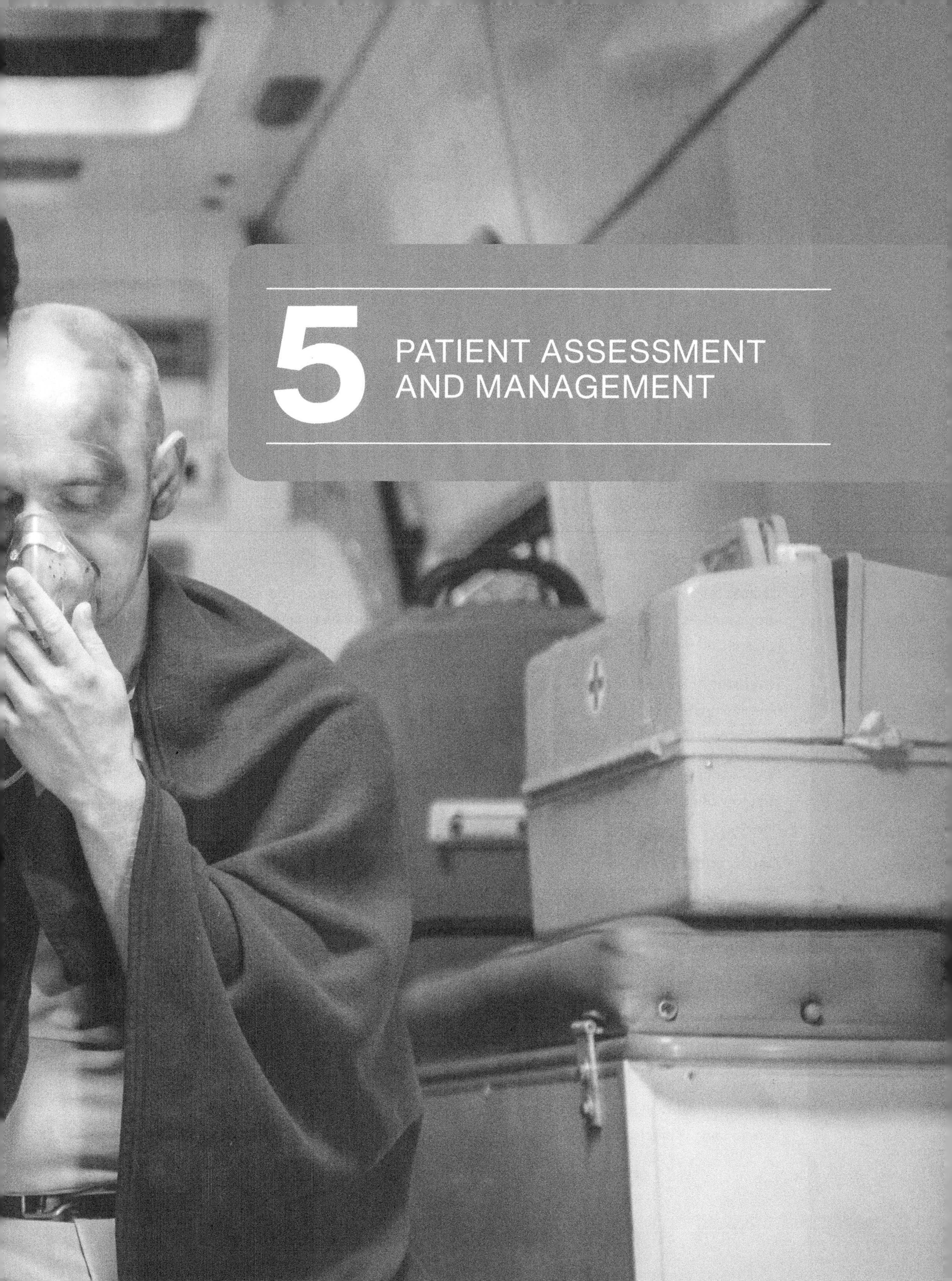

5 PATIENT ASSESSMENT AND MANAGEMENT

PATIENT ASSESSMENT AND MANAGEMENT

Vital signs are essential measurements used to assess a patient's immediate health status and guide treatment decisions. They include pulse, respiration, blood pressure, skin color, temperature, and level of consciousness. These indicators provide critical information about the body's condition and function.

The pulse represents the wave of blood moving through the arteries as the heart beats. It is typically assessed at several locations: the radial artery in the wrist, the carotid artery in the neck, and occasionally the femoral artery in the groin. Each of these sites provides valuable information about the patient's heart rate and blood circulation.

Rate: The number of beats per minute varies depending on the patient's age. For adults, a normal pulse rate is between 60 and 100 beats per minute. Children usually have a rate of 80 to 100 beats per minute, while infants have a rate of 100 to 120 beats per minute. Newborns typically have a pulse rate of 130 to 140 beats per minute. A pulse rate above these ranges indicates tachycardia, while a rate below suggests bradycardia.

Character: This describes the strength of the pulse. A strong pulse is referred to as full, whereas a very strong pulse is called bounding. Conversely, a weak pulse might be described as thready. Pulse strength can indicate the heart's efficiency and overall circulation.

Rhythm: The pulse rhythm is assessed by checking the regularity of the beats. A regular pulse has consistent intervals between beats, whereas an irregular pulse does not. Irregular rhythms can suggest various cardiovascular issues.

Respirations are measured by counting the number of breaths a person takes in one minute. Normal respiratory rates are between 12 and 24 breaths per minute for adults, and 30 to 50 breaths per minute for infants.

Depth and Ease: Respiratory depth refers to how much air is inhaled and exhaled with each breath. Breathing can be shallow or deep. Ease of breathing is assessed to determine if it is labored, which could indicate respiratory distress or illness.

Rhythm: Like pulse, respiratory rhythm can be regular or irregular. Regular respiration has consistent intervals between breaths, while irregular respiration varies.

Blood pressure measures the force of blood against the walls of the arteries. It consists of two readings: systolic and diastolic. Systolic pressure is the force when the heart's ventricles contract, and diastolic pressure is when the heart is at rest between beats.

Measurement: Blood pressure is recorded in millimeters of mercury (mm Hg). A typical blood pressure reading is presented as systolic/diastolic (e.g., 120/80 mm Hg). The pulse pressure, the difference between systolic and diastolic pressures, typically ranges from 30 to 40 mm Hg.

Techniques: Blood pressure can be measured using a sphygmomanometer (blood pressure cuff) and stethoscope or by palpation. Accurate measurements directly impact the diagnosis of hypertension or hypotension.

Skin color and temperature can provide additional clues about a patient's condition. Pale skin may suggest shock or poor circulation, while cyanosis (bluish skin) can indicate low oxygen levels. Redness may be associated with high blood pressure or fever. Normal skin should be warm and dry. Skin that is hot or cold can signal fever, shock, or environmental exposure.

Assessing a patient's level of consciousness helps determine their responsiveness and awareness. The AVPU scale is commonly used:

A - Alert: The patient is awake and aware of their surroundings.

V - Verbal: The patient responds to verbal stimuli.

P - Pain: The patient responds to painful stimuli but not to verbal prompts.

U - Unresponsive: The patient does not respond to any stimuli.

The pupil's reaction to light can reveal neurological issues. Normally, pupils constrict in bright light and dilate in low light. Unequal pupil reactions can indicate brain injury or other serious conditions.

History Taking: The SAMPLE Method

Obtaining a thorough medical history directly affects the ability to provide effective care. The SAMPLE acronym helps ensure that all relevant information is collected:

S - Signs and Symptoms: Document the patient's symptoms, which are subjective and based on their personal experience. Symptoms like pain or nausea cannot be measured directly but are critical for diagnosis.

A - Allergies: Determine if the patient has any known allergies, including to medications, foods, or environmental factors.

M - Medications: Find out what medications the patient is currently taking, including prescription, over the counter, and illegal drugs. This information is important for avoiding potential drug interactions and understanding the patient's condition.

P - Pertinent Medical History: Gather information about the patient's past medical issues, including chronic conditions, surgeries, and relevant family history. This can help in identifying possible underlying causes of the current problem.

L - Last Meal: Note when and what the patient last ate. This can be important for diagnosing gastrointestinal issues or if surgery is anticipated.

E - Events: Understand the events leading up to the patient's condition. Look for any medical alert bracelets or other indicators that might provide additional information (Hopper Institute, n/a).

Patient assessment is a valuable skill for emergency medical technicians and forms the core of their job. It is about systematically evaluating a patient's condition to provide the proper care. The first step in patient assessment is to assess the scene where the emergency has occurred. This is called the "scene size-up." It is essential to ensure safety before approaching the patient. Look for any potential hazards, such as traffic, fire, or hazardous materials. Also, determine the number of patients and whether additional resources are needed. This initial step helps you avoid risks and plan your response.

Once the scene is safe, check the patient's level of consciousness. This helps gauge how serious the situation is. To do this, approach the patient and see if they are awake and alert. If the patient is not fully responsive, you need to determine their level of awareness using the AVPU scale.

The next step is assessing the Airway, Breathing, and Circulation (ABCs):

Airway: Make sure the patient's airway is open. If it is blocked, you may need to perform maneuvers like tilting the head back or using airway adjuncts to clear it.

Breathing: Check if the patient is breathing. Count the number of breaths per minute and assess the quality of breathing. If the patient is not breathing effectively, provide oxygen or perform rescue breathing as needed.

Circulation: Evaluate the patient's pulse and look for signs of adequate blood circulation. Check the pulse rate, rhythm, and strength. Also, observe the patient's skin color and temperature. If the pulse is weak or absent, or if the skin is pale or cyanotic, immediate intervention might be necessary.

Next, conduct a thorough physical exam to check for injuries or abnormalities. Follow a systematic approach:

Head and Neck: Check for any signs of trauma or abnormal findings.

Chest: Look for chest injuries and listen for breath sounds.

Abdomen: Palpate the abdomen to identify tenderness, swelling, or other issues.

Pelvis: Gently assess for any signs of injury or deformity.

Extremities: Inspect the arms and legs for injuries, swelling, or changes in color.

Back: Assess the patient's back to see if it is safe and feasible.

Based on your assessment, begin the necessary treatments. This might include administering medications, performing first aid, or providing oxygen. Continuously monitor the patient's response to your interventions and adjust your care as needed.

Decide on the appropriate mode of transportation based on the severity of the patient's condition. Communicate clearly with your team to ensure that the patient is transported safely and efficiently.

Tips for Effective Patient Assessment:

Effective communication is crucial. Maintain clear and concise communication with your team members as well as with the patient. This helps in coordinating care and ensures that everyone involved is aware of the patient's condition and the actions being taken.

Staying calm under pressure is essential. Remain composed, even in stressful situations, to make informed and clear decisions. This calm demeanor helps manage the emergency effectively and provides reassurance to the patient.

Regularly reassess the patient's condition throughout the assessment process. Conditions can change quickly, so continuous evaluation ensures that you can adjust your interventions and care plan as needed.

Finally, adapt your approach to each individual situation. Be flexible and modify your assessment techniques based on the patient's specific needs and the emergency's circumstances. This adaptability enhances your ability to provide appropriate and effective care (Jugueta, 2024).

Overall, we covered the vital signs—pulse, respiration, blood pressure, skin color, temperature, and level of consciousness. The pulse indicates heart rate and circulation; respirations reveal breathing efficiency. Blood pressure measures arterial force, while skin color and temperature can indicate conditions like shock or fever. Level of consciousness is assessed using the AVPU scale. History is gathered using the SAMPLE method (Signs, Allergies, Medications, Medical history, Last meal, Events). Effective patient assessment involves ensuring scene safety, checking airway, breathing, and circulation, conducting a thorough physical exam, and maintaining continuous monitoring and communication.

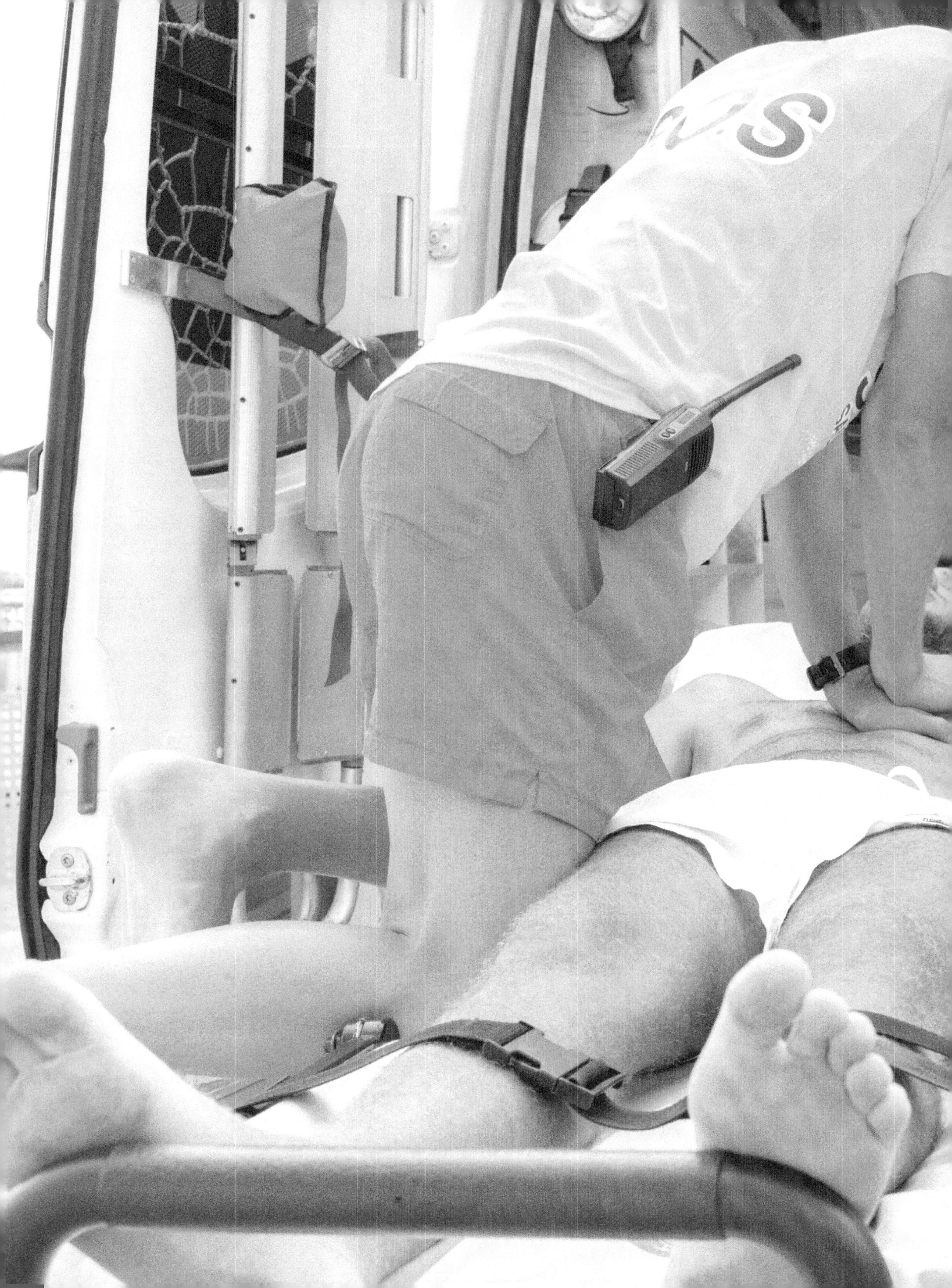

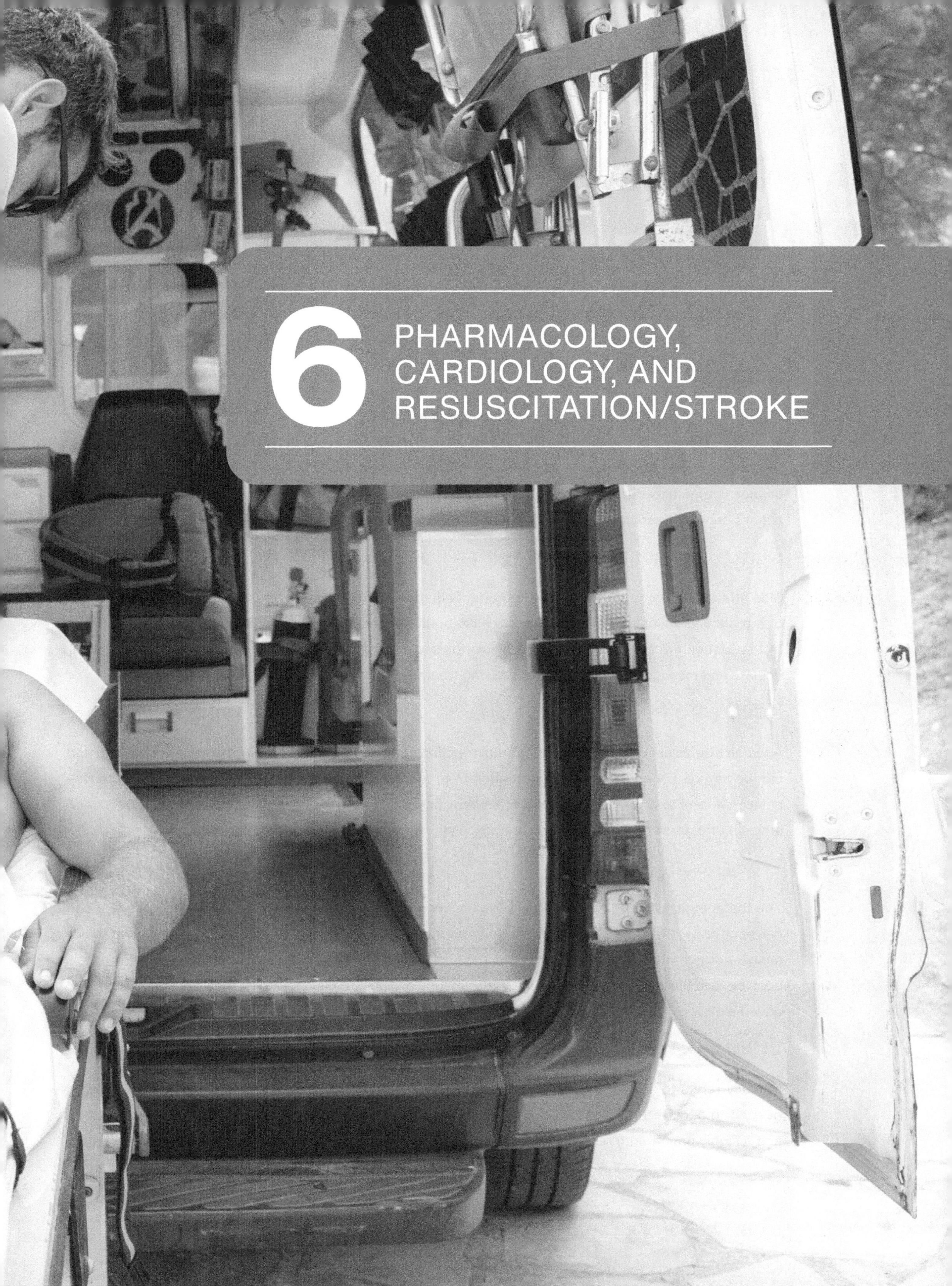

6 PHARMACOLOGY, CARDIOLOGY, AND RESUSCITATION/STROKE

PHARMACOLOGY, CARDIOLOGY, AND RESUSCITATION/ STROKE

Pharmacology is the study of the characteristics and effects of medications. Medications are chemical substances used to treat or prevent diseases and relieve pain. When discussing pharmacology, it is essential to understand various terms and concepts related to medications (EMSWorld, 2005).

Desired Effects

The primary goal of administering any medication is to achieve its desired effect. This is the specific therapeutic outcome that the drug is intended to produce. However, some drugs can have multiple effects, which can sometimes lead to confusion. For instance, epinephrine is used to increase heart rate and cardiac contractility during cardiac arrest but also helps open airways during anaphylaxis. These multiple actions can be beneficial in different clinical scenarios.

Side Effects

Side effects are unintended but expected effects that occur in addition to the desired therapeutic effects of a drug. For example, Albuterol, used to ease breathing in asthma or COPD patients, often causes an increased heart rate as a side effect. Knowing these potential side effects helps healthcare providers anticipate and manage them appropriately during treatment.

Adverse Effects

Adverse effects are unexpected and harmful reactions to a drug. These reactions are not anticipated and can be severe. For example, a drug intended to produce euphoria might also cause vomiting or, in rare cases, be fatal to a small percentage of users. Understanding the difference between side effects and adverse effects is important in pharmacology, as the latter can significantly harm the patient.

Therapeutic Index

The therapeutic index of a drug is the range between the minimum effective dose and the dose that can cause adverse effects. A wider therapeutic index indicates a safer drug. Healthcare providers aim to administer drugs within this range to achieve the desired effects without causing harm. Increasing a drug's dose beyond this range does not enhance therapeutic effects but can increase the risk of side effects and adverse effects.

Efficacy versus Potency

Efficacy refers to a drug's ability to produce the intended result, while potency is the amount of drug needed to achieve that result. For example, antibiotics have different efficacies in treating infections, and a highly potent drug requires a smaller dose to be effective. When choosing medications, healthcare providers consider both efficacy and potency to ensure the best outcomes for patients (Guardian Test Prep, n/a).

Medication Names and Routes of Administration

Medications can have multiple names: trade names, which are brand names given by manufacturers, and generic names, which are the original chemical names often used as the medication's name. For instance, ibuprofen is sold under trade names like Advil, Nuprin, and Motrin.

The trade names are capitalized as proper nouns, while the generic names are not. Medications can be either prescription medications, which require a physician's order and are distributed by pharmacists, or over the counter (OTC) medications, which can be purchased directly from retail sources.

The routes of medication administration are varied and include:

Intravenous (IV) injections: deliver medication directly into the bloodstream and are the fastest way to administer medication.

Oral administration: involves taking medication by mouth and absorption through the digestive system, which can take up to an hour.

Sublingual (SL) administration: places medication under the tongue for quick absorption through the oral mucous membrane.

Intramuscular (IM) injections: administered into the muscle, allowing quick absorption due to the muscle's blood vessels, though some medications may be slow-release.

Intraosseous (IO) injections: administered into the bone, entering the bloodstream through the bone marrow.

Subcutaneous (SC) injections: administered beneath the skin, in the tissue between the skin and muscle.

Transcutaneous administration: enters through the skin, producing a slow, long-lasting effect, as seen with nitroglycerin and nicotine patches.

Inhalation: involves medication being inhaled into the lungs for quick absorption, with some medications targeting the lungs specifically, minimizing effects on other body tissues. It comes in various forms, including aerosols, fine powders, and sprays.

Per rectum (PR) delivery involves delivering medication by the rectum, often used with children for easier administration and more reliable absorption.

Medication Forms and Their Characteristics

Medications come in various forms, including tablets and capsules, solutions and suspensions, metered-dose inhalers, topical medications, transcutaneous medications, gels, and gases for inhalation. Tablets and capsules are common forms for adult medications, with capsules being gelatin shells containing either powder or liquid. Tablets are compressed mixtures of medication and other substances, with some designed to dissolve quickly and others slowly in the digestive system.

Solutions are liquid mixtures where substances are evenly distributed and cannot be separated by filtering or standing. Suspensions, on the other hand, are mixtures where fine particles are distributed throughout a liquid but will settle if allowed to stand and must be shaken before use. Metered-dose inhalers administer small droplets or particles of medication through the lungs, delivering a consistent dose each time, and are commonly used in respiratory illnesses.

Topical medications are applied to the skin's surface and affect only the local area. They come in forms like lotions, creams, and ointments, with varying absorption rates. Transcutaneous medications are designed to be absorbed through the skin for systemic effects and can be applied using adhesive patches, such as nitroglycerin or nicotine patches.

Gels are semi-liquid substances administered orally and are clear, unlike the opaquer pastes or creams. Gases for inhalation, such as oxygen, are neither solid nor liquid and are meaningful in emergency medical settings.

Medications on Ambulances and Proper Administration Techniques

Medications commonly carried on ambulances include activated charcoal, ipecac, oral glucose, oxygen, and epinephrine auto-injectors. Activated charcoal to treat poisoning by mouth; it absorbs poisons and prevents them from being absorbed by the body. It is a suspension that must be shaken well before administration. Ipecac is used to induce vomiting in cases of ingested poisoning but has specific contraindications, such as ingestion of caustics or petroleum products.

Oral glucose is used for patients with altered mental status due to hypoglycemia. It is a simple sugar easily absorbed by the body, increasing blood sugar levels. Oxygen is administered to all medical and trauma patients to enhance cell function and prevent hypoxia. It is provided through various devices, such as nasal cannulas, Venturi masks, and non-rebreather masks, with different flow rates and oxygen concentrations.

Epinephrine auto-injectors are used for moderate to severe allergic reactions and severe asthma in pediatric patients. Epinephrine increases heart rate and blood pressure, decreases muscle tone of the bronchial tree, dilates lung passages, and constricts blood vessels. Proper administration involves ensuring the medication is not discolored, removing the auto-injector cap, placing the tip against the patient's thigh, and holding it in place for at least ten seconds.

Prescribed Medications Commonly Carried by Patients

Patients may carry prescribed medications like metered-dose inhalers, nitroglycerin, and epinephrine auto-injectors. Metered-dose inhalers, such as Albuterol, Proventil, and Ventolin, are used for respiratory distress and bronchospasms associated with asthma, chronic bronchitis, emphysema, and allergic reactions. They function as bronchodilators, enlarging constricted bronchial tubes, and have adverse effects like tachycardia, hypertension, and dizziness.

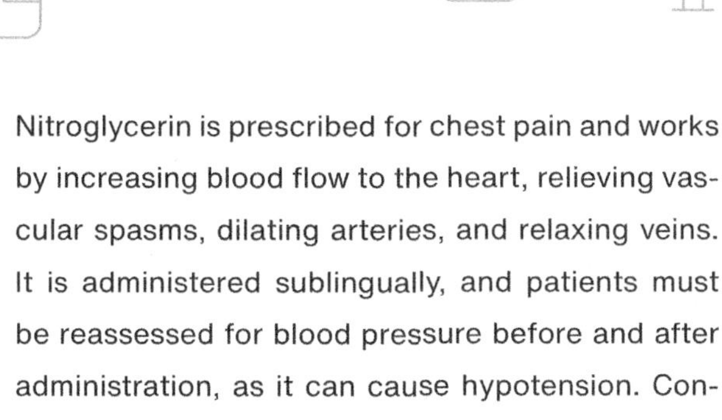

Nitroglycerin is prescribed for chest pain and works by increasing blood flow to the heart, relieving vascular spasms, dilating arteries, and relaxing veins. It is administered sublingually, and patients must be reassessed for blood pressure before and after administration, as it can cause hypotension. Contraindications include a blood pressure below 90 mm Hg systolic, heart rate less than 60, and recent ingestion of Viagra.

Epinephrine auto-injectors, as mentioned earlier, are urgent for allergic reactions and severe asthma. The administration technique is similar to that for ambulance-carried epinephrine auto-injectors, ensuring the medication is not discolored and following proper protocol for injection (EMSWorld, 2005).

The First Pass Effect

The first pass effect refers to the metabolism of a drug within the liver and kidneys before it reaches systemic circulation, reducing the drug's concentration and effectiveness. This concept is fundamental for dosing strategies, such as using loading doses to achieve therapeutic levels quickly, followed by maintenance doses to sustain the drug's effect.

Pharmacokinetics and Pharmacodynamics

Pharmacokinetics involves how the body absorbs, distributes, metabolizes, and excretes a drug. Pharmacodynamics describes how the drug affects the body, including the relationship between drug concentration and effect. These fields help understand timing, intensity, and duration.

Agonists and Antagonists

Agonists are drugs that activate receptors to produce a response, while antagonists block receptor activity. For example, Albuterol acts as an agonist to dilate airways, and Atrovent acts as an antagonist to prevent airway constriction. Understanding these mechanisms helps select the appropriate drug for specific conditions (Guardian Test Prep, n/a).

CARDIAC EMERGENCIES AND RESUSCITATION

Cardiac emergencies encompass a range of conditions that affect the heart's ability to function properly. These emergencies require prompt and efficient response to prevent serious outcomes, including death. Understanding the signs, symptoms, and appropriate responses to these conditions is useful for healthcare providers and first responders.

Recognizing Cardiac Compromise

Cardiac compromise refers to any heart-related problem that impacts its normal function. Patients experiencing cardiac compromise often present with a variety of symptoms. The most common complaint is chest pain, which can radiate to the left arm. Other symptoms include flu-like symptoms, dyspnea (difficulty breathing), palpitations, sudden sweating, nausea, vomiting, anxiety, and abnormal pulse or blood pressure.

When a patient exhibits these symptoms, it is essential to perform a focused history and physical examination, including OPQRST (Onset, Provocation, Quality, Radiation, Severity, Time) questions and obtaining a SAMPLE history (Signs/Symptoms, Allergies, Medications, Past medical history, Last oral intake, Events leading up to present illness).

Emergency Care for Cardiac Compromise

Immediate and appropriate care is vital for patients experiencing cardiac compromise. The following steps are typically taken:

Positioning: Place the patient in a comfortable position, usually sitting up.

Oxygen Therapy: Administer high-concentration oxygen through a nonrebreather mask.

Transport: Transport the patient immediately if they have no history of cardiac problems, have a history but no nitroglycerin, or if their systolic blood pressure is below 100.

Nitroglycerin Administration: Help administer nitroglycerin if the patient has chest pain, a history of cardiac problems, has their nitroglycerin with them, has a systolic blood pressure greater than 100, and if medical direction authorizes it. Repeat the dose every five minutes if there is no relief, the systolic blood pressure remains above 100, and medical direction authorizes it. A maximum of three doses can be administered.

Cardiovascular Disorders

Most cardiovascular disorders arise from changes in the arterial walls. Atherosclerosis involves the build-up of fatty deposits on the inner walls of arteries, leading to the formation of plaque. Over time, calcium may be deposited in the plaque, causing arteriosclerosis, which hardens the artery walls and increases blood pressure. Blood clots (thrombi) can form along plaque, potentially breaking off and causing occlusions in smaller vessels.

Coronary artery disease (CAD) is a significant cause of cardiac emergencies, characterized by reduced blood flow to the myocardium. The primary symptom of CAD is chest pain, known as angina pectoris. Electrical system malfunctions in the heart can result in arrhythmias (absent heartbeat) or dysrhythmias (irregular heartbeats), such as tachycardia (heart rate above 100 bpm) and bradycardia (heart rate below 60 bpm).

Acute Myocardial Infarction and Heart Failure

An acute myocardial infarction (AMI), commonly known as a heart attack, occurs when a portion of the heart muscle dies due to a lack of blood supply. This can lead to cardiac arrest, where the heart stops functioning altogether. Heart failure occurs when the heart cannot pump blood adequately, leading to fluid buildup in the lungs and other organs. Congestive heart failure (CHF) is a specific type of heart failure characterized by fluid accumulation due to poor heart function.

Signs and Symptoms of Congestive Heart Failure

- Patients with CHF may exhibit:
- Tachycardia (rapid heartbeat)
- Dyspnea (difficulty breathing)
- Normal or elevated blood pressure
- Cyanosis (bluish skin)

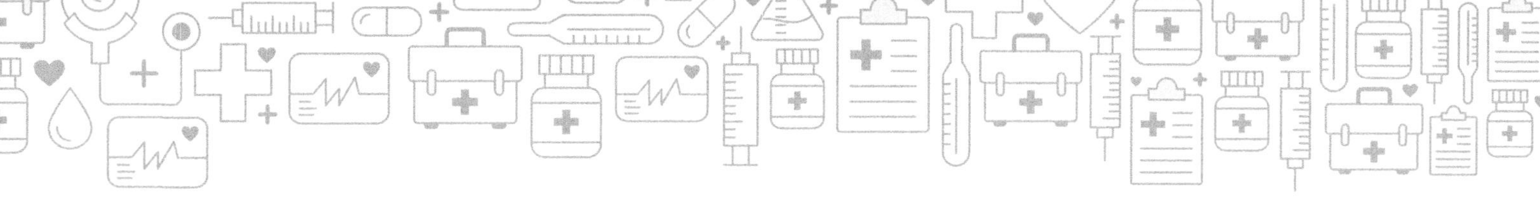

- Diaphoresis (sweating)
- Pulmonary edema (fluid in the lungs)
- Anxiety or confusion due to hypoxia
- Pedal edema (swelling in the feet)
- Engorged, pulsating neck veins (late sign)
- Enlarged liver and spleen; abdominal distension (late sign)

The Chain of Survival for Cardiac Arrest

Successful resuscitation from cardiac arrest depends on the "chain of survival," which includes:

- Timely access to emergency medical services (EMS)
- Early cardiopulmonary resuscitation (CPR)
- Early defibrillation
- Early advanced care

Defibrillation, the delivery of an electric shock to restore a normal heart rhythm, can be manual or automated. Manual defibrillation requires the operator to interpret the ECG and decide if a shock is needed. Automated external defibrillators (AEDs) analyze the heart rhythm and deliver shocks if necessary.

Shockable and Nonshockable Rhythms

Common shockable rhythms include ventricular fibrillation (v-fib) and ventricular tachycardia (v-tach). Nonshockable rhythms include pulseless electrical activity (PEA) and asystole. PEA is characterized by normal electrical activity without effective heart contractions, often due to severe illness or significant blood loss. Asystole indicates no electrical activity in the heart.

Coordinating CPR with AED

When using an automated external defibrillator, follow these steps:

- Stop CPR to verify the absence of a pulse and breathing.
- Resume CPR while preparing the patient for AED use.
- Attach electrode pads to the appropriate locations on the patient's chest.
- Clear the patient and wait for the AED to analyze the rhythm.
- Deliver a shock if advised, then resume CPR.
- Repeat the shock cycle as necessary, checking the pulse after each cycle.
- Transport the patient if a pulse is regained, six shocks have been delivered, or the AED advises no further shocks.
- If the patient goes back into cardiac arrest during transport, stop the vehicle, restart CPR, prepare the AED, and follow the shock cycle protocol again.

Special Considerations

Use AEDs only on adults who have not suffered trauma before collapse. Do not use AEDs on children under eight years old or on trauma victims. In trauma cases, the primary focus should be on preventing blood loss, which is often the root cause of nonshockable rhythms (Hopper Institute, n/a).

DETAILED GUIDE TO RESUSCITATION

Resuscitation, specifically cardiopulmonary resuscitation (CPR), is a critical emergency procedure performed to save lives in cases of cardiac arrest. This detailed guide outlines the systematic approach to performing resuscitation effectively, ensuring that every step is taken to optimize patient outcomes.

Initial Assessment and Response

When encountering a potential cardiac arrest scenario, the first step is to ensure the scene is safe for both the rescuer and the patient. Personal protective equipment (PPE) should be worn to maintain Body Substance Isolation (BSI). Upon approaching the patient, assess for a response by using both vocal and painful stimuli. Shout loudly, "Hey sir/madam, are you alright?" and if there is no response, proceed with a sternal rub, applying firm pressure to the patient's sternum. This is a painful stimulus intended to elicit a reaction if the patient is semi-conscious.

If there is no response, it is mandatory to call emergency medical services (EMS) immediately. If you are alone, call 911 and retrieve an Automated External Defibrillator (AED). If others are present, delegate these tasks to bystanders while you begin the next steps of resuscitation.

Airway Management

Once you have determined that the patient is unresponsive, the next step is to open the airway. This can be achieved using either the head-tilt chin-lift maneuver or the jaw-thrust technique. The head-tilt chin-lift is preferred unless spinal injury is suspected, in which case the jaw-thrust technique is used to minimize neck movement.

Breathing Assessment and Ventilation

With the airway open, check for breathing. This should be done within 5-10 seconds. Look for the rise and fall of the chest, listen for breathing sounds, and feel for air movement from the nose and mouth. If the patient is not breathing or is breathing inadequately, provide two rescue breaths. Each breath should be delivered over one second, just enough to see the chest rise, and avoid excessive force to prevent gastric inflation.

Various ventilation techniques can be used:

Mouth-to-Mouth: This method forms the most effective seal. Pinch the patient's nose and blow into their mouth.

Mouth-to-Mask: Using a mask that covers the nose and mouth, deliver breaths while holding the mask firmly to maintain a good seal.

Bag-Valve Mask (BVM): Squeeze the bag to ventilate through a mask that covers the nose and mouth. Ensure the mask is held firmly to maintain a proper seal.

Circulation Check and Chest Compressions

Next, check the carotid pulse for 5-10 seconds. If a pulse is present, provide one breath every 5-6 seconds and recheck the pulse every two minutes. If no pulse is detected, begin chest compressions immediately.

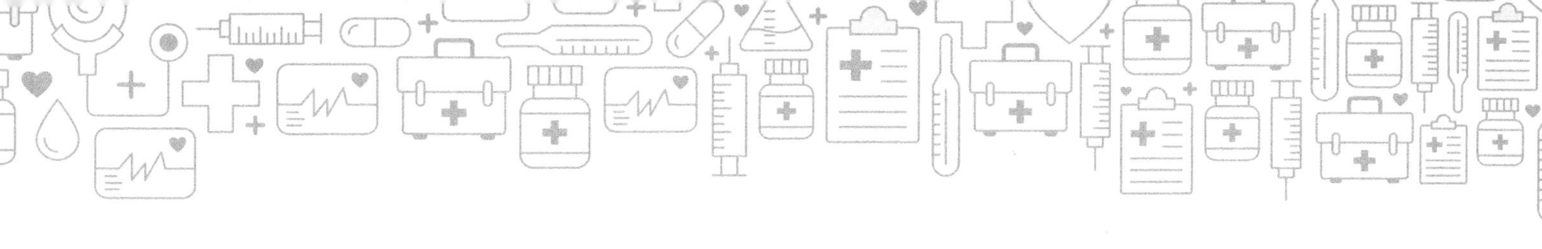

For effective chest compressions:

Ensure the patient is lying on a hard, flat surface.

Position yourself beside the patient.

Remove any clothing covering the chest.

Place the heel of one hand in the center of the chest, between the nipples. Place the other hand on top, interlocking the fingers.

Keep your arms straight and use your body weight to compress the chest at least 1½ to 2 inches deep.

Allow the chest to fully recoil between compressions.

Perform compressions at a rate of 100 per minute.

After 30 compressions, provide two breaths.

Defibrillation

Defibrillation is a critical component of resuscitation for patients in cardiac arrest due to shockable rhythms like ventricular fibrillation (V-fib). Upon arrival of an AED, attach the electrode pads to the patient's bare chest. Clear the area, ensuring no one touches the patient, and allow the AED to assess the heart rhythm. If a shockable rhythm is detected, clear the patient again and deliver the shock, then immediately resume CPR for five cycles before reassessing.

If the AED advises no shock, resume CPR immediately for five cycles before reassessing the rhythm. Continue this cycle as necessary.

Special Considerations for Infants and Children

Resuscitation techniques for infants and children vary slightly: if an infant or child's heart rate is below 60 bpm with signs of poor perfusion, initiate chest compressions. For children, the optimal compression-to-ventilation ratio is 15:2 with two rescuers, while infants require the two-thumb encircling hands technique for compressions. Provide ventilations at a rate of 1 breath every 3-5 seconds. In cases of witnessed cardiac arrest or arrest occurring within the past five minutes, apply the AED immediately.

Minimize Interruptions

It is essential to minimize interruptions to chest compressions, aiming for interruptions to last less than 10 seconds. If two rescuers are present, one should perform continuous chest compressions while the other provides ventilations at the appropriate rate (5-6 breaths per minute for adults and 3-5 breaths per minute for infants and children). Rescuers should switch roles every five cycles of compressions to maintain effectiveness and reduce fatigue.

UNDERSTANDING SHOCKABLE AND NONSHOCKABLE RHYTHMS

Ventricular fibrillation (V-fib) and ventricular tachycardia (V-tach) are shockable rhythms that can be treated with defibrillation. Nonshockable rhythms, such as pulseless electrical activity (PEA) and asystole, do not benefit from defibrillation. PEA indicates normal electrical activity without effective heart contractions, often due to severe illness or significant blood loss. Asystole shows no electrical activity and is often a sign of a severely compromised heart.

Continuous Monitoring and Adaptation

During resuscitation, continuous monitoring of the patient's condition is necessary. After each cycle of CPR, reassess the patient's pulse and breathing.

Adapt the resuscitation approach based on the patient's response and the guidance from the AED. Coordination with EMS is useful for providing advanced care as soon as possible.

Overall, effective resuscitation involves a systematic approach to ensure the best possible outcomes for patients experiencing cardiac arrest. By following these detailed steps, including initial assessment, airway management, breathing assessment, circulation check, and defibrillation, rescuers can provide critical care efficiently and effectively. Special considerations for different patient populations and minimizing interruptions to compressions further enhance the quality of resuscitation efforts. This comprehensive approach is decisive in saving lives and improving recovery rates in cardiac emergencies (EMT-training, n/a).

UNDERSTANDING AND TREATING STROKES

Stroke is a critical medical condition that EMS professionals often encounter. Accounting for about 2% of all EMS calls, strokes represent a massive portion of emergency responses. This guide delves into how EMTs and paramedics identify, treat, and care for stroke patients, emphasizing the importance of timely intervention and proper management.

Risk Factors and Statistics

Strokes are the fifth leading cause of death in the United States, responsible for over 137,000 deaths annually. Every 40 seconds, someone in the U.S. experiences a stroke, and every four minutes, someone dies from one (Unitek EMT, 2021). The main risk factor for stroke is high blood pressure, but other factors include smoking, obesity, high cholesterol, diabetes, previous transient ischemic attacks (TIA), end-stage kidney disease, and atrial fibrillation.

Identifying Stroke Symptoms

Early identification of stroke symptoms significantly influences the success of treatment. The acronym F.A.S.T. is a helpful tool:

Face Drooping: One side of the face droops or is numb. When asked to smile, the person's smile is uneven.

Arm Weakness: One arm is weak or numb. When asked to raise both arms, one arm drifts downward.

Speech Difficulty: Speech is slurred, or the person is unable to speak or hard to understand. They may have trouble repeating simple sentences.

Time to Call 911: If any of these symptoms are present, even if they go away, it is critical to call 911 immediately.

Other symptoms include sudden numbness or weakness, especially on one side of the body, confusion, trouble seeing in one or both eyes, difficulty walking, dizziness, and a sudden severe headache with no known cause.

Immediate Actions

When a stroke is suspected, quick action is essential. While waiting for EMTs or paramedics, the patient should lie down with their airway open. Check for breathing and pulse, and if necessary, perform CPR. If the person is breathing but unconscious, they should be rolled onto their side, unless there is a suspected spinal injury. Conscious patients should be reassured and kept comfortable, with any tight clothing or jewelry loosened. Importantly, do not give the patient anything to eat or drink, as they may have difficulty swallowing.

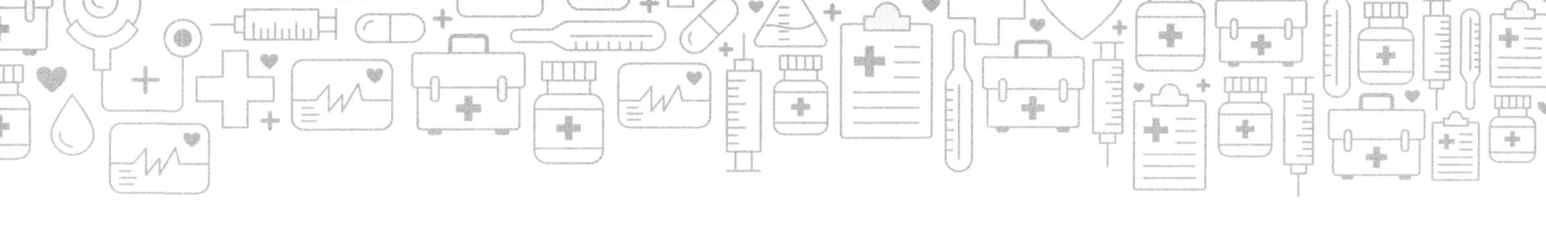

EMS Response and Treatment

Upon arrival, EMTs and paramedics conduct a rapid and systematic assessment using the ABCDE approach, which stands for Airway, Breathing, Circulation, Disability, and Exposure. This approach ensures a thorough initial evaluation, applicable in any emergency setting.

Airway and Breathing: The first step is to ensure the patient has an open airway and is breathing adequately. Oxygen may be administered to maintain saturation levels between 94-98%.

Circulation: EMTs check the patient's pulse and blood pressure. If the patient's heart is not beating, CPR is initiated immediately.

Disability: This involves assessing the patient's neurological status, often using validated prehospital stroke scales like the Cincinnati Prehospital Stroke Severity Scale or the Los Angeles Prehospital Stroke Screen (LAPSS). These tools help determine the extent of the stroke and guide treatment decisions.

Exposure: The patient's entire body is examined for additional signs of injury or illness, and pertinent medical history is gathered. This includes identifying any current medications, particularly anticoagulants, and noting recent illnesses, surgeries, or trauma.

Hospital Transport and Treatment

EMS personnel notify the receiving hospital of the incoming stroke patient, providing details about the patient's condition and the time they were last seen. This information is necessary for hospital staff to prepare and provide immediate care upon arrival. The patient's vital signs and neurological status are continually monitored during transport.

Upon reaching the hospital, a CT scan or MRI is typically performed to confirm the diagnosis and determine the type of stroke. An ischemic stroke happens when a blood vessel in the brain is blocked, usually by a blood clot, stopping blood flow to a part of the brain. A hemorrhagic stroke occurs when there is bleeding in or around the brain, either from a burst blood vessel or a leak in the brain's membranes.

For ischemic strokes, treatment may include medications such as tissue plasminogen activator (tPA), which can dissolve clots if administered within a few hours of symptom onset. Hemorrhagic strokes may require surgical intervention to stop the bleeding and relieve pressure on the brain.

Long-Term Management and Rehabilitation

After the acute phase, stroke patients often need long-term care and rehabilitation to recover lost functions. Stroke rehabilitation may involve physical therapy, occupational therapy, speech therapy, and support for managing daily activities. Rehabilitation aims to improve mobility, speech, and overall quality of life, helping patients regain as much independence as possible.

Preventive measures are also essential to reduce the risk of subsequent strokes. These may include lifestyle changes such as adopting a healthier diet, exercising regularly, quitting smoking, and controlling blood pressure and cholesterol levels. Medications such as aspirin or statins may be prescribed to help prevent future strokes (Unitek EMT, 2021).

UNDERSTANDING SYNCOPE: IDENTIFICATION, TREATMENT, AND CARE

Syncope, commonly referred to as fainting, is a sudden, temporary loss of consciousness often accompanied by a loss of muscle strength. This condition, characterized by a rapid onset, short duration, and spontaneous recovery, affects a significant number of individuals each year and accounts for nearly 8% of all EMS calls (Unitek EMT, 2021). Understanding the causes, symptoms, and appropriate responses to syncope is needed for effective management and treatment.

What is Syncope?

Syncope results from a temporary reduction in blood flow to the brain, which leads to a brief loss of consciousness. Various triggers can cause this reduction in blood flow, leading to fainting. Before losing consciousness, individuals may experience symptoms such as lightheadedness, sweating, pale skin, blurred vision, nausea, vomiting, or a sensation of warmth. In some cases, fainting may be preceded by muscle twitching. If these symptoms occur without a complete loss of consciousness, the condition is known as presyncope, and it is advised to treat it similarly to syncope.

Causes of Syncope

Syncope can be triggered by multiple factors ranging from benign to potentially fatal conditions. Broadly, the causes can be categorized into heart or blood vessel-related issues, vasovagal (or reflex) syncope, and orthostatic hypotension.

Heart or Blood Vessel-Related Syncope

Heart-related causes of syncope include abnormal heart rhythms, problems with heart valves or muscles, and blockages in blood vessels, such as those caused by a pulmonary embolism or aortic dissection. The most common heart-related cause is cardiac arrhythmia, where the heart beats too slowly, too rapidly, or irregularly, failing to pump sufficient blood to the brain. Conditions such as acute myocardial infarction (heart attack) can also lead to syncope, particularly in women, who may present fainting as a symptom of a heart attack. Recognizing heart-related syncope is necessary, as it often signals life-threatening conditions.

Vasovagal Syncope

Vasovagal syncope is the most common type and occurs in response to triggers such as fear, emotional trauma, severe pain, or prolonged standing. It results from a sudden drop in heart rate and blood pressure, reducing blood flow to the brain. The body's response to stress, pain, or other triggers can initiate a “fight-or-flight” reaction, where the heart rate initially increases but then drops suddenly, causing fainting. Symptoms leading up to a vasovagal episode, known as the prodrome, include lightheadedness, confusion, pallor, nausea, salivation, sweating, tachycardia, blurred vision, and a sudden urge to defecate.

Orthostatic Hypotension

Orthostatic hypotension syncope occurs when blood pressure significantly drops upon standing up from a lying or sitting position. This drop reduces blood flow to the brain, leading to fainting. Dehydration, medications, significant blood loss, or prolonged bed rest can trigger it. The elderly

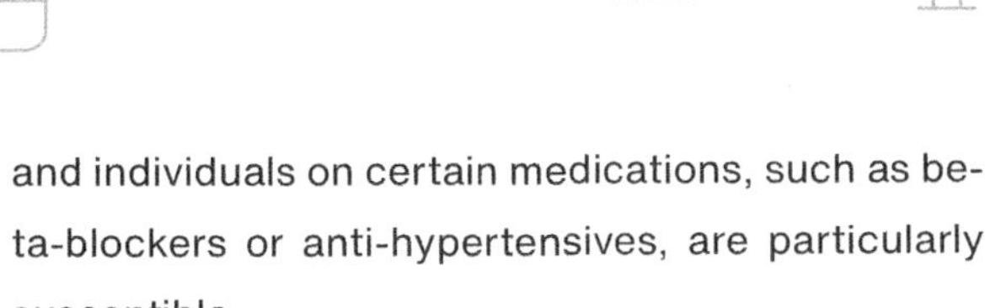

and individuals on certain medications, such as beta-blockers or anti-hypertensives, are particularly susceptible.

Treatment by EMTs and Paramedics

Upon arrival, EMTs and paramedics will perform a rapid and systematic assessment using the ABCDE approach. This approach, when accessed quickly, helps identify critical aspects of the patient's condition.

Preventing Future Episodes

Preventing recurrent syncope involves identifying and managing the underlying cause. For individuals with orthostatic hypotension, staying hydrated and avoiding rapid changes in posture can help. Those with vasovagal syncope might benefit from recognizing and avoiding triggers, such as stressful situations. Medications or treatments for underlying heart conditions can reduce the risk of heart-related syncope (Unitek EMT, 2021).

UNDERSTANDING SEIZURES

A seizure, formally known as an epileptic seizure, is a period of abnormal and excessive electrical activity in the brain. This sudden burst of electrical activity can result in a range of symptoms, from convulsions and shaking to more subtle signs like brief lapses in awareness or consciousness. Seizures vary significantly in their presentation, depending on the location of the abnormal electrical activity in the brain, the underlying cause, and individual patient factors such as age and overall health.

Causes of Seizures

Seizures can be triggered by a wide array of conditions. Common causes include head injuries, brain tumors, poisoning, genetic disorders, infections, and developmental issues. In some cases, high fevers can also provoke seizures, particularly in children. Despite these identifiable causes, around 70% of epilepsy cases have no known cause, suggesting a strong genetic component in many instances (Unitek EMT, 2021).

Types of Seizures

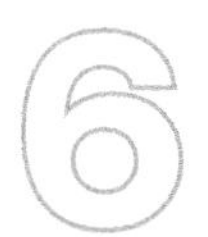

Seizures are broadly categorized into two types: focal and generalized. Focal seizures, also known as partial seizures, begin in a specific area of the brain. They can manifest as simple focal seizures, where the person remains conscious but experiences unusual sensations or movements, or as complex focal seizures, where there is a loss of awareness and strange behaviors, such as lip-smacking or hand movements.

Generalized seizures affect both sides of the brain and typically result in a loss of consciousness. They include several subtypes:

- **Tonic-clonic seizures** (grand mal) involve a mixture of muscle stiffness (tonic phase) and rhythmic jerking movements (clonic phase).
- **Absence seizures** (petit mal) are characterized by brief lapses in consciousness, often without any physical convulsions.
- **Myoclonic seizures** cause sudden muscle jerks.
- **Tonic seizures** involve sudden muscle stiffness.
- **Clonic seizures** are marked by repeated jerking movements.
- **Atonic seizures** lead to a sudden loss of muscle tone, causing the person to collapse.

Recognizing and Responding to Seizures

Witnessing a seizure can be alarming but understanding how to respond appropriately is crucial. During a tonic-clonic seizure, it is important to ensure the person's safety by clearing the area of any hazardous objects, cushioning the head, and turning them on their side to keep the airway clear. Contrary to some misconceptions, nothing should be placed in the person's mouth and attempts to restrain their movements should be avoided.

After the seizure, the person may experience a postictal period characterized by confusion, fatigue, and a headache. This period can last from a few minutes to several hours. During this time, it is important to offer reassurance and a calm environment.

Medical Intervention and Treatment

Emergency medical services play a leading role in managing seizures, especially if the seizure lasts longer than five minutes, known as status epilepticus, which is a medical emergency. Paramedics use the ABC-DE approach and ensure the airway is clear, providing oxygen, monitoring vital signs, and administering medications such as benzodiazepines to stop prolonged seizures.

For those with a known diagnosis of epilepsy, long-term treatment typically involves anti-seizure medications. The goal is to reduce the frequency and severity of seizures, improving the quality of life. In some cases, surgical intervention may be considered if medications are not effective.

Living with Epilepsy

Epilepsy, defined by the occurrence of two or more unprovoked seizures, affects about 3% of Americans by age 75, according to Unitek EMT. Living with epilepsy requires careful management, including medication adherence, lifestyle adjustments, and regular medical consultations. People with epilepsy are often advised to avoid triggers such as sleep deprivation, stress, and certain medications or substances.

Despite the challenges, many people with epilepsy lead fulfilling lives. Advances in medical treatment and increased awareness and understanding of the condition have significantly improved the prognosis for those affected. Support from healthcare professionals, families, and epilepsy organizations can provide invaluable assistance in managing the condition (Unitek EMT, 2021).

6

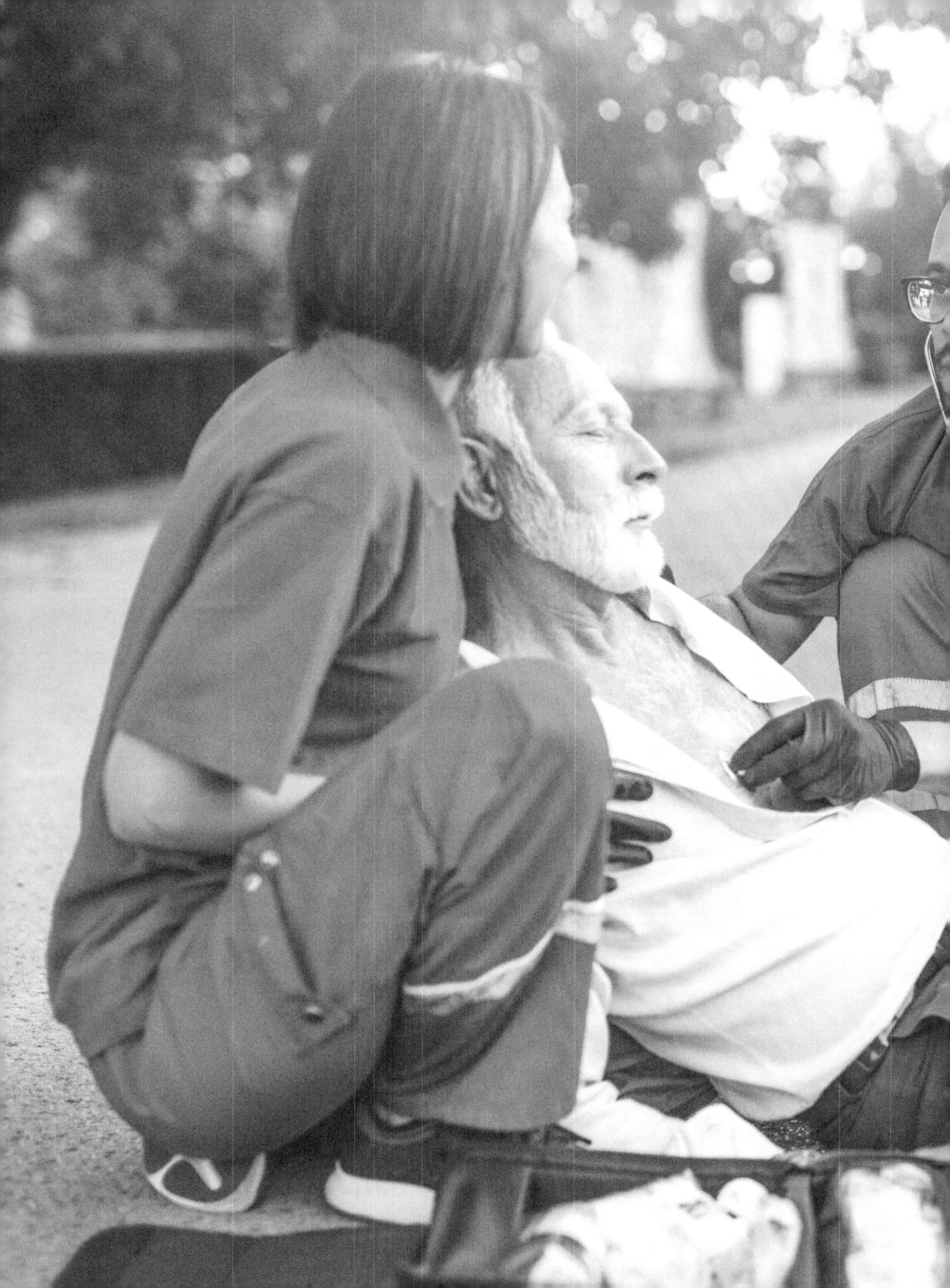

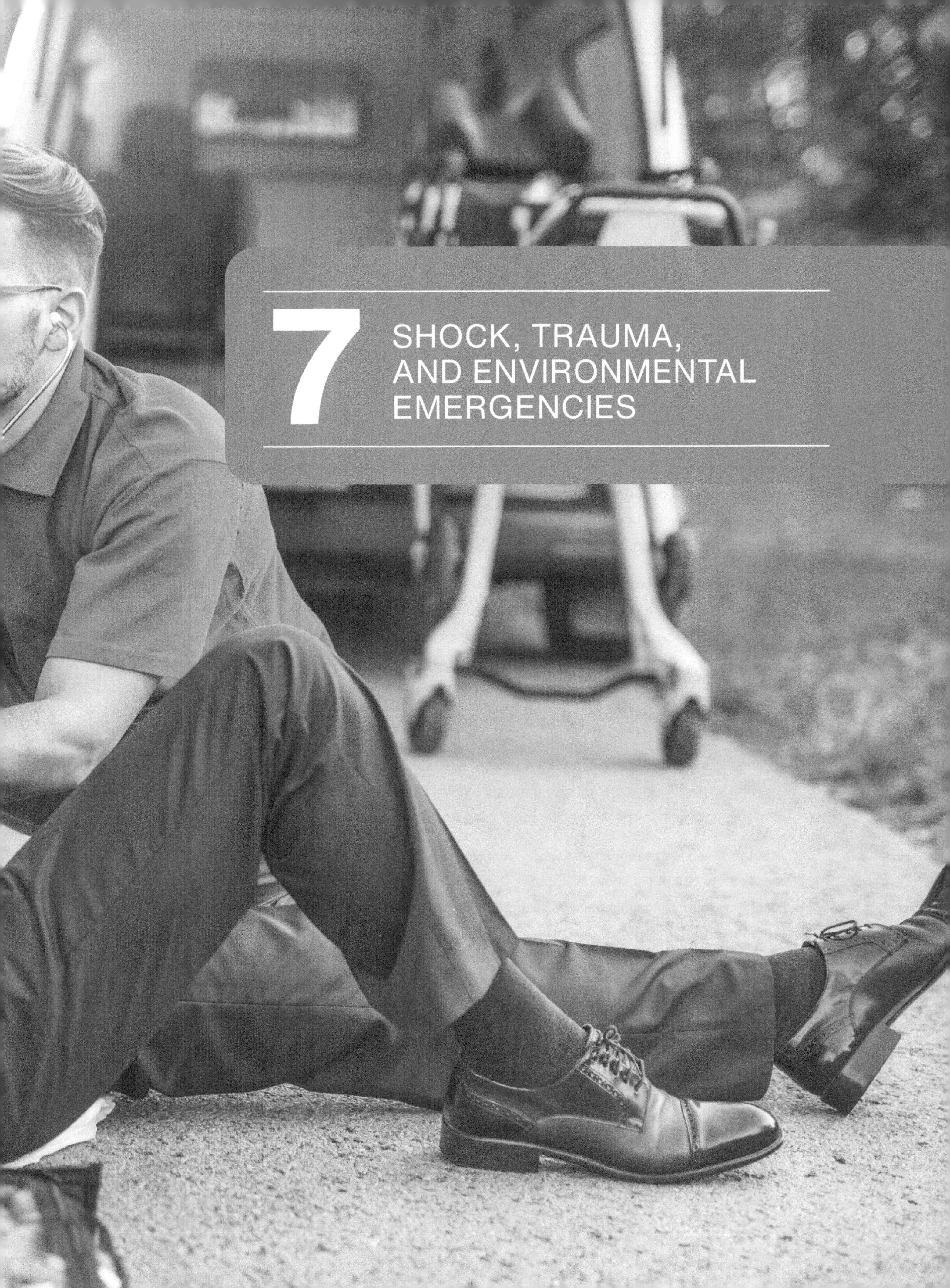

7 SHOCK, TRAUMA, AND ENVIRONMENTAL EMERGENCIES

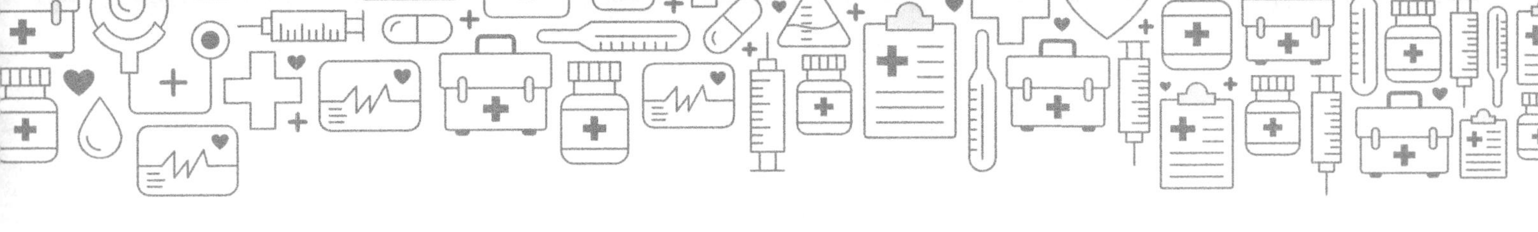

SHOCK, TRAUMA, AND ENVIRONMENTAL EMERGENCIES

Trauma encompasses both physical and psychological dimensions, each arising from highly stressful, frightening, or distressing events. Physical trauma refers to bodily injuries caused by external forces such as accidents, violence, or natural disasters. These injuries can range from minor cuts and bruises to severe conditions like fractures, burns, or internal damage, often requiring immediate medical attention (After Trauma, n/a).

Emotional trauma is the psychological response to stressful, frightening, or disturbing circumstances that are difficult to deal with or beyond one's control. These events can be one-time incidents or long-term circumstances. Trauma is subjective, and it affects people differently depending on their experiences and reactions. It can occur at any age and can immediately impact someone or manifest years later. Trauma can cause someone to feel terrified, threatened, embarrassed, rejected, abandoned, invalidated, unsafe, unsupported, trapped, ashamed, or powerless.

Traumatic experiences can arise from various situations, such as direct harm or neglect, witnessing harm to others, living in a traumatic environment, or being affected by familial or community trauma. Certain groups, such as people of color, military personnel, former or current prisoners, refugees, asylum seekers, LGBTQIA+ individuals, and those experiencing poverty, are more likely to encounter trauma and may find it more challenging to recover due to lack of support or societal stigma and discrimination (Mind, 2023).

TYPES OF EMOTIONAL TRAUMA AND THEIR CAUSES

Trauma is a complex response to distressing events that can manifest in various forms, significantly impacting an individual's mental and physical health. Understanding the different types of trauma—acute, chronic, and complex—can help in recognizing and addressing these experiences effectively.

Acute trauma is a response to a single, highly stressful event that poses a significant threat to an individual's safety or life. This type of trauma often results from incidents such as natural disasters, severe accidents, or witnessing violence. For example, experiencing a car accident or being present during a violent crime can trigger acute trauma. The immediate psychological response may include shock, anxiety, and confusion. If not addressed promptly, acute trauma can lead to acute stress disorder (ASD), characterized by intrusive memories, nightmares, and avoidance behaviors that typically arise within three days to a month after the event.

Chronic trauma arises from prolonged or repeated exposure to traumatic events. Unlike acute trauma, chronic trauma involves enduring stress over an extended period, often leading to long-lasting psychological effects. Common sources of chronic trauma include physical, sexual, and emotional abuse, as well as domestic violence. For instance, individuals subjected to ongoing physical abuse may suffer from chronic trauma, resulting in persistent fear, anxiety, and depression. Similarly, growing up in poverty, where

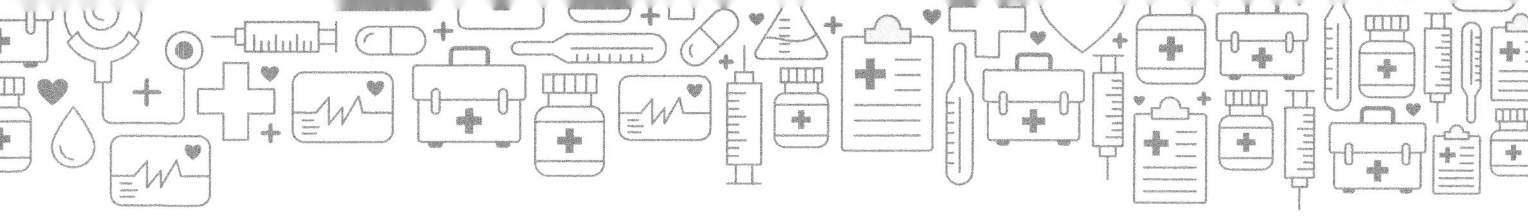

children are frequently exposed to violence, drug use, and inadequate living conditions, can cause chronic trauma, affecting their mental health and development.

Complex trauma involves multiple, prolonged, or repetitive exposure to traumatic events, often beginning in childhood. This type of trauma is more intricate, as it encompasses a range of experiences that cumulatively impact an individual's well-being. Examples include childhood abuse or neglect, long-term domestic violence, and war-related experiences. For children, experiencing repeated abandonment or neglect can lead to complex trauma, affecting their ability to form healthy relationships and causing long-term mental health issues like post-traumatic stress disorder (PTSD). Adults exposed to prolonged trauma, such as refugees fleeing war zones, may also develop complex trauma, struggling with trust and emotional regulation (Ertel, 2023).

Physical Trauma

Traumatic injuries are the biggest cause of death among people under the age of 40 in the United States (Sharp School, n/a). Proper pre-hospital examination and care can dramatically reduce pain, long-term damage, and mortality. Trauma emergencies result from physical forces acting on the body, whereas illnesses or diseases cause medical emergencies unrelated to external forces.

Evaluating the mechanism of injury (MOI) in trauma patients aids in the development of an index of suspicion for several forms of significant and potentially fatal underlying injuries. This level of suspicion is critical for detecting and being aware of potentially serious and undetected ailments.

Mechanism of Injury Profiles

Various MOIs produce different types of injuries. Nonsignificant injuries typically involve isolated body parts or falls without loss of consciousness. In contrast, significant injuries often involve multiple body systems, falls from heights, motor vehicle and motorcycle crashes, car versus pedestrian or bicycle accidents, gunshot wounds, and stabbings.

Blunt and Penetrating Trauma

Traumatic injuries are classified into blunt and penetrating trauma. Both types can result from various MOIs, and it is important to consider unseen as well as visible injuries. Blunt trauma results from force-causing injury without penetrating the soft tissues or internal organs. Penetrating trauma involves objects piercing the body, causing damage to internal organs and body cavities.

Blunt Trauma

Blunt trauma occurs when an object contacts the body. Common causes include motor vehicle crashes and falls. Skin discoloration and pain may be the only visible signs of blunt trauma, so a high index of suspicion for hidden injuries is necessary. Vehicular collisions, classified as frontal, rear-end, lateral, rollovers, and rotational, involve different directions of force impact. Significant MOIs in crashes include the death of an occupant, altered mental status, and ejection from the vehicle.

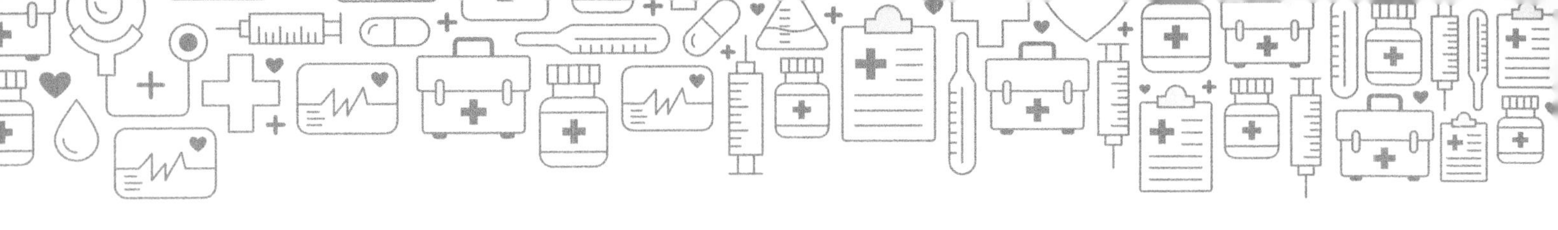

Penetrating Trauma

Penetrating trauma is the second leading cause of trauma death in the U.S. Low-energy penetrating trauma can result from accidental impalement or intentional stabbing. Medium- and high-velocity trauma typically involves bullets, whose unpredictable paths can cause extensive internal damage. The severity of penetrating injuries often depends on the projectile's speed rather than its mass, with high-velocity projectiles causing more severe damage.

Blast Injuries

Blast injuries, often seen in military conflicts and civilian incidents like terrorist activities, involve four mechanisms: primary blast injuries from the blast itself, secondary injuries from flying debris, tertiary injuries from being hurled by the explosion, and miscellaneous injuries such as burns or crush injuries. Organs containing air, such as the lungs and gastrointestinal tract, are particularly susceptible to pressure changes from blasts.

Multisystem Trauma

Multisystem trauma involves multiple body systems, such as head and spinal trauma, chest and abdominal trauma, or chest and extremity trauma. Rapid transport and alerting medical control are essential, with on-scene time ideally limited to less than ten minutes. Surgical intervention is often required for definitive care in such cases (Sharp School, n/a).

EMT and Trauma Care

Emergency Medical Technicians play an essential role in providing initial care for traumatic injuries, which are serious and often life-threatening. Trauma can affect various parts of the body, and usually, the symptoms are similar to those associated with any severe injury:

- Profuse bleeding
- Bruising
- Bone fractures
- Mutilation
- Dismemberment
- Burns
- Extreme pain

When responding to a trauma call, EMTs use the ABCDE approach to systematically assess and stabilize patients. This method helps ensure that no critical aspect of the patient's condition is overlooked, even in the chaotic environment of an emergency scene.

Traumatic injuries can result from various incidents like car accidents, falls, or violence. Each situation requires specific first-aid measures before EMS providers arrive. For instance, if someone is bleeding heavily, applying pressure to the wound is necessary. In cases where there is a potential spinal injury, such as in car accidents, avoid moving the victim unless there is an imminent danger.

One of the challenges in treating traumatic brain injuries may appear immediately after the injury or take weeks to manifest. When assessing a potential brain injury, an EMT should ask several critical questions to gather comprehensive information. They should inquire about how the injury occurred and if the person lost consciousness, including the duration of unconsciousness.

It is important to note any changes in the patient's alertness, speech, or coordination. The EMT should also ask about other signs of injury and the specific parts of the body affected. In cases of head injury, determining the exact point of impact is necessary. Additionally, understanding the force of the injury,

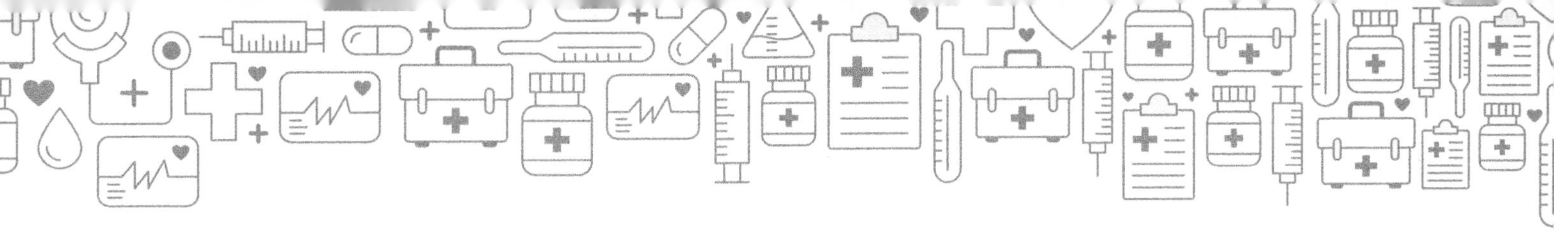

such as the speed of a car in an accident, the height of a fall, or the time elapsed since the incident, can provide valuable context for the EMT's assessment.

Once EMTs arrive, they prioritize rapid assessment and transport to the appropriate medical facility. Depending on the nature and severity of the injury, patients might be taken to specialized centers. For example, burn victims are transported to burn centers, while head injury patients are taken to hospitals with neurological expertise.

Training for EMTs involves realistic simulations to prepare them for the unpredictability of trauma calls. These simulations mimic real-life scenarios, complete with actors, props, and the chaos typical of emergency scenes. This firsthand training helps EMT students develop the confidence and skills needed to handle actual emergencies effectively.

In summary, EMTs are essential in managing traumatic injuries and providing critical care during the crucial moments after an injury occurs. Their training, which includes systematic assessment techniques and realistic simulations, ensures they are well-prepared to save lives and minimize the long-term impact of traumatic injuries (Unitek EMT, 2020).

BLEEDING AND SHOCK MANAGEMENT

Emergency Medical Technicians play a critical role in the initial management of patients experiencing bleeding and shock. The swift and efficient management of these conditions is key to improving the patient's survival rate and prevent further complications. EMTs must quickly identify the type of bleeding to apply the appropriate treatment effectively.

Bleeding can be classified into three primary types:

- Hemorrhage bleeding
- Internal bleeding
- External bleeding (Limmer and O'Keefe, 2020)

External Bleeding

External bleeding is the visible loss of blood from the body. It can be life-threatening based on the volume and flow of the blood. The volume refers to the amount of blood lost, where significant loss can be critical, especially in small children or infants. The flow indicates the movement of blood; continuous or spurting blood suggests severe bleeding (Red Cross, n/a).

External bleeding can be classified into three main categories:

1. ***Arterial bleeding*** is the most severe, characterized by bright red blood that spurts with each heartbeat.
2. ***Venous bleeding*** is less forceful but involves a steady flow of dark red blood.
3. ***Capillary bleeding*** is the least severe and it involves slow oozing of blood from minor cuts or abrasions.

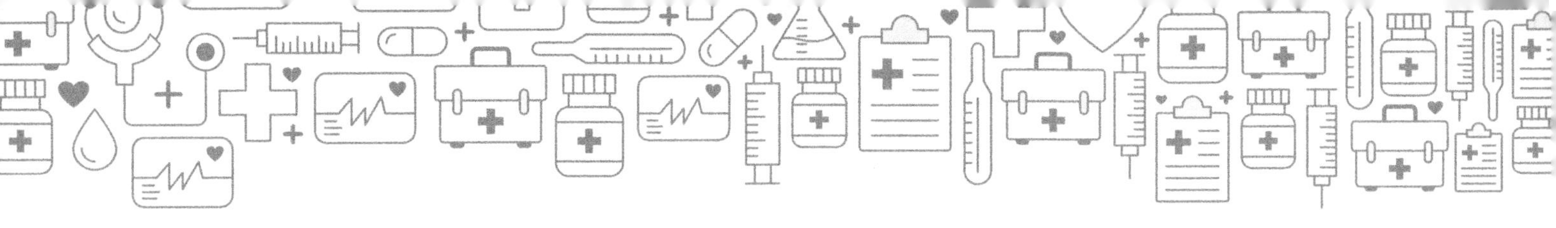

Controlling External Bleeding

- Direct pressure
- Elevation
- Hemostatic agents
- Tourniquet
- Splinting
- Cold application

Direct pressure is the primary way to stop external bleeding. EMTs should use a gloved hand and gauze bandage to apply firm pressure to the wound and keep it there until the bleeding stops. If the gauze becomes soaked, add more dressings on top without removing the soaked ones to maintain constant pressure. Once bleeding is controlled, secure the dressing with a bandage, checking for a distal pulse to make sure it is not too tight.

In some cases, elevating the injured extremity above the heart while applying direct pressure can help reduce blood flow to the wound. However, elevation should be avoided if a musculoskeletal injury, an impaled object in the extremity, or a spine injury is suspected, as it might cause further harm.

Hemostatic agents are another tool for managing severe external bleeding. These agents, which can be in the form of powders, dressings, or gauze bandages, work by promoting clotting at the wound site. They absorb the liquid portion of the blood, leaving the larger elements to clot. Despite the use of hemostatic agents, manual pressure is still necessary to ensure effective bleeding control.

For bleeding that cannot be controlled by direct pressure or hemostatic agents, particularly in extremity injuries, a tourniquet may be used. The tourniquet must be used according to the manufacturer's instructions. Once in place, it should not be removed or loosened, and a notation should be attached to the patient to inform other healthcare providers of its application.

Splinting can help stabilize the sharp ends of broken bones, reducing further tissue damage and bleeding. Cold applications can also be used to minimize swelling, constrict blood vessels, and reduce pain, although these should be used alongside manual pressure techniques for optimal effectiveness.

Special situations, such as head injuries and nosebleeds, require specific approaches. For head injuries with increased intracranial pressure, which refers to elevated pressure within the skull, stopping the external bleeding can increase this pressure, so drainage should be allowed to flow freely, using a gauze pad to collect it. For nosebleeds, patients should sit and lean forward while applying direct pressure to the nostrils. They should remain calm and quiet, and if they lose consciousness, place them in the recovery position with readiness for suction (Limmer and O'Keefe, 2020).

Internal Bleeding

Internal bleeding refers to the loss of blood that occurs inside the body, such as within the stomach or brain. This type of bleeding is typically the result of trauma or injury, although it can also stem from conditions like gastritis, organ damage, or bleeding disorders. Unlike external bleeding, internal bleeding is not visible and can be challenging to diagnose. It can indicate a serious, potentially life-threatening condition that requires immediate medical attention (Holland, 2023).

Patient assessment for internal bleeding involves looking for specific signs and symptoms. Injuries to the body's surface, such as bruising, swelling, or pain over vital organs, can indicate internal bleeding. Painful, swollen, or deformed extremities, and bleeding from the mouth, rectum, or vagina are

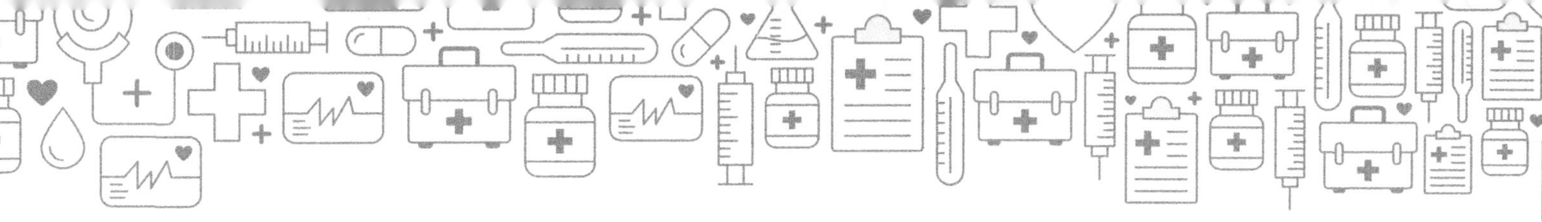

also common signs. Other indicators include a tender, rigid, or distended abdomen, vomiting a coffee-ground-like substance or bright red vomitus, dark, tarry stools, or bright red blood in the stool.

In managing internal bleeding, EMTs must maintain the patient's airway, breathing, and circulation (ABCs). Administering high-concentration oxygen via a nonrebreather mask is essential to ensure the patient receives adequate oxygen. Any external bleeding should be controlled to prevent further blood loss. Steps should also be taken to preserve the patient's body temperature, as hypothermia can exacerbate shock. Prompt transport to an appropriate medical facility is required for definitive care (Limmer and O'Keefe, 2020).

Blood vessel injury is one of the most common causes of internal bleeding. Even tiny tears from an injury might cause bleeding throughout the body. This is often exacerbated by problems with clotting factors, which are proteins required to stop bleeding. If the body does not make enough of these proteins, bleeding can become serious, even from little wounds.

Certain medications also contribute to internal bleeding risks. Blood thinners, prescribed to prevent clotting, can lead to excessive bleeding if an accident occurs. Over-the-counter medications like aspirin can damage the stomach lining, increasing the risk of gastrointestinal bleeding.

Chronic high blood pressure is another important risk. Elevated pressure weakens blood artery walls over time, increasing the risk of aneurysms—bulging areas that can rupture and cause internal bleeding. In addition, genetic bleeding diseases such as hemophilia, where blood does not clot properly, can result in severe bleeding from minor accidents.

Gastrointestinal (GI) issues are also a notable cause of internal bleeding. The following conditions can lead to bleeding within the abdomen:

- Colon polyps
- Colitis
- Crohn's disease
- Gastritis
- Esophagitis
- Peptic ulcers

Internal bleeding can also result from more severe causes. Trauma, such as car accidents, falls, or heavy objects falling on the body, can cause damage to organs, blood vessels, and bones, potentially leading to internal bleeding without visible external wounds.

Complications from surgery can result in internal bleeding. Despite a surgeon's efforts to control bleeding before closing an incision, some cases may still experience ongoing bleeding if an issue was overlooked (Holland, 2023)

Shock (Hypoperfusion)

Shock is a serious medical condition where the body's tissues and organs do not get enough oxygen and nutrients, leading to their failure and potentially death if not treated. It happens when the heart is not pumping blood effectively, when there's not enough blood in the body, or if the blood vessels are too wide or leaky. Sometimes, even if the heart is pumping well, shock can occur if the body's demand for oxygen and nutrients is so high that the blood cannot keep up. This can happen in situations such as:

- Severe infections
- High fevers
- Breathing problems
- Extreme pain (Summa Health, n/a)

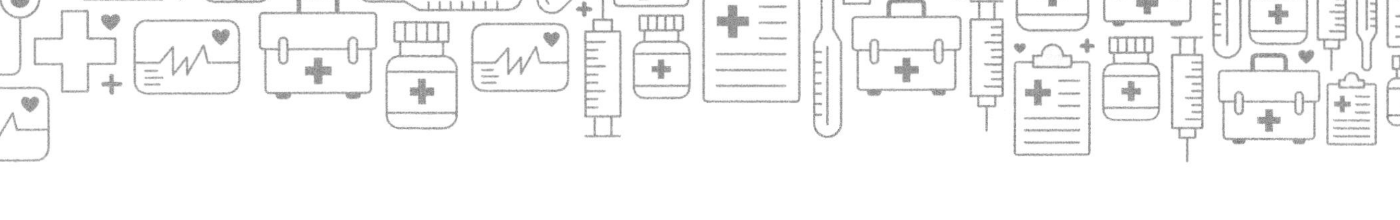

There are three main types of shock:

1. **Hypovolemic shock** occurs when there is a significant decrease in the amount of circulating blood and plasma. This type can be due to severe bleeding, either internal or external, as seen in trauma or major injuries.
2. **Cardiogenic shock** is associated with heart problems, particularly myocardial infarction, where the heart muscle is damaged and struggles to pump blood effectively.
3. **Neurogenic shock** arises from a different mechanism involving the nervous system. It happens when there is uncontrolled dilation of blood vessels due to nerve paralysis, causing blood vessels to widen excessively.

When managing a patient in shock, EMTs must act fast and methodically to improve the chances of survival. First, they need to assess the patient's condition, looking for signs such as altered mental status, pale and clammy skin, nausea, and vital sign changes. Late indicators like thirst, dilated pupils, and cyanosis around the lips and nails can suggest worsening shock.

Immediate intervention includes maintaining an open airway and evaluating the patient's breathing. If breathing is insufficient, it should be addressed urgently. For patients who are breathing adequately, administering high-concentration oxygen using a nonrebreather mask is essential. Controlling external bleeding is critical.

In cases of suspected pelvic fractures, EMTs should use a pelvic binding device to stabilize the injury and reduce further bleeding. All suspected bone or joint injuries should be splinted to prevent additional damage. EMTs must also work to prevent heat loss, which can exacerbate shock.

Rapid transportation to a medical facility is needed; the goal is to minimize the time spent at the scene to enhance the patient's chances of recovery. Throughout the process, maintaining calm and reassuring communication with the patient is important for their comfort and cooperation (Limmer and O'Keefe, 2020).

SOFT TISSUE AND BURN INJURIES

Soft tissue injuries are common and include abrasions, lacerations, punctures, bites, and eye injuries. These wounds, while often appearing superficial, can sometimes hide more severe underlying conditions that require immediate and effective management. EMTs manage the initial assessment and treatment of these injuries to prevent complications such as infection and bleeding.

Abrasions occur when the outermost layer of the skin is scraped off, often due to friction against a rough surface. This type of injury exposes the underlying, sensitive nerve endings, making the wound particularly painful. Although these injuries rarely bleed excessively once dressed, they must be cleaned and covered with sterile gauze to prevent infection.

Lacerations, on the other hand, are cuts caused by sharp objects that result in rough or jagged wounds. The severity of bleeding depends on the depth and involvement of larger blood vessels. EMTs should control bleeding by applying direct pressure and sterile dressings and monitor for signs of deeper damage.

Puncture wounds are caused by objects penetrating the skin, potentially creating a path between an entrance and an exit wound. These injuries are particularly prone to infection and require careful

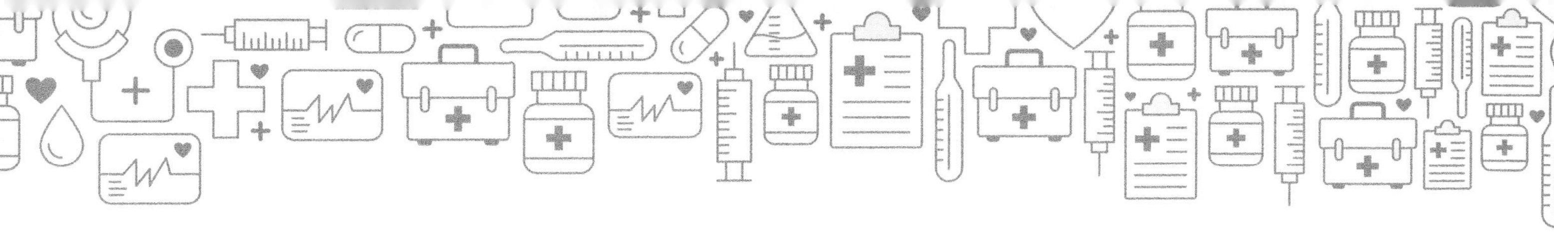

assessment for any exit wounds and impaled objects. EMTs should stabilize impaled objects with bulky dressings rather than removing them, as removal could worsen bleeding.

Bites from insects, animals, or humans pose significant risks of infection and disease transmission. Human bites are considered emergencies due to the elevated risk of infection and should be transported promptly.

Animal bites, depending on the animal and the severity, may require treatment for potential diseases such as rabies. In all bite cases, cleaning the wound and applying sterile dressings is critical.

Eye injuries, a unique category of soft tissue injuries, can be caused by foreign bodies like grit or chemicals. EMTs should lay the patient flat, tilt the head to the affected side, and flush the eye with water or saline for at least 15 minutes to prevent further damage (MedicTests, n/a).

Burn Injuries

Burns are categorized based on their depth and the percentage of body surface area affected. Immediate assessment includes identifying the type and severity of the burn and associated injuries. EMTs must prioritize stopping the burning process by removing any heat-retaining materials and cooling the burn with water briefly. For significant burns, the ABCs are essential.

For first and second-degree burns, EMTs should cover the area with clean, dry sheets, and use saline-soaked gauze for pain relief. Third-degree burns, involving deeper tissue damage, require more extensive care, including the administration of high-flow oxygen and intravenous fluids to prevent hypovolemic shock.

Additionally, EMTs should monitor for signs of airway compromise, especially with facial burns or inhalation injuries. In such cases, you should provide high-flow oxygen and consider advanced airway management. For chemical burns, copious irrigation, and specific treatments like calcium gluconate for hydrofluoric acid burns are necessary.

Transporting burn patients to specialized burn centers or high-level trauma centers is critical for optimal recovery. Burn centers offer specialized care that can significantly improve outcomes for severe burn injuries. EMTs must also be vigilant for other injuries, such as fractures or inhalation of toxic gasses, ensuring comprehensive initial treatment and timely transfer to appropriate facilities (Ebright, 2022).

ENVIRONMENTAL EMERGENCIES

Environmental emergencies include a wide range of conditions such as heat-related illnesses, cold exposure, water-related incidents, and altitude sickness. Effective EMT response involves quick assessment, stabilization, and appropriate treatment to prevent further harm and improve patient outcomes.

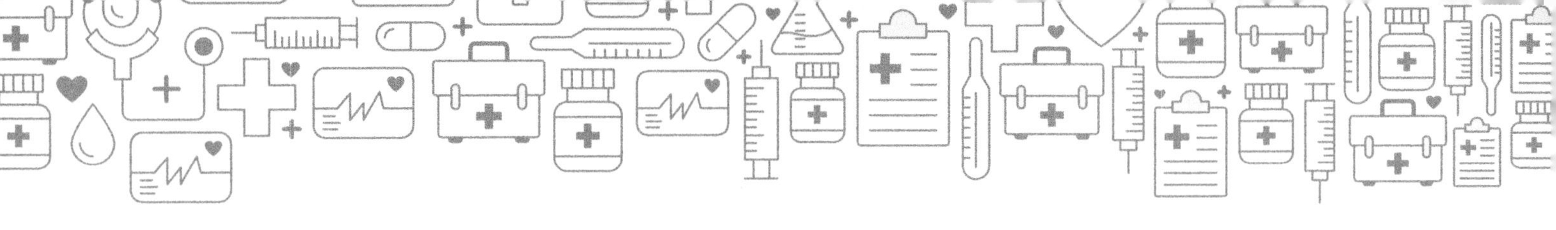

Heat-Related Illnesses

Heat-related illnesses range from mild conditions like heat cramps to severe conditions such as heat exhaustion and heat stroke. EMTs must recognize the signs and symptoms of these conditions to provide timely and effective care.

Heat Cramps are muscle spasms resulting from loss of salt and water through heavy sweating. EMTs should help the patient rest in a cool environment and provide water or electrolyte solutions.

Heat Exhaustion symptoms include heavy sweating, weakness, dizziness, nausea, and headache. EMTs should move the patient to a cooler place, lay them down, and elevate their legs. Cool the patient with damp cloths and provide sips of water.

Heat Stroke is a life-threatening condition marked by a high body temperature, altered mental state, and unconsciousness. Rapid cooling is critical. EMTs should remove the patient's clothing, apply cool packs to the neck, armpits, and groin, and fan the patient while misting with water. Immediate transport to a medical facility is essential.

Cold Exposure

Cold-related emergencies include hypothermia and frostbite, both of which require prompt and careful management.

Hypothermia: This occurs when the body temperature drops below normal (98.6 F). Symptoms include shivering, slurred speech, and confusion. Severe hypothermia can lead to unconsciousness and death. EMTs should remove any wet clothing, insulate the patient with blankets, and provide warm, non-alcoholic, non-caffeinated beverages if the patient is conscious (Pearson, n/a). Smoking reduces blood flow to the extremities, whereas caffeine causes the heart to beat faster and pump more cold blood. Alcohol can make one feel warm, so this may seem odd, but in reality, causes the body to lose heat (Travelers Risk Control, n/a).

Frostbite: This affects extremities such as fingers, toes, ears, and nose. It causes the skin to become white, hard, and numb. EMTs should protect the affected areas from further exposure, avoid rubbing or massaging the skin, and provide gentle rewarming using warm (not hot) water. Ice crystals are located at the capillary level, and scratching the area where the injury has occurred could inflict further harm to the already damaged tissues. Pain management and rapid transport to a hospital are crucial.

Water-Related Incidents

Drowning and near-drowning incidents require immediate intervention to prevent brain damage or death due to hypoxia.

Drowning: EMTs should focus on rescuing the victim safely and provide airway management. Rescue breathing and chest compressions may be necessary. Monitoring for hypothermia and secondary complications like pulmonary edema (illness caused by an excess of fluid in the lungs) is essential.

Near-Drowning: Survivors may still experience respiratory distress or other complications. Continuous monitoring, oxygen administration, and rapid transport to a hospital are necessary for comprehensive evaluation and treatment.

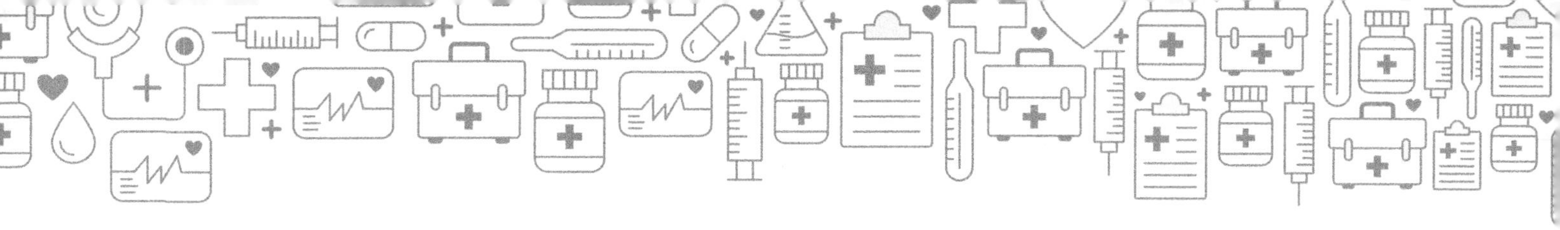

Altitude Sickness

High altitudes can cause a range of symptoms due to reduced oxygen availability, known as altitude sickness.

Acute Mountain Sickness (AMS): Symptoms include headache, nausea, fatigue, and dizziness. EMTs should advise descent to lower altitudes, rest, and hydration.

High-Altitude Pulmonary Edema (HAPE): A severe form of altitude sickness. It involves fluid accumulation in the lungs, causing breathlessness and cough.

High-Altitude Cerebral Edema (HACE): Another severe form, HACE involves swelling in the brain, causing confusion and loss of coordination. Both conditions require immediate descent and supplemental oxygen. Rapid evacuation to a lower altitude and medical facility is critical.

General Management

For all environmental emergencies, EMTs must follow these general management principles:

Assessment: Conduct a thorough primary and secondary survey to identify life-threatening conditions and gather information about the patient's history and symptoms.

Stabilization: Ensure the patient's airway, breathing, and circulation are stable. Address any immediate life threats.

Temperature Regulation: Whether the patient is suffering from heat or cold exposure, regulating body temperature is mandatory. Use appropriate techniques to either cool or warm the patient as needed.

Hydration and Nutrition: Administer fluids carefully, considering the patient's condition. Avoid giving food or drink if the patient is unconscious or has an altered mental status.

Transport: Promptly transport the patient to an appropriate medical facility. Continuously monitor the patient's condition during transport and provide necessary interventions (Pearson, n/a).

MUSCULOSKELETAL INJURIES

The musculoskeletal system is fundamental to movement and stability, consisting of:

- Bones
- Joints
- Muscles
- Cartilage
- Ligaments
- Tendons

Bones provide the framework, while joints facilitate bending. Muscles, classified as skeletal (voluntary), smooth (involuntary), and cardiac (myocardial), enable movement. Cartilage offers flexibility, and ligaments connect bones, providing joint stability. Tendons link muscles to bones, allowing for joint movement.

Bone fractures cause soft tissue swelling and blood clots, leading to cell death at the injury site. New tissue forms, eventually becoming a new bone. Compartment syndrome, a severe condition caused by swelling from fractures or crush injuries, can lead to cellular damage and loss of blood flow, risking limb loss if untreated.

In emergency care, you need to quickly identify life-threatening conditions, assess distal circulation, sensation, and motion, and apply proper splinting. The six Ps of assessment (pain, pallor, paresthesia, pulses, paralysis, pressure) guide the evaluation of musculoskeletal injuries (Limmer and O'Keefe, 2020).

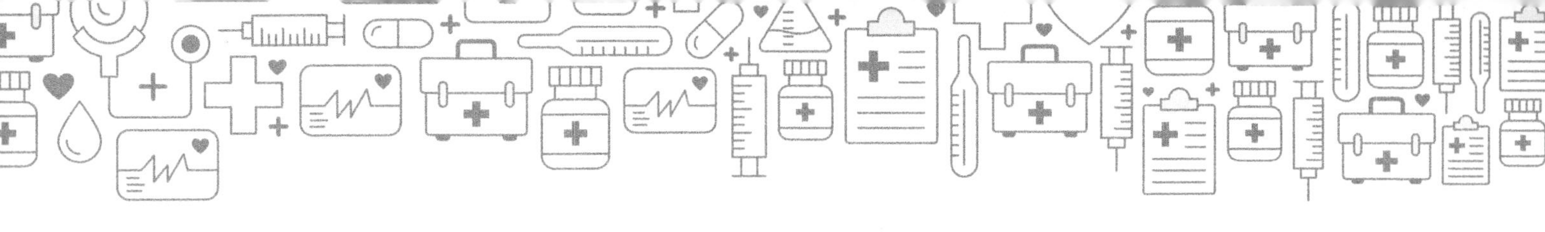

Musculoskeletal injuries are among the most frequent cases managed by EMTs, often stemming from blunt force trauma such as vehicle collisions, sports accidents, falls, and assaults. These injuries, affecting connective tissues, ligaments, tendons, muscles, and bones, can result in significant pain and necessitate proper management to prevent further injury and long-term damage.

Fractures can result in embolisms, particularly from fat entering the bloodstream from damaged bone marrow. Crush injuries can lead to rhabdomyolysis, where damaged muscles release harmful myoglobin. Improper splinting can exacerbate pain and tissue damage, leading to complications like ischemia (Collopy, 2012). Ischemia is a serious condition where a part of the body is not getting enough blood flow, leading to a lack of oxygen. It often results from blockages in the arteries and can cause life-threatening issues like heart attacks or strokes (WebMD Editorial Contributors, 2023).

EMTs must limit on-scene time but ensure interventions like splinting to stabilize injuries and reduce pain. Effective assessment of musculoskeletal injuries involves managing life-threatening hemorrhages, visually inspecting and palpating the injury, and documenting any swelling, deformity, or crepitus (grinding sensation from bone ends). It is important to check circulation, sensation, and motion distal to the injury, noting any deficits before splint application.

The primary goal is to realign bones and joints to reduce pain and protect soft tissues. Traditionally, EMTs are taught to splint injuries in the position found unless distal circulation is compromised. Realignment involves gentle traction to reposition bones, while joint injuries are splinted in the position found unless distal circulation is impaired. Proper splinting reduces pain, bleeding, and tissue damage and must be complete, compact, and comfortable.

To manage musculoskeletal injuries, you should administer analgesia, which is pain relief medication. While realignment can reduce pain significantly, the administration of narcotics like morphine or fentanyl, and sedatives for severe cases, is essential. Studies show that prehospital analgesia is often underutilized, especially in pediatric cases, despite its proven benefits.

Effective splints must be complete, immobilizing joints above and below the injury, compact to avoid additional pressure on the injury, and comfortable with adequate padding to prevent tissue damage. Different splint types, like vacuum splints or SAM Splints, offer varying benefits, but EMTs should practice their application to ensure proper use.

Femur fractures, often resulting from high-impact trauma, require careful management due to their association with internal injuries. Mid-shaft fractures are treated with traction splints, which realign bone ends, control bleeding, and reduce pain. However, applying these splints can be challenging in multi-system trauma cases, necessitating careful assessment and proper technique (Collopy, 2012).

7

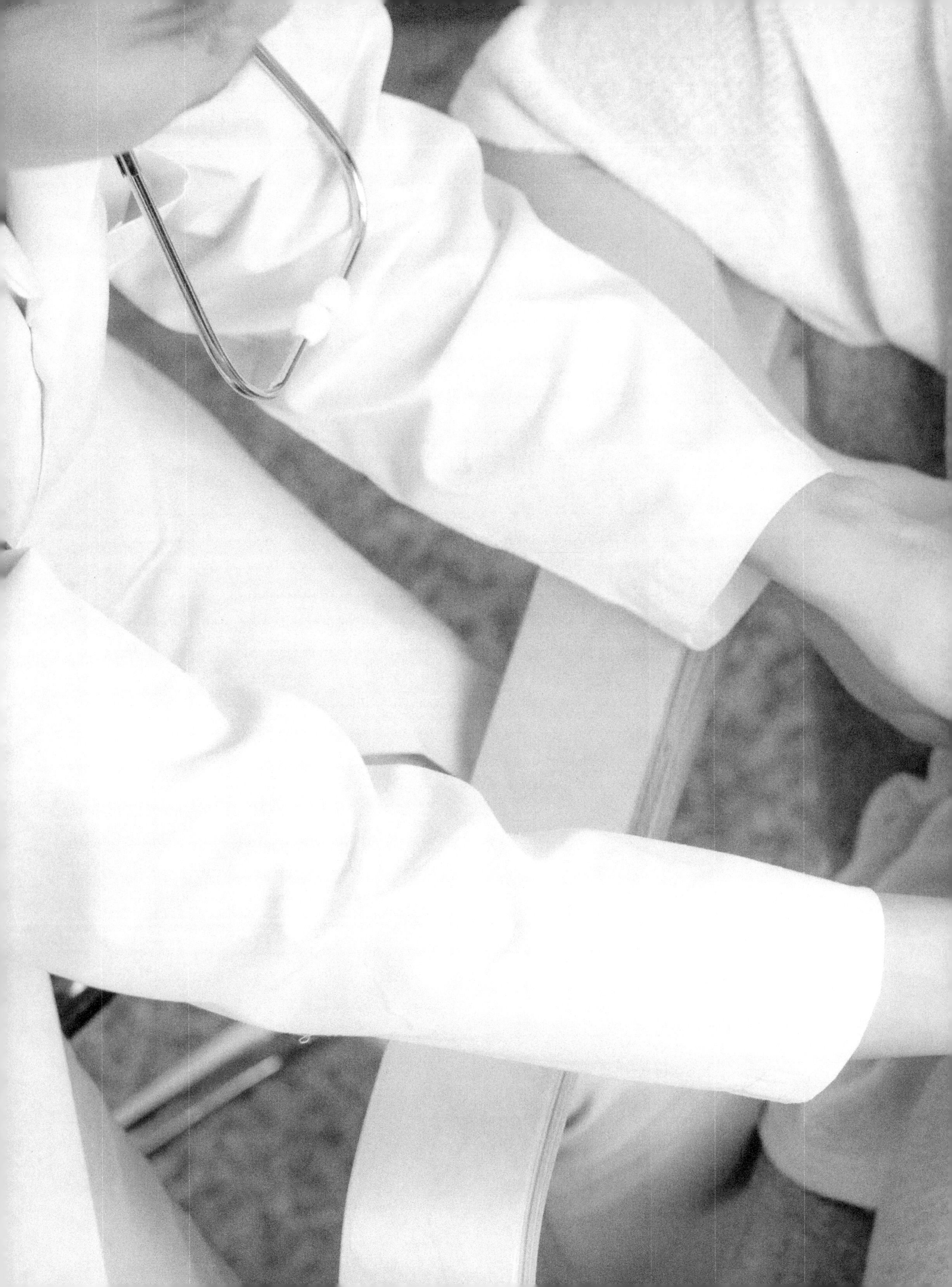

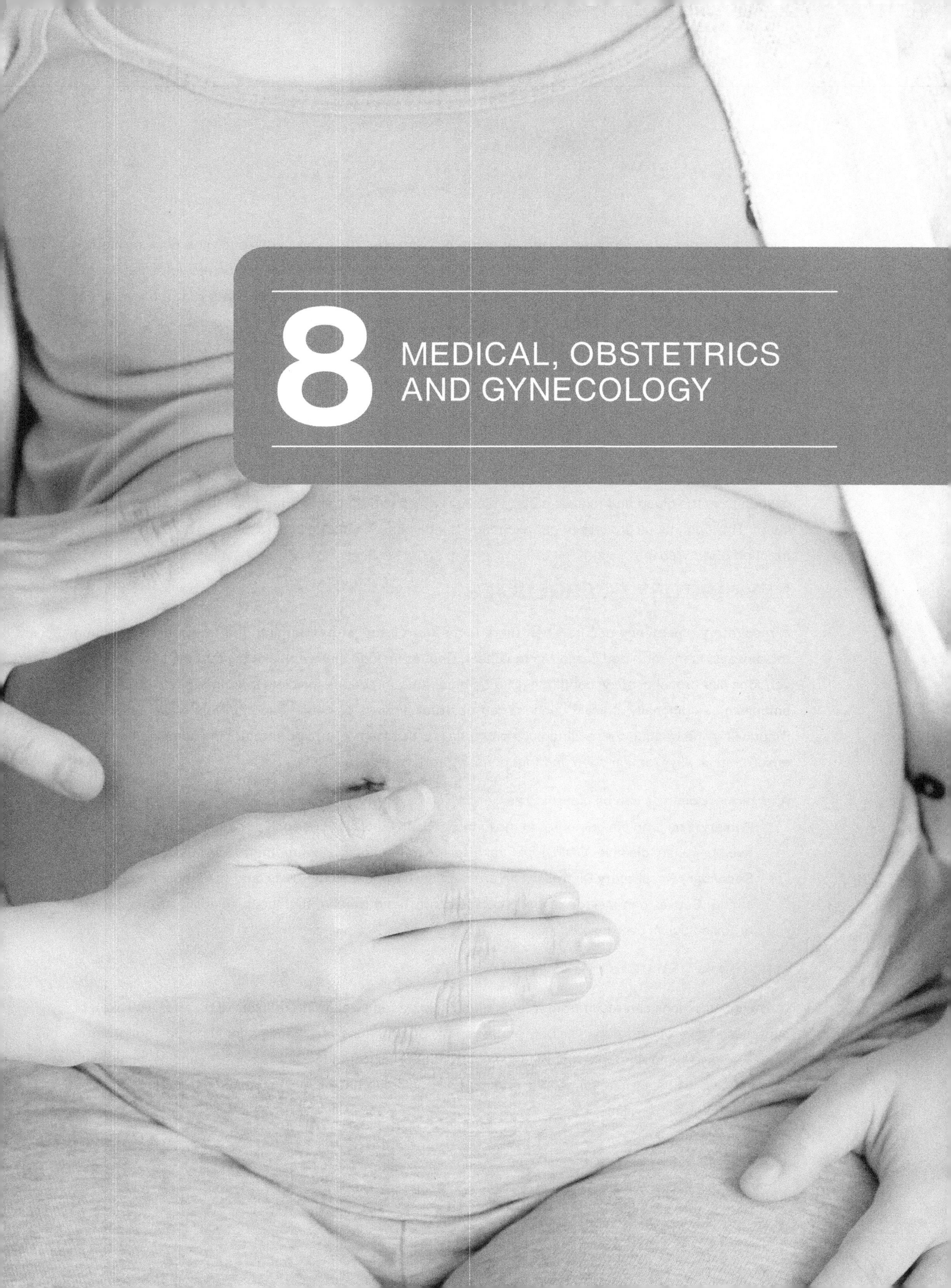

8 MEDICAL, OBSTETRICS AND GYNECOLOGY

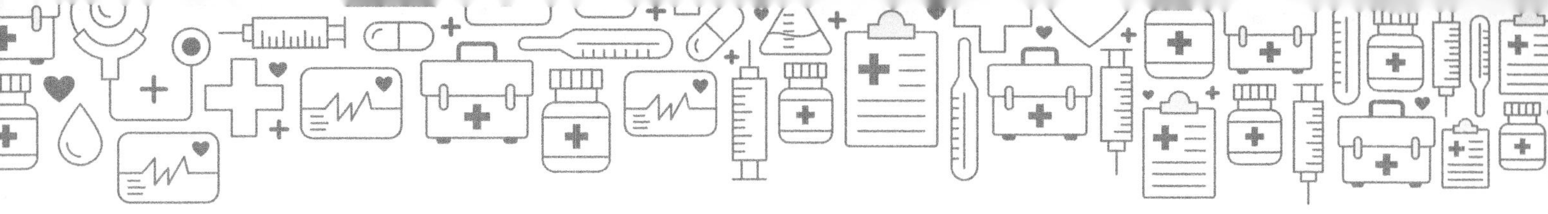

MEDICAL, OBSTETRICS AND GYNECOLOGY

The respiratory system enables breathing and gas exchange. Air comes in through the nose or mouth, goes down the pharynx and past the voice box (larynx), protected by a flap called the epiglottis that keeps food out of the trachea. Air comes in through the nose or mouth, goes down the throat (pharynx) and past the voice box (larynx), protected by a flap called the epiglottis that keeps food out of the windpipe (trachea).

Inhalation involves the diaphragm and intercostal muscles contracting, expanding the chest cavity, and creating negative pressure to pull air into the lungs. During exhalation, these muscles relax, reducing the chest cavity's size and pushing air out.

Oxygenated blood from the alveoli travels to the heart, which pumps it throughout the body. Cells receive oxygen from the blood and release carbon dioxide, which is then transported back to the lungs for exhalation. This continuous process of gas exchange is indispensable for cellular respiration and overall bodily function (EMS Web Info, n/a).

RESPIRATORY EMERGENCIES

A respiratory emergency occurs when there is a severe issue with breathing due to diseases affecting the airways, lungs, or blood vessels in the chest. Causes include airway blockages that might need interventions like bronchoscopy, conditions like asthma, lung infections, or clots in lung vessels (pulmonary embolism). Additionally, certain cancers can obstruct airways or cause superior vena cava syndrome. Diagnosing and treating these conditions promptly is crucial to prevent life-threatening complications and ensure the airways remain open and functional (Aurora et al., n/a).

A respiratory distress can be classified as:

Primary: The problem originates in the lungs, caused by conditions such as asthma, chronic obstructive pulmonary disease (COPD), pleural effusion, pneumonia, pneumothorax, or pulmonary edema.

Secondary Respiratory Distress: The problem is elsewhere in the body, and the lungs are compensating. Causes can include diabetic ketoacidosis, head trauma, metabolic acidosis, stroke, sepsis, or toxicological overdose.

Airway Obstruction

Airway obstructions can result from foreign objects, impaired swallowing reflexes (e.g., after a stroke), or suppressed gag reflexes due to alcohol or drugs. Mild obstructions where the patient is coughing forcefully may resolve without intervention. Severe obstructions, indicated by silent cough, cyanosis, or inability to speak or breathe, require immediate intervention, including back blows, abdominal thrusts, or a finger sweep if the object is visible.

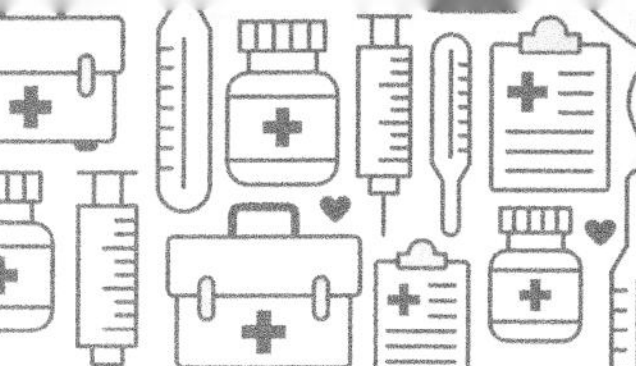

Asthma

Asthma involves chronic inflammation of the airways, triggered by allergens, infections, exercise, or smoke. During an asthma attack, bronchioles constrict, swell, and fill with mucus, hindering airflow. EMTs should calm the patient, manage the airway, provide oxygen therapy, and assist with prescribed inhalers.

COPD (Chronic Obstructive Pulmonary Disease)

COPD includes diseases like emphysema and chronic bronchitis, characterized by the slow dilation and disruption of airways and alveoli. Symptoms include shortness of breath, fever, and increased sputum. Treatment often involves high-flow oxygen and medications such as prednisone, Proventil, and Atrovent.

Congestive Heart Failure (CHF)

CHF causes fluid accumulation in the lungs, leading to breathing difficulties. It results from weakened heart ventricles, often due to heart attack, coronary artery disease, hypertension, or valve disease. Symptoms include shortness of breath, sweating, and cyanosis (Unitek EMT, 2021). Cyanosis is when your skin, lips, and/or nails turn a bluish tone due to a lack of oxygen in your blood reaching the tissues in your body (Cleveland Clinic, 2022).

Treatment involves seating the patient upright, providing high-flow oxygen, and positive pressure ventilation with a bag-valve-mask (BVM).

Inhalation Injuries

Inhalation of chemicals or smoke can cause bronchial irritation and symptoms like shortness of breath, coughing, hoarseness, and chest pain. EMTs should administer high-flow oxygen and assist breathing with a BVM if respiratory effort is insufficient.

Pneumonia

Pneumonia presents with fever, chills, cough with yellowish sputum, and chest pain. Emergency care includes oxygen therapy to alleviate breathing difficulties.

Pneumothorax and Tension Pneumothorax

A pneumothorax is air in the pleural space, causing lung collapse. It can occur spontaneously or from trauma. Symptoms include sharp chest pain and diminished breath sounds. Treatment involves high-flow oxygen and cautious use of positive-pressure ventilation. A tension pneumothorax is a severe form, compressing the lungs and other organs, requiring needle decompression and occlusive dressing over chest wounds.

Pulmonary Embolism (PE)

PE is caused by a blood clot or other particles blocking a pulmonary artery, leading to sudden shortness of breath, rapid breathing, and chest pain. Treatment involves high-flow oxygen and rapid transport to the hospital.

EMTs use the ABCDE method for assessment and intervention in respiratory emergencies. They

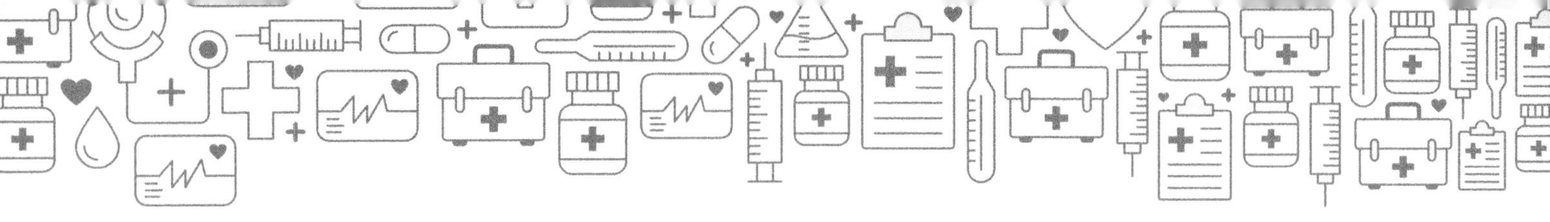

should ensure that the airway is open and clear. Next step is assessing the respiratory rate, effort, and quality of breath sounds. Then, checking pulse, blood pressure, and signs of shock is mandatory. Neurological status should also be evaluated followed by exposing and examining the chest for injury or abnormalities (Unitek EMT, 2021).

Pediatric Considerations

When addressing pediatric respiratory distress, EMTs must consider unique anatomical and physiological factors that differ significantly from adults. These variations influence assessment, intervention, and equipment choices, emphasizing the need for specialized training and competency maintenance in pediatric care.

Anatomical Differences and Implications

Pediatric airways are narrower and more flexible than adult airways, making them more susceptible to obstruction, and require careful management during intubation and ventilation. The smaller diameter of the trachea and increased propensity for airway edema necessitate the use of appropriately sized equipment to prevent trauma and ensure effective airway management. Additionally, the larger tongue and higher positioning of the larynx in children complicate visualization and insertion of airway devices.

Accurate assessment of respiratory distress in pediatric patients involves careful observation of the respiratory rate, effort, and oxygenation. Signs such as nasal flaring, grunting, retractions, and cyanosis are critical indicators of severe distress. EMTs should utilize tools like pulse oximetry and capnography to monitor oxygen saturation and ventilation status continuously. Given the higher metabolic rate in children, hypoxemia can develop faster, necessitating prompt intervention.

Noninvasive ventilation techniques, such as bag-valve mask ventilation are fundamental in pediatric respiratory management. Proper BVM technique, including a secure mask seal and appropriate ventilation rate, is key to avoid gastric insufflation and barotrauma. EMTs must be adept at selecting and using supraglottic airway devices (SGAs) as primary airway tools, given their effectiveness and ease of placement compared to endotracheal intubation (ETI) (Harris et al., 2022).

Geriatric Considerations

As individuals age, their respiratory system undergoes significant structural and functional transformations. Structurally, the lungs lose weight and surface area, accompanied by a change in color from yellowish pink to gray due to dark pigmentation patches. The development of emphysema is common, characterized by the loss of tissue elasticity and destruction of alveolar walls, reducing the lung's efficiency. Additionally, aging lungs experience a loss of functional pulmonary capillaries, further diminishing respiratory efficiency.

The chest anatomy also changes with aging. Conditions such as kyphosis, an abnormal curvature of the spine, increase due to changes in posture and muscle tone. The rib cage becomes more rigid due to muscle loss, calcification of bones, and arthritic changes. This increased rigidity extends to the trachea and connecting airways, impairing the overall mechanics of breathing. Consequently, elderly patients often present with an increased anterior/posterior chest diameter, leading to a barrel chest appearance, especially in those with COPD (University of Texas Medical Branch, 1994).

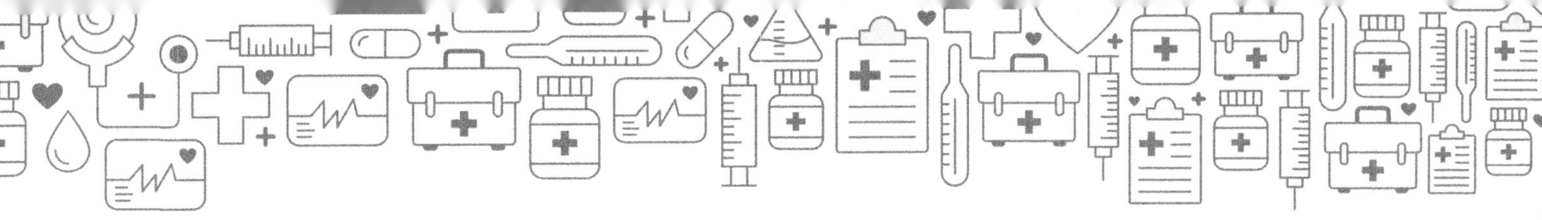

When treating elderly patients with respiratory distress, EMTs must consider several unique factors to ensure effective and compassionate care. Primarily, communication is critical. Elderly patients should be spoken to in a respectful and clear manner, with explanations provided about the procedures being performed. Encouraging them to express their concerns can help alleviate anxiety and foster cooperation.

One of the main technical considerations is the increased risk of airway injuries due to decreased lubrication and muscle tone in the elderly. When performing airway suction, EMTs should use a catheter half the size of the internal diameter of the endotracheal tube and limit suction duration to about seven seconds. It is crucial to be gentle and attentive to prevent laryngeal injuries and other complications.

Physiologically, elderly patients may exhibit transient hypertensive and tachycardic responses to endotracheal intubation, especially if multiple attempts are necessary. EMTs should be prepared to manage these responses and monitor the patient closely throughout the procedure.

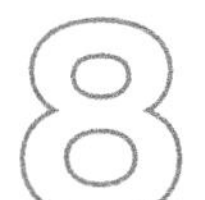

Additionally, training and preparedness are mandatory. EMT teams should regularly rehearse real-world scenarios in high-stress environments to build proficiency and confidence. Selecting the right equipment, such as portable suction units, can enhance the efficiency and effectiveness of care in the field (Say, 2022).

ENDOCRINE AND HEMATOLOGIC EMERGENCIES

The endocrine system is composed of tissues, primarily glands, which produce and release hormones. These hormones are chemical messengers that travel through the bloodstream to organs, skin, muscles, and other tissues, coordinating various functions in the body. The signals carried by hormones instruct the body on what to do and when to do it, playing a basic role in maintaining health and supporting life.

The primary function of the endocrine system is to release hormones into the bloodstream and continuously monitor their levels. Hormones interact with target cells to relay messages, influencing every aspect of health. This includes:

- Regulating metabolism
- Maintaining homeostasis (such as blood pressure, blood sugar levels, fluid balance, and body temperature)
- Promoting growth and development
- Controlling sexual function and reproduction
- Managing the sleep-wake cycle (Cleveland Clinic, 2022)

Among the most common endocrine emergencies are those associated with diabetes, a disorder affecting glucose metabolism and insulin function. Diabetes mellitus encompasses both Type 1 and Type 2 diabetes, both of which can lead to serious complications. Type 1 diabetes, often diagnosed in childhood, results from the body's inability to produce insulin, necessitating lifelong insulin therapy. Type 2 diabetes, typically emerging later in life, involves inadequate insulin production or ineffective insulin action.

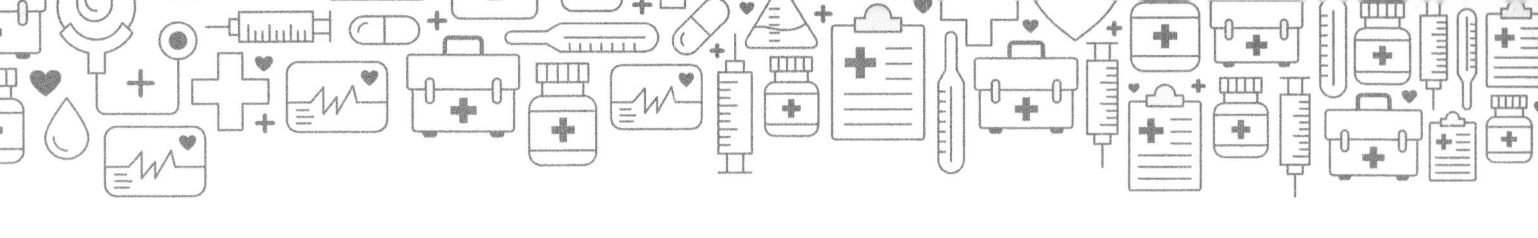

Hyperglycemia occurs when blood glucose levels exceed normal limits, often due to insufficient insulin. Signs include rapid, deep breathing (Kussmaul respirations), fruity breath odor, and dehydration. Conversely, hypoglycemia arises from low blood glucose levels, potentially due to excessive insulin or inadequate food intake. Symptoms include pale, cool skin, rapid shallow breathing, and altered mental status, potentially progressing to unconsciousness if not promptly addressed.

EMTs should take immediate action based on their assessment. For hyperglycemic emergencies, treatment focuses on managing dehydration and insulin levels. This may include administering fluids and ensuring prompt transport to medical facilities where insulin and intravenous fluids can be administered. In hypoglycemic emergencies, EMTs should quickly provide oral glucose to conscious patients, who can safely swallow. For unconscious patients or those at risk of aspiration, EMTs must prepare for rapid transport, ensuring airway protection and potential glucose administration by advanced providers if necessary.

During any endocrine emergency, EMTs should prioritize a thorough primary assessment, focusing on the patient's airway, breathing and circulation. It is essential to identify any signs of insulin-related issues and distinguish between hyperglycemia and hypoglycemia. Accurate blood glucose measurement using a glucometer can guide treatment decisions. EMTs must also be prepared for secondary complications, such as seizures or altered mental status, by providing appropriate interventions and maintaining clear communication with medical facilities (Sharp School, n/a).

Hematologic emergencies involve critical disorders related to bleeding or clotting that necessitate immediate medical intervention to prevent severe outcomes or death. These emergencies can be due to either inherited conditions or acquired factors. Symptoms may include spontaneous bleeding, jaundice, and skin manifestations such as petechiae or purpura (Jones et al., 2024).

Purpura is red, pink, or purple patches larger than two millimeters, formed when tiny blood vessels burst and leak blood under the skin, resulting in pooled blood that can change color as it heals. Petechiae are similar but smaller, less than two millimeters, and result from broken capillaries, appearing as flat spots that change color over time (Huizen, 2021).

The initial response begins with a scene size-up to ensure safety. This involves wearing appropriate personal protective equipment like gloves and eye protection and assessing the scene for potential trauma or multiple patients. It is essential to determine if advanced life support (ALS) may be necessary, such as administering pain relief for patients in vaso-occlusive crises.

Following scene safety, EMTs should conduct a primary assessment to identify key symptoms and signs. For patients of African American or Mediterranean descent, who may be at risk of conditions like sickle cell disease, a detailed evaluation is crucial.

Initial observations should include checking the patient's level of consciousness, airway, and breathing. If the patient shows signs of inadequate breathing or altered mental state, high-flow oxygen should be provided immediately. Additionally, for those with respiratory difficulties, the EMT must open the airway, use airway adjuncts if necessary, and assist with ventilation.

Assessment of circulation is another crucial step. Patients with sickle cell crises might present a rapid pulse as their bodies attempt to push the sickled cells through narrowed blood vessels. For those with hemophilia or other bleeding disorders, signs of acute blood loss such as pallor, weak pulse, and hypotension should be monitored closely.

Having a comprehensive history is required as well. EMTs should gather information about the patient's condition, including previous crises, any recent illnesses, or unusual stressors. The OPQRST mnemonic can help assess pain characteristics and associated symptoms like nausea or shortness of breath. Additionally, understanding past medical history, including the frequency and resolution of previous crises, provides valuable context for treatment.

A secondary assessment involves thorough physical examination and vital signs monitoring. These signs may include normal to rapid respirations, pale clammy skin, and low blood pressure. It is important to use a pulse oximeter to check oxygen saturation, though readings might be affected by anemia. Frequent reassessment is key to monitoring changes in the patient's condition, ensuring that interventions are effective and adjusting them as needed.

Emergency care is primarily supportive and symptomatic. For patients with inadequate breathing or altered mental status, rapid transport to a hospital with high-flow oxygen and positioning for comfort is essential. Hospital care may involve analgesics, antibiotics, IV fluids, or blood transfusions based on the severity of the condition. Coordination with medical teams and accurate documentation are key to ensuring continuity of care (Sharp School, n/a).

ANAPHYLAXIS AND TOXICOLOGY

Anaphylaxis is a severe, potentially fatal allergic reaction that occurs rapidly after exposure to an allergen, such as peanuts or bee stings. This reaction triggers the immune system to release a surge of chemicals, leading to a dramatic drop in blood pressure and constriction of the airways, which can obstruct breathing. Symptoms typically include a fast, weak pulse, skin rash, nausea, and vomiting. Immediate treatment with an injection of epinephrine is critical to counteract the reaction and prevent serious complications or death (Mayo Clinic Staff, 2021).

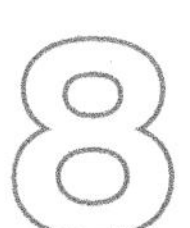

There are four types of allergic reactions:

- **Type 1 reactions** are anaphylactic, where histamines cause inflammation and can lead to severe complications like anaphylactic shock and blocked airways.
- **Type 2 reactions** are cytotoxic, occurring when antibodies bind to cell surfaces, leading to conditions like autoimmune hemolytic anemia and Graves' disease.
- **Type 3 reactions** are immunocomplex, where antibodies form complexes that damage tissues and organs, causing conditions such as rheumatoid arthritis and lupus.
- **Type 4 reactions** are cell-mediated and typically manifest 48 hours after exposure, resulting in conditions like chronic asthma and contact dermatitis.

Upon arriving at the scene, EMTs should first assess the patient's condition by checking vital signs and evaluating symptoms. Key indicators of anaphylaxis include a sudden drop in blood pressure, difficulty breathing, and a rapid, weak pulse. The presence of rash, swelling, or gastrointestinal symptoms like

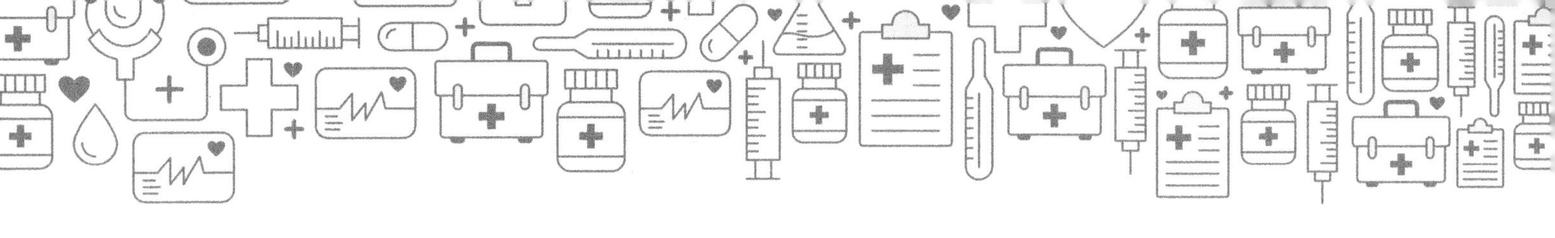

nausea and vomiting also supports the diagnosis. EMTs should ensure the scene is safe and use appropriate personal protective equipment, such as gloves and eye protection, to avoid exposure to allergens or bodily fluids.

If anaphylaxis is suspected, the EMT's primary action is to administer epinephrine. This medication, typically delivered via an auto-injector like an EpiPen, works rapidly to reverse the effects of the allergic reaction. Epinephrine constricts blood vessels to raise blood pressure and relaxes the muscles in the airways to facilitate breathing. EMTs should be prepared to use this device if the patient has one or administer it if it is part of their protocol.

Following the administration of epinephrine, EMTs must monitor the patient closely. This includes observing for any signs of improvement or deterioration. Vital signs should be regularly checked to ensure that the patient's blood pressure, heart rate, and oxygen levels are stable. An oxygen saturation monitor can be used to assess the patient's oxygen levels, which may drop during anaphylaxis. If the patient is experiencing respiratory distress, EMTs should provide supplemental oxygen and consider airway management techniques, such as using an oxygen mask or inserting an airway adjunct if necessary.

In addition to epinephrine, EMTs might administer antihistamines to alleviate symptoms like itching and hives. However, antihistamines should not replace epinephrine but rather complement it in managing allergic reactions. If the patient's condition is severe or if there are signs of deterioration, transport to the nearest hospital is essential for further treatment. EMTs should alert the receiving facility about the patient's condition and any treatments administered (Unitek EMT, 2023).

EMTs also play a leading role in managing toxicology emergencies by providing immediate and effective care. Their responsibilities include identifying the toxin involved, assessing the patient's condition, and initiating appropriate interventions. EMTs begin by determining the type and route of exposure, which can be inhalation, ingestion, injection, or absorption. They perform a thorough assessment of the patient's vital signs, level of consciousness, and symptoms, which might include:

- Nausea
- Vomiting
- Seizures
- Respiratory distress

When a patient inhales poison, EMTs should take them outside right away to provide them with more oxygen. If necessary, they must disinfect the patient by taking off any contaminated clothing and use a self-contained breathing apparatus for protection. The patient must be taken to the emergency room as soon as possible, with supplies for suctioning and ventilator support ready in case they become necessary.

When it comes to ingested toxins, 80% of poisoning is by mouth. EMTs might administer activated charcoal if it is indicated and within the appropriate time frame. Activated charcoal is a suspension that binds to the toxin in the stomach and transports it out of the system, making it more effective and less harmful than ipecac syrup.

In case of injected poisons, which usually happen because of drug abuse, such as heroin or cocaine, EMTs should monitor the airway, provide high-flow oxygen, and be alert for nausea and vomiting. Immediate transport to the emergency department is essential, as injected poisons are quickly absorbed and can cause severe local tissue damage, making dilution or removal impossible.

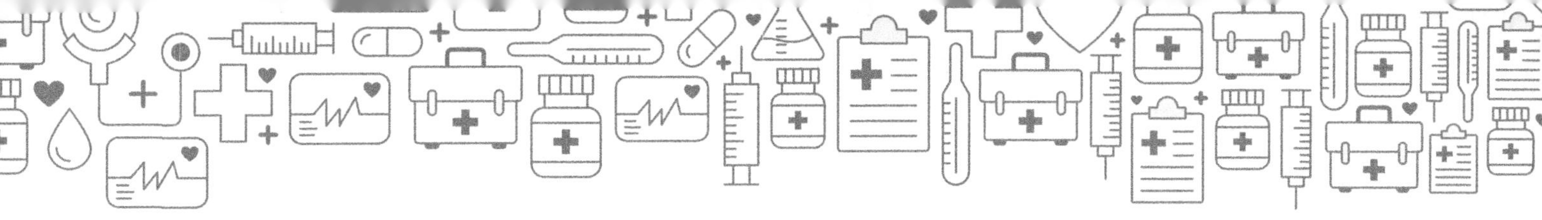

Absorbed and surface contact poisons can cause various effects on the patient, including skin damage, chemical burns, rashes, lesions, and systemic effects. It is relevant to differentiate between contact burns and contact absorption. Signs of absorbed poisoning include a history of exposure, visible liquid or powder on the skin, burns, itching, irritation, and characteristic odors.

Emergency treatment involves avoiding contamination, promptly removing the substance from the patient, and removing all contaminated clothing. The affected skin should be flushed and washed thoroughly; if a large amount of material is spilled, flood the area for at least 20 minutes. For chemical agents in the eyes, irrigate for at least 5-10 minutes for acids and 15-20 minutes for alkalis, ensuring the fluid runs from the bridge of the nose outward.

In industrial settings, do not try to neutralize substances with other chemicals; instead, wash them off with plenty of water and transport material safety data sheets with the patient to the hospital. The only exception to using water is when the poison reacts violently with it; in such cases EMTs should:

- Brush the chemical off
- Remove contaminated clothing
- Apply a dry dressing
- Transport the patient promptly to the emergency department
- Always wear appropriate protective gear during these procedures (Sharp School, n/a)

OBSTETRICS AND NEWBORN CARE

An obstetrician is a medical specialist who cares for individuals during preconception, pregnancy, childbirth, and the postpartum period. They manage and treat conditions associated with pregnancy to ensure the health of both the parent and baby. Obstetricians provide prenatal care, diagnose, and treat pregnancy complications, and deliver babies. They use various tools like ultrasounds and lab tests to monitor the pregnancy, manage labor and delivery, and provide postpartum care for up to six weeks after childbirth. Their responsibilities include prenatal screenings, evaluating fetal development, detecting anomalies, and treating health conditions that could affect the pregnancy (Cleveland Clinic, 2022).

The female reproductive system plays a valuable role in sexual activity, fertility, pregnancy, and childbirth. It consists of several key components. The ovaries, located on each side of the uterus, produce hormones and store eggs. Each month, an egg is released in a process called ovulation. The fallopian tubes connect the ovaries to the uterus, allowing the egg to travel. The uterus, or womb, thickens its lining monthly to prepare for potential pregnancy. If fertilization occurs, the egg implants in the uterine lining and develops into a fetus. If not, the lining is shed during menstruation. The cervix connects the uterus to the vagina, a muscular tube that leads to the outside of the body. Together, these structures facilitate reproduction and the menstrual cycle (Health Direct, n/a).

Pregnancy introduces numerous physiological changes in the body, which EMTs must understand to provide effective care. These changes primarily affect the respiratory, cardiovascular, and musculoskeletal systems, and are crucial for ensuring both maternal and fetal health.

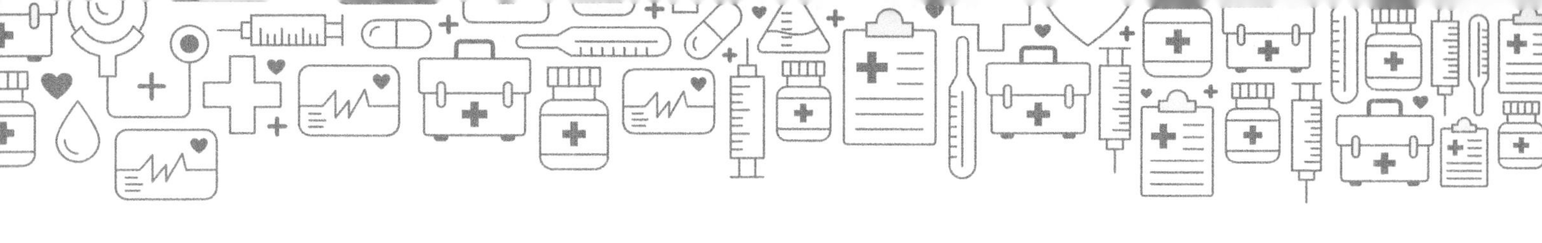

During pregnancy, hormonal fluctuations prepare the body for childbirth and support fetal development, increasing the risk of complications from trauma and medical conditions. For instance, as the fetus grows, the uterus expands significantly, displacing abdominal organs and potentially compromising respiratory and cardiovascular functions.

By the second trimester, the growing uterus pushes up on the diaphragm, reducing respiratory capacity and increasing breathing rates. Additionally, blood volume rises by up to 50% by the end of pregnancy to meet the needs of the fetus and prepare for blood loss during delivery. This increased blood volume necessitates a higher heart rate and cardiac output, which can complicate the management of trauma patients.

The third trimester brings additional challenges. The displacement of the stomach and changes in gastrointestinal motility increase the risk of vomiting and aspiration, especially in trauma scenarios. Weight gain and altered body mechanics also elevate the risk of slips and falls due to a shifted center of gravity and joint laxity caused by hormonal changes. These factors, combined with the increased workload on the heart, necessitate careful assessment and management by EMTs.

Labor progresses through three stages: dilation of the cervix, delivery of the infant, and delivery of the placenta. The first stage starts with contractions and ends with full dilation of the cervix, typically lasting longer for first-time mothers. EMTs need to recognize signs of true labor, such as regular contractions and the rupture of the amniotic sac.

In cases of premature rupture, supportive care and transport are essential if labor does not commence immediately. During the second stage, as the fetus moves through the birth canal, EMTs must decide whether to assist with delivery on-site or transport the patient to a hospital. Crowning, or the appearance of the baby's head at the vaginal opening, signals the imminent delivery of the infant. The third stage concludes with the delivery of the placenta, requiring EMTs to ensure that it separates completely from the uterine wall.

Pregnancy complications that EMTs might encounter include hypertensive disorders, bleeding, and diabetes. Preeclampsia, or pregnancy-induced hypertension, often develops after the 30th week and can lead to eclampsia, characterized by seizures. Treatment involves positioning the patient on her left side, providing supplemental oxygen, and rapid transport to medical facilities. In cases of internal bleeding, such as from an ectopic pregnancy or placental abruption, you must act swiftly.

Vaginal bleeding in early pregnancy might indicate a miscarriage, while bleeding later in pregnancy can signal serious placental conditions. Gestational diabetes, which typically resolves after childbirth, requires management like that of diabetes in non-pregnant patients, often involving dietary changes, medication, or insulin.

Trauma involving pregnant patients presents unique challenges. EMTs must consider both the mother and the fetus, as trauma can significantly affect both. Common traumatic incidents include motor vehicle crashes and assaults. Pregnant women are at a higher risk of falls due to altered balance and joint instability.

Increased blood volume and heart rate mean that significant hemorrhage might not immediately show signs of shock, necessitating vigilant monitoring. In cases of severe trauma, such as a motor vehicle crash, EMTs should be alert for signs of placental abruption and manage any resulting shock with high-flow oxygen and positioning the patient on her left side (Sharp School, n/a). Placing a pregnant patient on her left side or tilting a spine board to the left helps prevent compression of the vena cava, ensuring proper blood flow and oxygenation to both the mother and fetus (Medic Tests, n/a).

Assessment and management of pregnant trauma patients involve several key considerations. EMTs should maintain an open airway, administer high-flow oxygen, and assess circulation meticulously. Rapid transport to a trauma center is essential for severe cases. Special attention is needed to manage vomiting and airway management to prevent aspiration. If the patient is in labor, EMTs must prepare for an imminent delivery, ensuring a safe and appropriate environment for childbirth.

Finally, cultural values and teenage pregnancy add additional layers of complexity. Respecting cultural differences is essential in providing care that aligns with the patient's beliefs and preferences. Teenage pregnancies often come with challenges related to both physical and psychological development. EMTs should manage these situations with sensitivity and respect for the young patient's privacy and autonomy (Sharp School, n/a).

Emergency Medical Technicians provide indispensable support in obstetrics and newborn care, especially during emergencies involving pregnant patients. Pregnancy introduces numerous physiological changes in the body, which EMTs must understand to provide effective care. These changes primarily affect the respiratory, cardiovascular, and musculoskeletal systems, and are crucial for ensuring both maternal and fetal health.

Delivering a child as an EMT in the absence of a sterile OB kit can be challenging but manageable with proper precautions. Even without an OB kit, essential protective equipment such as eye protection, gloves, and a mask should always be used to safeguard both the patient and the responder. When delivering the baby, using clean sheets or towels, which should be fresh and not previously used, helps maintain some degree of cleanliness. Immediately after birth, you must clear the baby's mouth of any blood or mucus using a gloved finger.

Avoid cutting or tying the umbilical cord; instead, focus on wrapping the placenta in a clean towel or placing it in a plastic bag for transport. Maintain the placenta and the infant at the same level, or slightly elevate the placenta if possible. Keeping the infant warm is critical to prevent hypothermia (Sharp School, n/a).

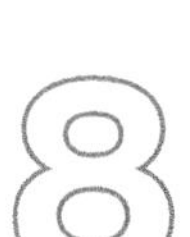

ABDOMINAL AND GYNECOLOGICAL EMERGENCIES

In dealing with abdominal and gynecological emergencies, EMTs must approach each situation with a blend of clinical expertise and compassionate care. These emergencies can range from acute abdominal pain to complex gynecological conditions, requiring both immediate medical attention and sensitivity to the patient's emotional state.

When assessing abdominal emergencies, the EMT's primary objective is to identify and address any life-threatening conditions. Abdominal pain can stem from various sources, including appendicitis, gastrointestinal issues, or trauma. The EMT should start with a thorough patient history and physical examination, focusing on pain location, onset, and severity. It is crucial to inquire about any associated symptoms, such as vomiting, diarrhea, or fever, as these can provide important clues to the underlying cause. Immediate interventions might include stabilizing the patient's airway, breathing, and circulation, and providing analgesia if needed.

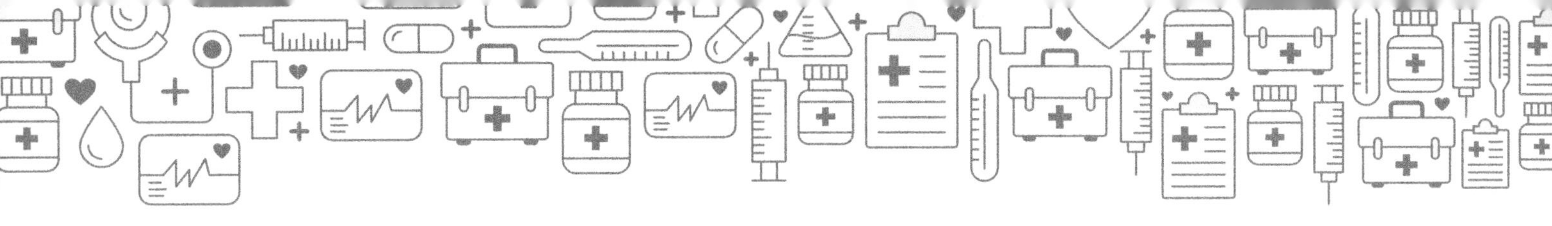

In cases of trauma, especially involving penetrating injuries or severe blunt force, EMTs must be vigilant for signs of internal bleeding or organ damage. Rapid transport to an appropriate medical facility is essential for further diagnostic work and treatment. For abdominal trauma, it is important to minimize movement and avoid applying direct pressure to the injured area, as this could exacerbate internal injuries.

Gynecological emergencies encompass a range of conditions that can affect women at various stages of life, from menstrual issues to pregnancy-related complications. One demanding area is the management of sexual assault or rape. In these cases, the EMT's role extends beyond immediate medical care to include psychological support and evidence preservation. It is essential to approach these situations with the utmost professionalism, sensitivity, and respect. Providing the option for a female EMT when can help the patient feel more comfortable and supported.

The EMT should be aware of the potential for drugs used to incapacitate individuals during sexual assaults and be cautious about preserving evidence. You must advise the patient against cleaning herself, changing clothes, or urinating, as these actions can destroy important evidence. Instead, focus on providing immediate medical care, addressing any life-threatening injuries, and facilitating a supportive environment. If appropriate, offer to contact local rape crisis centers to provide additional support and resources.

In cases involving gynecological emergencies such as ectopic pregnancies or spontaneous abortions, EMTs must assess the severity of bleeding and pain, and monitor for signs of shock. Ectopic pregnancies, where the embryo implants outside the uterus, can cause severe internal bleeding if the fallopian tube ruptures. Symptoms typically include sharp abdominal pain, vaginal bleeding, and sometimes shoulder pain due to referred pain from internal bleeding. You need to transport the patient rapidly to an emergency facility to manage these potentially life-threatening conditions.

Spontaneous abortions, or miscarriages, require careful management to ensure the safety and well-being of the patient. EMTs should be prepared to manage heavy vaginal bleeding and support the patient emotionally, as this can be a distressing experience. Providing comfort, maintaining a calm demeanor, and ensuring that the patient is transported safely to a medical facility are key aspects of care (Studocu, n/a).

BEHAVIORAL AND PSYCHIATRIC EMERGENCIES

Behavioral and psychiatric emergencies are significant challenges for EMTs and paramedics, accounting for about 8% of all EMS calls (Unitek EMT, 2021). These emergencies involve patients exhibiting severe behavioral or mental patterns that cause substantial distress or impair their ability to function. The primary goal in such situations is to ensure the safety of both the patient and others while providing appropriate care.

A psychiatric emergency is identified by several key signs. The patient may pose a danger to themselves or others or exhibit severe impairment in their ability to care for themselves and perform daily functions. Additionally, there might be significant property damage or violent behavior involved. In such cases, the patient's situation often escalates to a point where immediate intervention becomes necessary to ensure safety and address the crisis effectively.

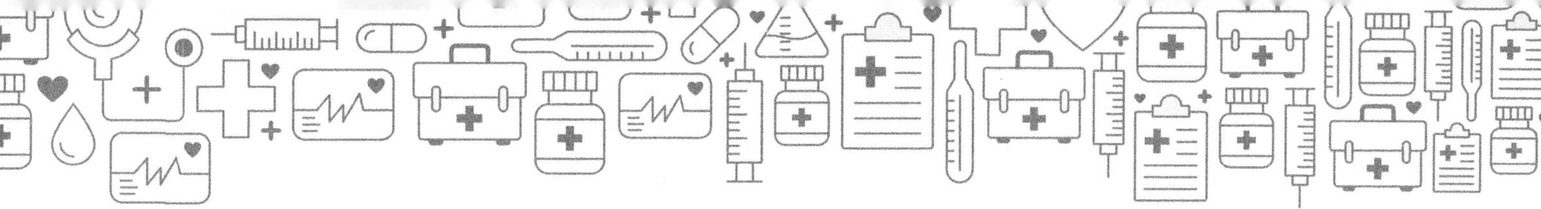

Common conditions leading to psychiatric emergencies include:

- » Schizophrenia
- » Bipolar disorder (especially mania)
- » Depression
- » Anxiety states
- » Substance intoxication
- » Withdrawal
- » Delirium
- » Dementia

Managing behavioral emergencies involves effective de-escalation techniques to ensure safety and calm. Key methods include maintaining a calm demeanor by speaking in a relaxed, clear voice and avoiding confrontational language. It is important to respect personal space by keeping a safe distance to prevent further agitation. Establishing verbal contact by introducing yourself and explaining your role can help build trust. Being concise in communication, using simple language and short sentences, ensures clarity. Identifying the patient's needs and feelings involves acknowledging their concerns and emotions. Setting limits by establishing clear boundaries and offering choices helps guide behavior. Finally, listen actively, pay close attention to the patient's words, and respond empathetically to achieve effective de-escalation.

8

In managing psychiatric emergencies, a structured approach is essential. A typical protocol often follows "Zeller's Six Goals" of emergency psychiatric care. These goals include:

Excluding medical causes for the symptoms
Rapidly stabilizing the acute crisis
Avoiding coercion
Treat in the least restrictive environment.
Create a therapeutic alliance.
Develop an appropriate disposition and aftercare strategy to ensure continued support and recovery (Unitek EMT, 2021).

The focus is also on treating the patient in the least restrictive environment possible, forming a therapeutic alliance, and developing an appropriate disposition and aftercare plan to ensure continued support and recovery.

In extreme cases, EMTs may need to restrain a patient to ensure the safety of both the patient and the crew. This situation typically arises when a patient poses a risk to themselves or others due to severe agitation or violent behavior. Restraint must always comply with local regulations and protocols, which often require law enforcement involvement for legal authorization. However, EMTs frequently assist in the physical restraint process alongside police officers.

Effective restraint requires careful planning and coordination. Ideally, a team of four or five individuals should be involved to manage each extremity and the patient's head, ensuring safety and effectiveness.

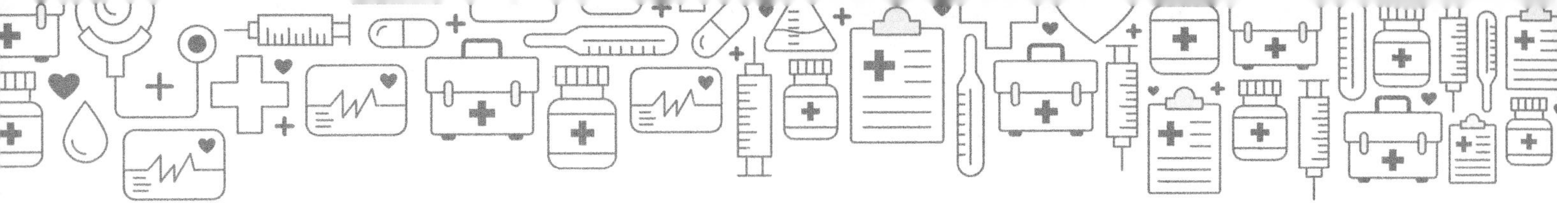

Using soft, humane restraints is crucial; options like handcuffs or flex-ties are avoided to prevent injury. The patient should be restrained in a face-up position to reduce the risk of positional asphyxia, avoiding a prone position despite any provocations or verbal abuse.

It is important to position the patient so they cannot use their major muscle groups to resist. Continuous monitoring is essential, especially watching for sudden changes in the patient's condition, such as becoming unusually quiet, which could indicate a serious deterioration in their health (EMS World, 2006).

We covered respiratory emergencies, detailing critical interventions for acute breathing issues. We addressed endocrine and hematologic crises, including diabetes and blood disorders. Anaphylaxis and toxicology sections highlight severe allergic reactions and poisoning management. The obstetrics and newborn care segment focuses on childbirth complications and neonatal care. We discussed abdominal and gynecological emergencies, emphasizing urgent female reproductive health issues. Finally, we explored behavioral and psychiatric emergencies, offering insights into acute mental health crisis management.

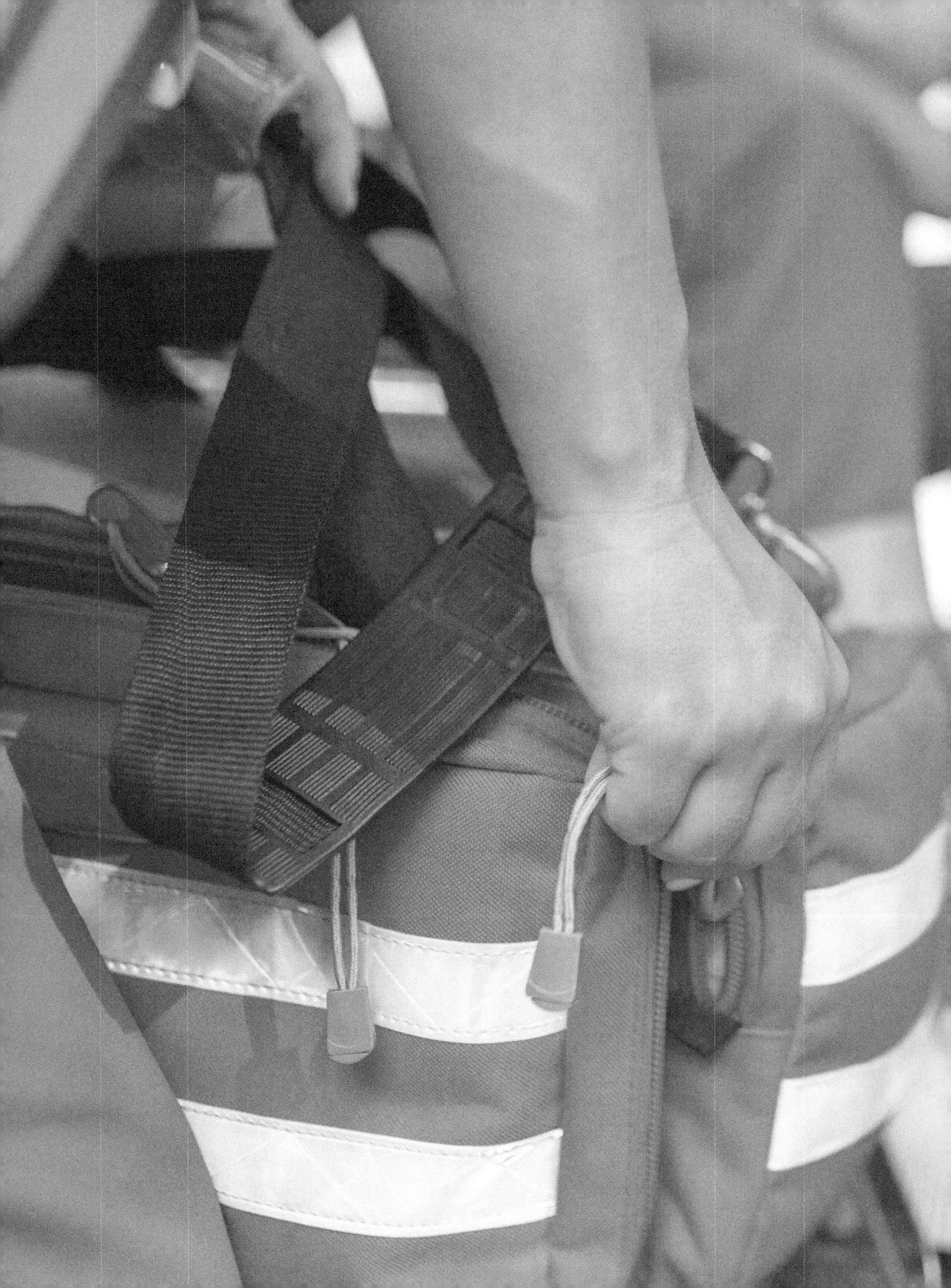

9 EMS OPERATIONS

EMS OPERATIONS

The evolution of ambulance services reflects a dramatic shift from basic transport to sophisticated emergency medical response. Originating in Ancient Rome with simple carts for injured soldiers and evolving through medieval times with rudimentary horse-drawn carts, ambulance services took a significant leap in the 18th century with Dominique-Jean Larrey's 'flying ambulances' during the Napoleonic Wars. This early innovation emphasized rapid medical transport.

The 19th century saw the establishment of civilian ambulance services and the first hospital-based ambulances in the US, enhancing the integration of medical care with transport. The early 20th century introduced motorized ambulances, significantly improving response times and efficiency. World War II further advanced these services with air ambulances and radio communication.

The 1960s marked a turning point with the advent of paramedic programs and advanced prehospital care, laying the groundwork for modern EMS. By the 1970s and 1980s, standardized training and advanced equipment, including defibrillators and ALS units, became commonplace.

Today, integrating technologies like GPS and telemedicine in ambulances underscores the ongoing evolution of EMT transport operations, enhancing both the speed and quality of pre-hospital care (GoAid, 2024).

TRANSPORT OPERATIONS

Proper sanitation of emergency vehicles is necessary to prevent the spread of infection and maintain a safe environment for both patients and medical personnel. The process begins with removing used linens and medical waste following each call. Used linens are placed in designated receptacles, and medical waste is discarded properly. After removing waste, the vehicle's contaminated areas are washed with soap and water.

Non-disposable equipment used during patient care must be disinfected, and the stretcher should be cleaned with an EPA-registered germicidal or virucidal solution or a bleach and water mixture diluted at 1:100. Routine cleaning of the emergency vehicle should be scheduled to ensure thorough sanitation. Additionally, each piece of equipment should be cleaned according to the manufacturer's recommendations, and these procedures should be documented in a written policy.

Basic medical supplies are mandatory for effective emergency response. Sterile gloves are essential for infection control and must always be available to ensure procedures are conducted hygienically. You need oxygen supplies, including portable tanks, masks, and regulators, for patients experiencing respiratory distress. Additionally, a well-stocked jump kit containing various tools and supplies that EMTs might need immediately upon arriving at a scene is required. This kit typically includes basic medications, bandages, splints, and a stethoscope, providing the necessary resources for prompt and effective patient care.

The next category is stabilization and transport equipment, important for ensuring patient safety and effective care during emergency responses. Various types of splints, such as padded and rigid, are necessary for immobilizing broken limbs and stabilizing injured body parts. Backboards should be used for patients with suspected spinal injuries, as they provide stability and support during transport. Additionally, stabilization equipment, including cervical collars and other devices, is designed to keep patients secure and minimize movement, further enhancing safety and reducing the risk of additional injury during transport.

The emergency obstetric kit is specifically designed for childbirth situations. It includes items like sterile towels, umbilical tape or sterilized cord, and a small rubber bulb syringe.

The cleaning and sanitation supplies should include disinfectants such as wipes and sprays to maintain hygiene by effectively cleaning non-disposable equipment and surfaces. Additionally, proper receptacles for medical waste and contaminated linens are essential to prevent contamination and ensure safe disposal, thereby upholding a clean and sanitary environment in the ambulance.

Medical equipment is necessary for monitoring patient vital signs and includes devices such as blood pressure cuffs, thermometers, and pulse oximeters. EMTs need a portable suction unit to clear the airway of fluids or obstructions and ensure that the patient's breathing is not compromised.

Patient care report forms are necessary for EMTs to document patient information, treatment provided, and any changes in the patient's condition. Moreover, communication devices such as radios or mobile dispatch terminals are valuable for coordinating with dispatch and other emergency services, ensuring efficient and effective response and transport.

Defensive Driving Techniques

Driving an emergency vehicle involves significant responsibility and requires a set of defensive driving techniques to ensure safety. The frequency of ambulance crashes in the United States, over 6,000 annually, underscores the importance of these techniques (Sharp School, n/a).

Training is essential for emergency vehicle operators, with some states mandating the completion of approved emergency vehicle operations courses. Drivers must be physically fit and alert, avoiding the operation of vehicles if they are under the influence of drowsy medications, alcohol, or are fatigued from extended shifts. Furthermore, managing stress and maintaining emotional maturity are crucial for the safe operation of emergency vehicles.

Speed alone does not enhance patient care; proper care and attention are more important than driving at high speeds. All passengers must always wear seat belts and shoulder restraints, and if an EMT removes their seatbelt to provide care, they must fasten it again as soon as possible.

Drivers should be familiar with their vehicle's acceleration, braking characteristics, and handling under various conditions. They must understand how the vehicle maneuvers, including cornering, swaying, and stopping. On multilane highways, staying in the extreme left lane allows other drivers to move over safely. The activation of sirens and lights should be based on local protocols, the patient's condition, and anticipated clinical outcomes.

Helicopter Medical Evacuation

Helicopter medical evacuation, commonly known as medivac, is performed exclusively by helicopters, and provides rapid transport for patients in critical conditions. Medivac protocols and capabilities vary across EMS services, tailored to specific needs and regional resources.

Medivac is often called upon when ground transport to a hospital is too lengthy, or when road, traffic, or environmental conditions make ground transport impractical. It is also utilized when a patient requires advanced medical care that EMTs cannot provide, or in situations involving multiple patients that could overwhelm nearby hospitals accessible by ground.

Patients receiving medivac often have time-dependent injuries or illnesses, such as strokes, heart attacks, serious spinal cord injuries, trauma, or conditions like near-drownings or severe wilderness accidents. Notifying the dispatcher is the first step in initiating a medivac, and in some areas, EMS personnel may directly communicate with the flight crew to coordinate the response (Sharp School, n/a).

RESCUE OPERATIONS AND HAZARDOUS MATERIALS

Hazardous materials, often termed as hazmat, encompass a range of agents, including chemical, biological, and nuclear substances, which pose significant risks to human health and the environment. While the media sometimes portrays hazmat incidents in the context of bioterrorism, most exposures result from accidental or natural chemical spills. Although these events are rare and typically localized, they require thorough preparation and response strategies to effectively mitigate their impact.

According to data from the United States Department of Transportation Office of Hazardous Material Safety, between 12,000 to 18,000 hazmat events occur annually. These incidents range from roadway spills and industrial leaks to lab chemical exposures and naturally occurring toxic releases. Notably, many hazmat incidents go unreported, as they are managed locally without the need for escalation (Berry and Perera, 2022).

HazMat EMTs

Rescue operations involving hazardous materials are critical components of emergency response services. These operations are conducted out by highly trained professionals known as Hazardous Materials Emergency Medical Technicians (HazMat EMTs).

These specialized EMTs possess the knowledge and skills necessary to provide emergency medical care in environments contaminated by hazardous substances, such as chemical spills, radioactive material exposures, and biological contaminants. The multifaceted role of a HazMat EMT extends beyond the typical duties of an EMT, focusing on identifying, assessing, and mitigating risks associated with hazardous materials to safely treat and transport affected patients.

A critical aspect of a HazMat EMT's role is executing decontamination procedures for both patients and responders. This involves removing or neutralizing contaminants from individuals and medical equipment to prevent the spread of hazardous materials.

Effective decontamination is essential for ensuring the safety of patients, medical personnel, and the wider community. HazMat EMTs must be well-versed in the use of personal protective equipment (PPE), selecting and correctly using the appropriate level of protection for various hazardous environments.

Effective communication and coordination with hazmat response teams and other emergency services are key components of a HazMat EMT's duties. These professionals collaborate closely with other responders to manage the scene of a hazardous materials incident. They provide essential medical insights into the management of the incident, helping guide the actions of the hazmat team, particularly in assessing the severity of exposures and advising on necessary medical interventions. Clear and concise communication ensures seamless interagency coordination and operational efficiency during hazardous materials incidents.

Training and Preparedness

Becoming a HazMat EMT requires extensive training and certification. The journey typically begins with completing an EMT-Basic course, which provides foundational knowledge in emergency medical care. After obtaining EMT-Basic certification, individuals may choose to advance their skills by enrolling in EMT-Advanced (or Intermediate) training, which includes more in-depth medical training, such as administering intravenous fluids and using advanced airway devices.

Specialized hazmat training is the next step, starting with awareness-level training and progressing to operations-level and technician-level training, depending on the desired role and responsibilities. This training covers the fundamentals of hazardous materials response, including recognizing and identifying hazardous substances, using PPE, and performing basic control, containment, and confinement operations. Continuous education is key for HazMat EMTs to stay updated on the latest practices, technologies, and regulations in hazardous materials management.

Situational Awareness and Safety Protocols

HazMat EMTs must continually assess the environment for new or escalating hazards to make informed decisions quickly. This ability to anticipate changes in the situation, including potential secondary incidents or worsening conditions, allows for proactive adjustments to response strategies. Adhering to established safety protocols is equally important, as these guidelines are designed to protect not only the HazMat EMTs but also the victims and the public (Unitek EMT, 2024).

Decontamination and Stabilization

The foremost priority during a hazmat incident is safety. Establishing an incident command system is critical for organized response management, designating hot, warm, and cold zones to control and isolate the scene.

Hot Zone: This area immediately surrounds the source of contamination and is strictly controlled. Only personnel with full protective equipment should enter to rescue victims and prevent further exposure. The extent of the hot zone depends on the type of hazmat involved, and all items within this area are considered contaminated until properly decontaminated.

Warm Zone: Decontamination occurs in this zone, just outside the hot zone. Initial medical management, such as airway support, may also take place here. The primary decontamination method involves removing contaminated clothing and using water to thoroughly rinse the skin. This linear process ensures systematic and efficient decontamination, minimizing the risk of secondary contamination.

Cold Zone: Located upwind and uphill from the warm zone, the cold zone serves as the command and support area. Here, decontaminated patients receive further triage and stabilization, including administering oxygen, bronchodilators, and intravenous fluids if needed. EMTs need to ensure effective decontamination because patients interact with numerous responders en route to medical facilities (Berry and Perera, 2022).

INCIDENT MANAGEMENT AND MASS CASUALTY INCIDENTS

A mass casualty incident (MCI) occurs when the number of patients exceeds the capacity of local emergency resources. The scale of an MCI can vary based on the resources available in a given area. In the US, nearly 10,000 MCIs happen annually, often from incidents like multi-vehicle crashes rather than high-profile disasters. These events can overwhelm facilities, hindering effective care. Notable events like the September 11, 2001, attacks and the Boston Marathon bombing have heightened public awareness and driven improvements in MCI management. Preparation involves understanding potential causes, expected injuries, and strategies for resource mobilization. When local resources fall short, national emergency response systems provide additional support (Binkley and Kemp, 2022).

EMTs' responsibilities extend from initial on-scene assessment to patient stabilization and transport. Effective incident management requires EMTs to adhere to structured protocols and work seamlessly within the established incident command system.

Upon arrival at an MCI, EMTs must quickly identify the type of incident to tailor their response appropriately. Each type demands specific safety measures and treatment protocols. MCIs can be categorized into various types, such as:

- Planned events (e.g., large sporting events)
- Conventional incidents (e.g., transportation accidents or severe weather)
- Chemical
- Biological
- Radiological
- Nuclear (CBRN) events
- Catastrophic health events (e.g., pandemics)

Managing an MCI effectively involves organizing the response according to the five S's: scene safety assessment, scene size-up, send information, scene set-up, and START (Simple Triage and Rapid Treatment).

Scene Safety Assessment: Ensuring the scene's safety is the first priority. EMTs must identify potential hazards and ensure the area is secure before proceeding.

Scene Size-Up: EMTs must evaluate the scale of the incident, estimate the number of casualties, and determine the resources required.

Send Information: Communicating with dispatch and other responding agencies is critical to ensure additional resources are promptly mobilized.

Scene Set-Up: Establishing a command center and delineating zones (hot, warm, and cold) helps organize the scene and ensure efficient operations. The hot zone is where the incident occurred and is the most dangerous area, while the warm zone is for decontamination, and the cold zone is for treatment and transport.

START Triage: This involves quickly categorizing patients based on the severity of their injuries using the START method. Patients are tagged as minor (green), delayed (yellow), immediate (red), or expectant (black) based on their condition and the urgency of their need for medical intervention.

The authority to declare an MCI varies by region but includes incident commanders, local hospitals, EMS personnel, and emergency management agencies. Early activation of MCI protocols ensures a coordinated response and efficient resource allocation.

Communications and Incident Management

Effective communication is key in MCI management. A command center equipped with multiple radios and communication devices helps coordinate efforts. Scene commanders use headsets, microphones, and checklists to maintain a clear and continuous flow of information. This ensures that all responders are updated on the scene dynamics and can adjust their strategies accordingly.

On-Scene Control and Hierarchical Approach

On-scene control is critical to managing the chaos of an MCI. Various roles must be established early to ensure an organized response. The incident commander oversees the entire operation, while the safety officer assesses hazards and ensures responder safety. The radio officer coordinates communications, and the medical supervisor manages triage, treatment, and patient transportation.

METHANE Protocol

To quickly assess the extent of an MCI, EMTs use the METHANE mnemonic. This structured approach helps in providing a comprehensive initial report and facilitates a swift and effective response:

- **M:** Major incident declaration
- **E:** Exact location
- **T:** Type of incident
- **H:** Hazards present
- **A:** Access routes
- **N:** Number of casualties
- **E:** Emergency services required
- Triage and Treatment

Triage is a critical component of MCI management. The START method helps EMTs prioritize patients based on the severity of their injuries. Those categorized as immediate (red) require urgent medical attention, while delayed (yellow) patients have serious but stable conditions. Minor (green) patients have non-life-threatening injuries, and expectant (black) patients are either deceased or unlikely to survive, given the available resources.

Resource Allocation and Inventory

Efficient resource allocation is essential in MCIs. EMTs must manage limited resources effectively, prioritizing the most critical patients. The Federal Emergency Management Agency's Incident Resource Inventory System can help track and allocate resources. This system allows for consistent identification and inventory of resources, facilitating mutual aid operations based on mission needs.

Challenges and Solutions

Several factors, termed “MCI Multipliers,” can complicate the response to an MCI. These include limited scene accessibility, biohazard contamination, self-deploying responders, and communication gaps. Early role establishment and clear communication can mitigate these challenges. For example, designating a staging area for ambulances and setting up triage zones with color-coded tarps can streamline operations and ensure that resources are used efficiently.

Specific Considerations for Mass Shootings

In the case of MCIs caused by mass shootings, the American College of Surgeons and the FBI recommend the THREAT protocol. This protocol emphasizes the need for rapid intervention to control bleeding and quickly move patients to safe areas for further assessment and treatment:

- **T:** Threat suppression
- **H:** Hemorrhage control
- **RE:** Rapid Extrication to safety
- **A:** Assessment by medical providers
- **T:** Transport to definitive care (DeNolf and Kahwaji, 2022)

TERRORISM AND WEAPONS OF MASS DESTRUCTION

A weapon of mass destruction (WMD) is a powerful weapon capable of causing massive death and destruction. These weapons are so devastating that their mere existence in a hostile nation's arsenal poses a severe threat. WMDs include nuclear, biological, and chemical weapons, often collectively referred to as NBC weapons. The term "weapons of mass destruction" has been in use since at least 1937, initially describing large-scale bomber aircraft. However, the true destructive potential of WMDs became evident during World War II with the atomic bombing of Hiroshima, resulting in immense loss of life and widespread devastation (The Editors of Encyclopaedia Britannica, 2024).

Chemical weapons are designed to cause harm through toxic effects. They are categorized into several types, each with its own clinical presentation and treatment requirements:

Blood Agents (e.g., Hydrogen Cyanide) interfere with cellular respiration, leading to symptoms like respiratory distress and anxiety. Immediate treatment often involves antidotes like Sodium Thiosulfate.

Vesicants (e.g., Sulfur Mustard) cause painful blisters and damage to the skin and respiratory system. Decontamination is crucial, and treatment includes supportive care and antibiotics if lewisite is involved.

Pulmonary Agents (e.g., Phosgene) primarily affect the respiratory system, causing pulmonary edema. Treatment focuses on removing the agent and providing respiratory support.

Nerve Agents (e.g., Sarin) cause severe symptoms like salivation, lacrimation, urination, and defecation. These require rapid administration of antidotes such as atropine and pralidoxime.

Biological weapons involve microorganisms or toxins that can cause disease. Biological agents include:

Anthrax: Characterized by flu-like symptoms and progressing to severe respiratory issues, treatment requires antibiotics like ciprofloxacin.

Botulism: Causes paralysis and requires antitoxin and supportive care.

Plague: Can present as pneumonic plague

with severe respiratory symptoms; it is managed with antibiotics.

Viral Hemorrhagic Fevers: Such as Ebola, leads to severe multi-system failure and hemorrhage, requiring specialized treatment and isolation.

Radiological/nuclear weapons involve radiation exposure, which can be external or internal. Responders must focus on:

Time, Distance, and Shielding: Minimize exposure by reducing time near the source, increasing distance, and using appropriate protective gear.

Decontamination: Removing radioactive materials from the body and environment without delaying essential medical treatment.

Explosive weapons create various injuries through blast effects, which include:

Primary Blast Injuries: Caused by blast waves and affects organs such as the lungs.

Secondary Injuries: Result from flying debris.

Tertiary Injuries: Due to the blast wind throwing victims.

Quaternary Injuries: Includes burns and crush injuries.

EMS Response and Protocols

Personal Protective Equipment ensures the safety of EMT personnel. Appropriate PPE must be used to protect against the specific type of WMD. For example, chemical incidents may require full-body suits, while radiological events need protective clothing and monitoring equipment.

The process of removing harmful substances from victims is essential. Decontamination can be performed through:

Gross Decontamination: Initial, rapid removal of contaminants using water or other agents.

Technical Decontamination: More thorough cleaning performed by specialized teams.

Definitive Decontamination: Detailed and thorough washing, often conducted in a dedicated decontamination corridor.

EMTs should identify and prioritize patients based on the severity of their condition. The START (Simple Triage and Rapid Treatment) system is often used for triage during mass casualty incidents, including those involving WMDs (Reed-Schrader et al., 2023).

Terrorism

Terrorism is a method of using violence or threats to create fear, aiming to achieve political goals by intimidating a wide audience, not just the immediate victims. The term originated during the French Revolution in the 1790s, describing the Reign of Terror led by the Jacobin party, which used mass executions to suppress opposition.

Unlike conventional warfare, which focuses on military strength, terrorism seeks to influence or destabilize governments through fear and psychological impact. It is often used when direct military victory is unattainable, making it a tool for those with limited power to challenge or coerce larger entities. Terrorism is about creating widespread fear to push for political change or disrupt existing power structures (Jenkins, 2024).

The first priority for EMTs arriving at a scene is safety. They must wait for confirmation from police or bomb disposal experts that the area is secure before entering, especially if there's a risk of secondary explosions. In cases involving shootings or other high-risk scenarios, EMTs should not approach unless trained in tactical medicine and equipped with protective gear. For incidents involving chemical, biological, or radiological threats, specialized PPE is necessary.

In the aftermath of a blast, EMTs deal with multiple types of injuries. Primary blast injuries result from the shockwave of the explosion, causing damage to air-filled organs like the lungs and ears. Secondary blast injuries occur from flying debris and shrapnel, which can penetrate the body and cause severe trauma. Tertiary blast injuries are due to being thrown by the blast, leading to blunt trauma and amputation. Lastly, quaternary blast injuries include burns and exposure to hazardous materials, requiring immediate care.

EMTs must also be prepared for specific types of terrorist attacks. For stabbings, they often involve multiple, deep wounds, particularly in the upper body, and require prompt treatment. Targeted Automobile Ramming Mass Casualty (TARMAC) attacks involve vehicles used to run over people, causing blunt trauma to various body parts (Alpert and Grossman, 2023).

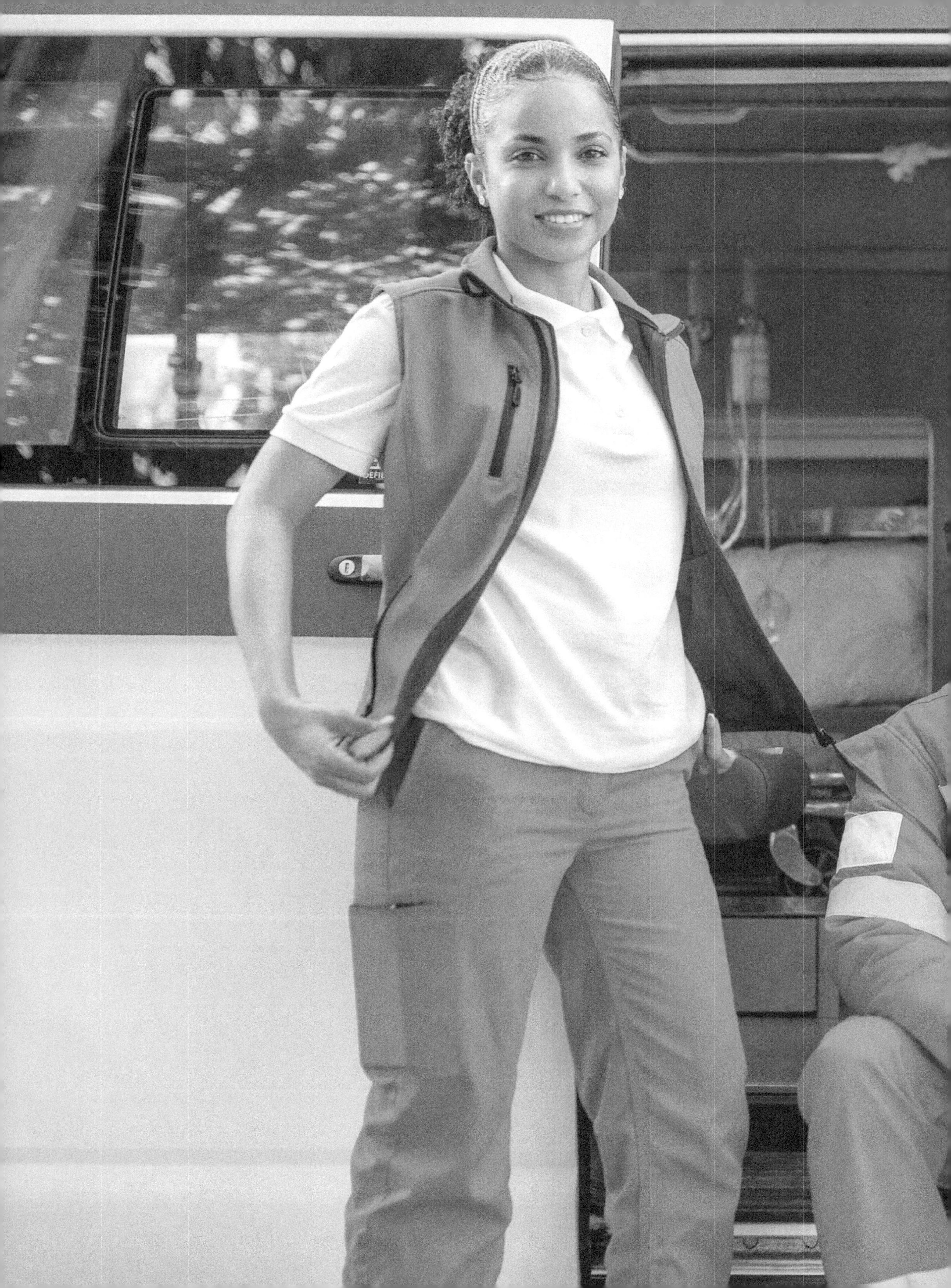

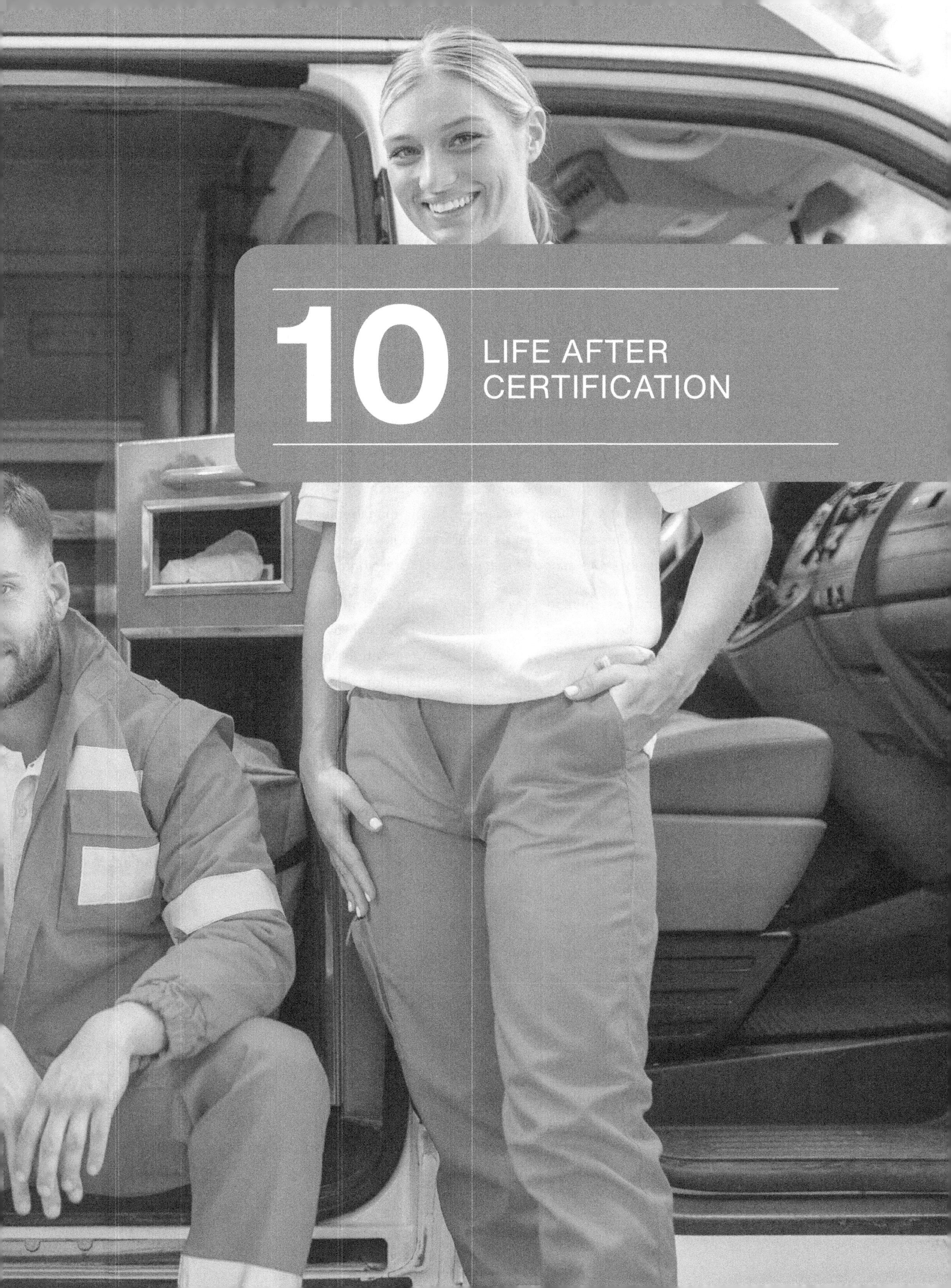

10 LIFE AFTER CERTIFICATION

LIFE AFTER CERTIFICATION

Career advancement opportunities for EMTs and Emergency Room Technicians (ERTs) are abundant, with multiple paths for growth and specialization available to those who wish to further their careers beyond initial certification.

ADVANCED CERTIFICATION AND SPECIALIZATION

For EMTs, advancing their careers typically involves moving up to roles with greater responsibilities and advanced skills. The most common progression is from a basic EMT to an Advanced EMT (AEMT) or paramedic. AEMTs receive additional training in areas such as advanced airway management, medication administration, and more complex patient assessments.

Paramedics, the highest level of prehospital care providers, undergo extensive education covering advanced medical procedures, including advanced airway management, intravenous therapy, and critical care techniques. Achieving certification as a paramedic involves rigorous training and examination but significantly expands an EMT's scope of practice and professional opportunities.

Continuing education is essential for EMTs to stay current with medical advancements and maintain their certifications. Most states require completion of recertification by continuing education units (CEUs). Beyond these requirements, enrolling in advanced courses, attending workshops and seminars, and participating in professional conferences can provide valuable knowledge and skills.

Professional organizations, such as the National Association of Emergency Medical Technicians (NAEMT) and the National Association of Emergency Medical Technicians and Emergency Room Technicians (NAEMT/ERT), offer resources and networking opportunities that can further enhance career development.

Experience in various settings can significantly contribute to career growth. EMTs should seek opportunities to work in different environments, such as urban and rural areas, and participate in community outreach and special events. This varied experience helps them develop a broader skill set and adapt to different challenges.

Building a strong professional network is essential for career advancement. EMTs can expand their networks by joining professional organizations, attending industry events, and connect with colleagues on platforms like LinkedIn. Networking provides access to support, guidance, and new career opportunities. Mentorship from experienced professionals can offer invaluable insights and advice, helping EMTs navigate their career paths more effectively.

Several paths are available for those interested in specializing further. Critical Care Paramedics (CCPs) receive training to manage critically ill patients during transport. Tactical EMS providers work with law enforcement and military units, offering medical support during high-risk operations. Flight paramedics provide care during air medical transport, which requires additional certification and the ability to operate under high-pressure conditions.

Community paramedicine focuses on delivering preventive and chronic care services in patients' homes, aiming to reduce hospital readmissions and improve patient outcomes. ERTs may specialize in pediatric emergency care, trauma care, or take on leadership roles within the emergency department.

Transition to Other Healthcare Roles

Many EMTs and ERTs transition to other roles within healthcare due to their extensive experience in emergency care. Some become Registered Nurses (RNs) by completing an accredited nursing program and passing the NCLEX-RN exam. Others may pursue careers as Physician Assistants (PAs), which involve diagnosing illnesses and prescribing treatments, requiring a master's level PA program, and passing the PA National Certifying Exam (PANCE).

For those aspiring to become Medical Doctors (MDs) or Doctors of Osteopathic Medicine (DOs), the path involves significant education and training, including medical school and residency. Alternatively, transitioning to healthcare administration involves managing healthcare facilities, improving patient care, and overseeing budgets and policies, requiring a degree in healthcare administration and relevant experience (Cotroneo, 2024).

You learned about the various paths for advancement and the traits necessary for success. The pros and cons of the profession, along with the differences between a paramedic and an EMT, provided a foundational understanding of your career choice.

We focused on preparing you for the NREMT exam, detailing eligibility requirements, registration processes, fees, retake policies, recertification, and tips for exam day success. You are well-prepared to tackle the certification exam with confidence.

Then we explored the roles and responsibilities of an EMT, covering the history of EMT services, the public health role of EMTs, and important medical, legal, and ethical issues. Communication and documentation skills were also highlighted as key components of the job.

We emphasized workforce safety and wellness, including proper lifting and moving techniques and patient restraint methods, ensuring you are equipped to handle the physical demands of the job safely.

An in-depth understanding of anatomy, physiology, and medical terminology was provided in Chapter 4, forming the backbone of your medical knowledge, and enabling accurate assessment and communication in emergency situations.

We also delved into patient assessment and management, teaching history taking, vital signs monitoring, and patient assessment techniques to ensure thorough and effective care.

Pharmacology, cardiology, resuscitation, stroke, seizures, and syncope were also covered, offering a deep dive into these critical areas, and equipping you with the skills to manage life-threatening emergencies.

We explored shock, trauma, and environmental emergencies, learning to manage trauma, bleeding, shock, soft tissue and burn injuries, and various environmental emergencies.

We focused on medical, obstetrics, and gynecologic emergencies, covering respiratory, endocrine, hematologic, anaphylaxis, toxicology, obstetrics, newborn care, and abdominal and gynecological emergencies, ensuring you are prepared for a wide range of medical scenarios.

We discussed transport operations, rescue operations, hazardous materials, incident management, mass casualty incidents, terrorism, and weapons of mass destruction. You are prepared for the operational aspects of the job and large-scale emergencies.

Finally, we explored life after certification, highlighting career advancement opportunities, specialization paths, the importance of continuing education, and the potential for transitioning to other healthcare roles. Building a strong professional network and seeking mentorship were emphasized as essential for career growth.

Congratulations on completing this comprehensive guide to your EMT certification journey. This book has equipped you with the essential knowledge and skills to excel in the field of emergency medical services.

As you begin your career as an EMT, remember that constant learning, gaining various experiences, and developing a professional network are critical to your success. Use the knowledge and abilities you learnt from this book, stay committed, and strive for success in your job. Best of luck with your qualification and future endeavors!

Dear Reader,

We understand that preparing for the NREMT exam can feel like a challenging task, and that's why we want to provide you with additional tools to support your journey toward success.

As a valued customer, you have exclusive access to our advanced e-learning platform, "Learnik," designed to enhance your study experience and offer targeted resources to help you excel in the NREMT exam. By scanning the QR code below, you'll unlock a wealth of supplementary learning resources directly related to the topics covered in this book.

On Learnik, you'll find a variety of interactive features to optimize your preparation:

Scenario-Based Quizzes: The platform generates personalized quizzes based on real-life scenarios and the content of the book you've purchased. These quizzes are designed to reinforce your understanding of key concepts and skills essential for the NREMT exam and help you track your progress.

But there's more! Learnik also offers a wide range of bonus content to enrich your learning experience:

Audiobooks: Study on the go with our professionally narrated audiobooks, allowing you to learn during your commute or downtime.

Flashcards: An effective tool for quickly memorizing essential medical terminology, procedures, and guidelines. Our flashcards are structured to present critical facts in a clear and concise format.

These resources are designed to complement your study routine, making your preparation more comprehensive and efficient. They are available exclusively to our valued customers like you, helping to maximize your chances of success in the NREMT exam.

So why wait? Scan the QR code below and embark on your learning journey with Learnik. It's the perfect way to elevate your NREMT exam preparation. We're here to support you every step of the way as you work toward your goals.

Thank you for choosing our educational materials, and we wish you all the best in your NREMT exam preparation!

For any issues, feel free to contact us at info@learnik.com

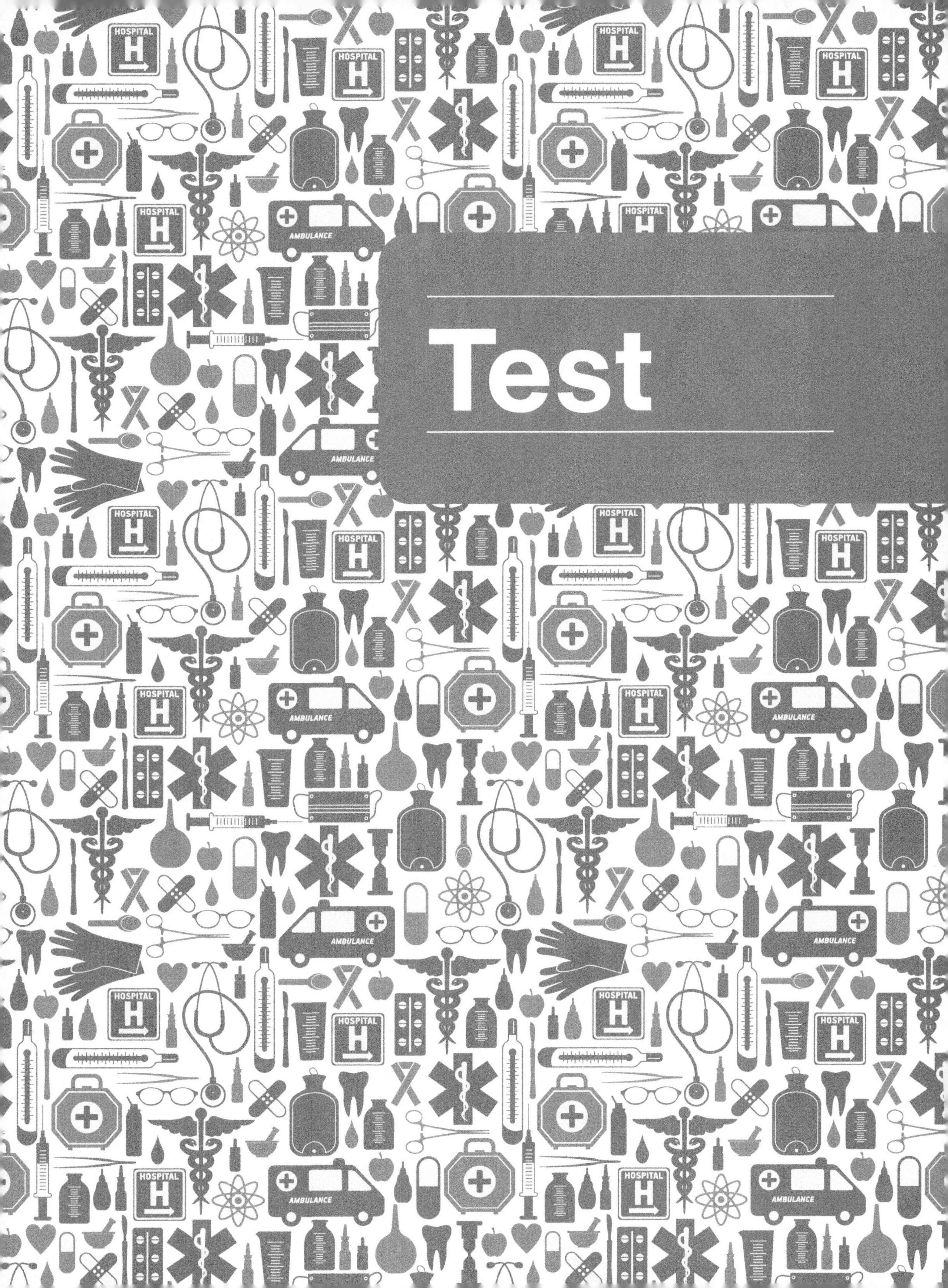
Test

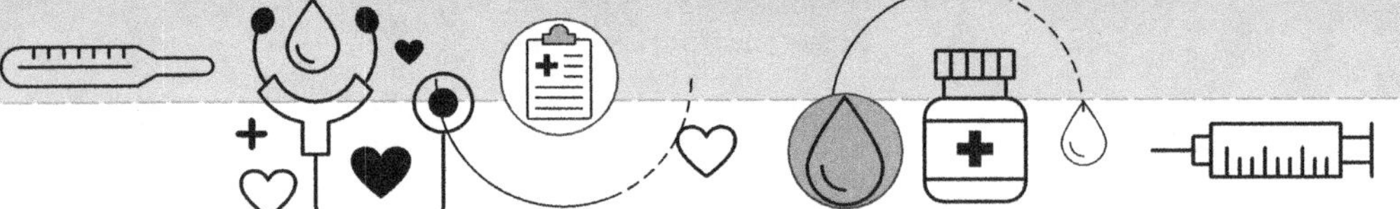

TRAUMA

Question 1

A male patient in his 20s presents with an open fracture on the lateral aspect of his lower leg. Which bone is most probably fractured?

- ☐ Fibula
- ☐ Tibia
- ☐ Radius
- ☐ Ulna

Question 2

Which position is optimal for a patient experiencing shock?

- ☐ Prone with legs elevated
- ☐ A position of comfort
- ☐ Modified Fowler's position
- ☐ Supine with legs elevated

Question 3

In the context of using a traction splinting apparatus, complete the following statement: Fasten the splint's support straps around the limb and disengage the ______________ once the __________________ is achieved.

- ☐ Mechanical traction / PMS
- ☐ Manual traction / mechanical traction
- ☐ Pressure / manual traction
- ☐ Ankle / PMS

Question 4

An extensive physical assessment ought to be performed __________________

- ☐ Subsequent to executing vital emergency interventions
- ☐ Immediately for an unresponsive individual before proceeding with other actions
- ☐ To ascertain the cause and nature of the injury
- ☐ Solely by healthcare professionals within a clinical environment

Question 5

Which of the following options does not categorize a mechanism of injury associated with penetrating trauma based on velocity?

- ☐ Medium velocity
- ☐ Low velocity
- ☐ Vital velocity
- ☐ High velocity

Question 6

In the context of the AVPU scale utilized to evaluate a patient's consciousness, what does the letter 'V' denote?

- ☐ Vasodilation
- ☐ Veins
- ☐ Visceral
- ☐ Responsive to verbal stimuli

Question 7

In the context of performing an initial evaluation on a patient with a substantial mechanism of injury (MOI), which option listed below is not pertinent to evaluating their respiratory function?

- ☐ Conduct a quick neurological assessment

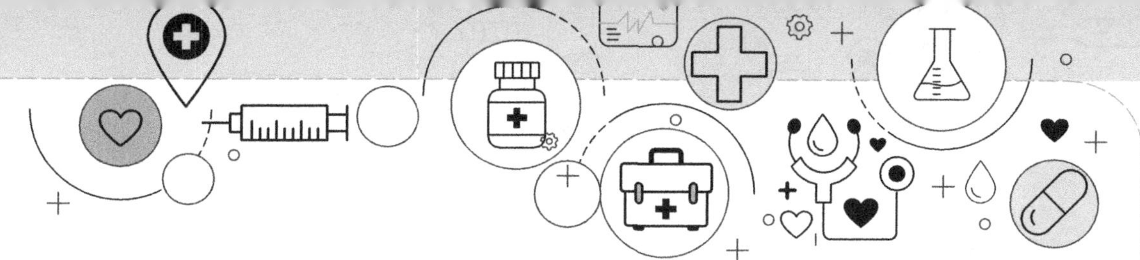

☐ Inspect the thorax and neck
☐ Evaluate the ventilation
☐ Auscultate breath sounds

Question 8

The prefix 'cost-' denotes which anatomical structure?

☐ Ribcage
☐ Shinbone
☐ Carpus
☐ Currency

Question 9

In which of the following scenarios is it necessary to don gloves, a gown, mask, and protective eyewear?

☐ Performing oral or nasal suctioning
☐ Administering an injection
☐ Arterial bleeding control
☐ Carrying out endotracheal intubation

Question 10

In which part of the human body can the radius be found?

☐ Adjacent to the thumb in the arm
☐ Next to the little toe in the leg
☐ Adjacent to the big toe in the leg
☐ Next to the little finger in the arm

Question 11

Initial shock is known as ________________; in contrast, advanced shock is referred to as ________________.

☐ Decompensated / recompensated
☐ Recompensated / decompensated
☐ Compensated / decompensated
☐ Compensated / recompensated

Question 12

Which of the following actions are advisable when managing traumatic vaginal bleeding?

☐ Check if the patient is pregnant
☐ Insert gloved fingers into the vagina
☐ Utilize a sterile absorbent pad
☐ Identify the cause of the injury

Question 13

Thermal health conditions are classified into which two primary categories?

☐ 'cold-related'; 'heat-related'
☐ 'cool-related'; 'warm-related'
☐ 'cold-related'; 'warm-related'
☐ 'heat-related'; 'cool-related'

Question 14

Individuals exhibiting discrepant pupil sizes are likely to have what condition?

☐ Have experienced head trauma
☐ Commonly also have meningitis
☐ All aforementioned conditions apply
☐ Could be a normal variant

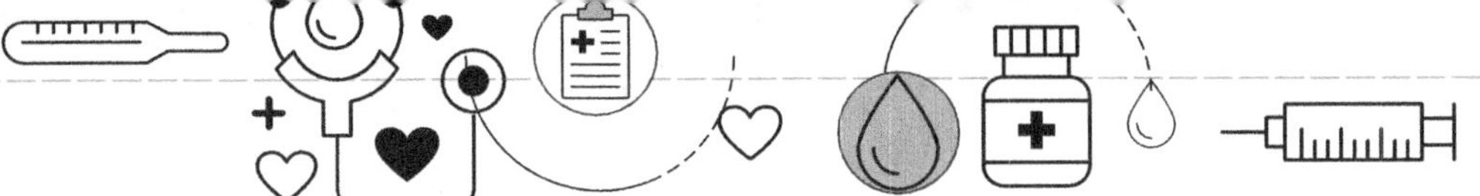

Question 15

In the study of trauma kinematics, all of the following represent types of blunt trauma collisions except:

- ☐ Organs impacting external to the body
- ☐ Organs impacting each other within the body
- ☐ Patient impacting a portion of the vehicle
- ☐ Vehicle impacting another object

Question 16

What is your initial assessment of the patient?

- ☐ An evaluation that helps determine the severity of the patient's condition
- ☐ An observation of their state after interventions and transit
- ☐ An interpretation of their vital signs to gauge their condition
- ☐ An unreliable measure of consciousness

Question 17

In the acronym DCAPBTLS, to what does the letter 'S' refer?

- ☐ Swelling
- ☐ Systole
- ☐ Signs
- ☐ Severity

Question 18

Under what circumstances would you extract a foreign object embedded in the cheek?

- ☐ It penetrates only one side of the cheek
- ☐ It poses a threat to the airway
- ☐ It does not conflict with religious beliefs
- ☐ It extends into the mandibular region

Question 19

What is the most recommended position for transporting a patient experiencing shock?

- ☐ Modified Trendelenburg position
- ☐ Lying flat with legs raised
- ☐ Any position that ensures the patient's comfort
- ☐ Face down with legs elevated

Question 20

In the AVPU scale utilized to evaluate a patient's responsiveness, what does the letter 'P' denote?

- ☐ Prevention
- ☐ Provocation
- ☐ Pertinent medical history
- ☐ Pain

Question 21

In the context of the SAMPLE acronym in medical history taking, the query "Have you previously experienced any cardiac issues?" corresponds to which letter?

- ☐ A
- ☐ M
- ☐ P
- ☐ L

Question 22

Which of the following does not describe a typical injury mechanism in orthopedic trauma?

- ☐ Torsional force
- ☐ Indirect force
- ☐ Rotational force
- ☐ Direct impact

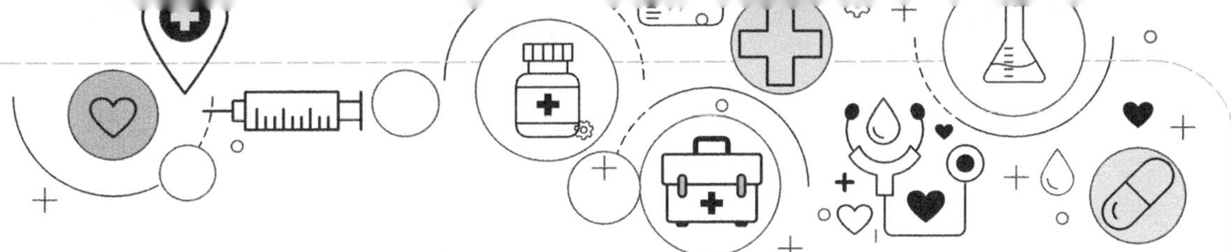

Question 23

Identify the option that does not belong to the upper limb anatomy.

- ☐ Ulna
- ☐ Patella
- ☐ Humerus
- ☐ Radius

Question 24

Upon arriving at a mass casualty incident along with your colleague Jermain, you initiate treatment for a severe arterial hemorrhage on a woman who had been ejected from a vehicle. As you provide her with a trauma dressing to hold and ask her to apply pressure, you hear an infant crying nearby. You proceed to investigate the source of the distressing sound coming from the car. What actions have you taken?

- ☐ Conducted scene triage
- ☐ Acted in the best interest of both patients
- ☐ Abandoned the patient
- ☐ Adhered to the principles of the Good Samaritan Law

Question 25

Which of the following is not a factor to consider in cases of electrical emergencies?

- ☐ Lightning strikes may cause cardiac arrest
- ☐ Superficial skin injuries may not signify the severity of burns
- ☐ Presence of entrance and exit wounds
- ☐ Lightning rarely leads to cardiac arrest

Question 26

During exposure to cold environments, which of the following does NOT contribute to an increased risk of cold-related injuries?

- ☐ Consumption of alcohol
- ☐ Existing medical conditions or injuries
- ☐ Reduction in local blood circulation
- ☐ Age of the individual

Question 27

You respond to a situation involving a postal service vehicle that has lost control on a dirt track and overturned. Eyewitnesses have indicated that the vehicle ignited, and the postal worker is outside attempting to recover scattered mail. Upon your arrival, the fire brigade has just extinguished the flames, and the driver is observing the smoldering debris from a distance. Your immediate course of action should be:

- ☐ Conduct a SAMPLE history assessment for the driver
- ☐ Perform a detailed physical examination on the driver
- ☐ Implement cervical spine stabilization using a standing backboard
- ☐ Request the driver to complete a refusal of transport form

Question 28

In the context of the SAMPLE assessment, the observation of a patient's pallor is classified as _________.

- ☐ A sign
- ☐ A symptom
- ☐ Syncope
- ☐ Dermis

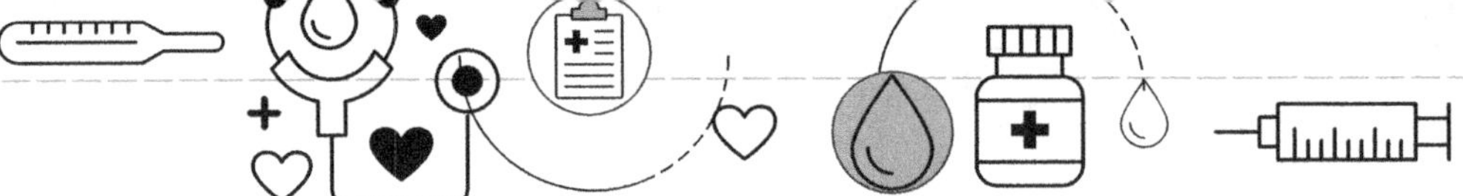

Question 29

What is a common consequence of a scalp laceration?

- ☐ Lead to meningitis
- ☐ Severe bleeding
- ☐ Minimal bleeding
- ☐ All of the listed options

Question 30

Which response alternative does not fall under the distinctive anatomical, physiological, and pathophysiological considerations for injured elderly patients?

- ☐ Brain enlargement heightening the risk of cerebral hemorrhaging after head trauma
- ☐ The utilization of multiple medications could influence assessment, especially vital signs
- ☐ Decreased strength leading to a higher propensity for falls
- ☐ Pulmonary system changes making older individuals more vulnerable to trauma

Question 31

Your colleague proposes that the patient may have sustained a zygomatic fracture. This would imply injury to which region of the body?

- ☐ Thoracic region
- ☐ Dorsal area
- ☐ Cervical region
- ☐ Facial area

Question 32

You and your colleague have been dispatched to an ATV incident. Upon arrival, you find a 60-year-old male lying adjacent to the roadway. He reports that he lost control of the four-wheeler, resulting in it overturning multiple times. Which of the following options represents the MOST accurate procedural sequence?

- ☐ BSI - Direct assistant to align the head in an inline position - Apply cervical collar - Instruct placement of patient onto board
- ☐ BSI - Direct assistant to maintain manual head immobilization - Assess circulation, motor, and sensory functions - Apply cervical collar
- ☐ Assess circulation, motor, and sensory functions - Direct assistant to align head in inline position - Direct movement to backboard
- ☐ Direct assistant to maintain manual head immobilization - Direct assistant to align head in inline position - Assess CMS functions - Make transport decision

Question 33

The term 'evisceration' refers to which of the following conditions?

- ☐ The presence of a flap of tissue due to a laceration
- ☐ An avulsion injury with exposure of a long bone
- ☐ A superficial skin abrasion
- ☐ An internal organ extending through a bodily opening

Question 34

You and your colleague Mary have been dispatched to a motor vehicle accident involving a single car and a moose. What should be your initial priority?

- ☐ Extricate the patient from the vehicle and move them away from the moose
- ☐ Ensure the scene is safe
- ☐ Contact wildlife authorities

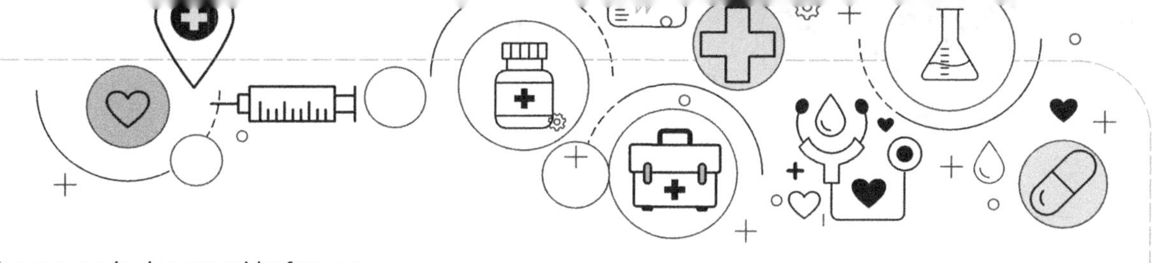

☐ Confirm the moose is deceased before approaching

Question 35

What does the letter 'R' signify in the OPQRST acronym?

☐ Radiate
☐ Rapid breathing very shallow
☐ Radial
☐ Refraction

Question 36

In the mnemonic DCAPBTLS, to what does the letter 'P' refer?

☐ Penetrations
☐ Pupillary responses
☐ Pain
☐ Pleural edema

Question 37

Upon arriving at the scene where an individual has been involved in a vehicular collision, you note significant damage to the front of the car. The individual is positioned upright in the driver's seat, reporting pain in the back and chest, which limits their ability to breathe deeply. What is the appropriate method to extricate this individual from the vehicle?

☐ Apply a traction splint to any fractures and slide the patient out on a backboard
☐ Utilize the Jaws of Life to cut through the vehicle's B posts and remove the roof
☐ Employ a KED or similar device and then secure the patient to a spine board
☐ With two EMTs inside the car and two outside the car

Question 38

Which of the following is NOT typically part of the standard protocol for burn treatment?

☐ Remove jewelry and clothing
☐ Transport to appropriate facility
☐ Airway management
☐ Apply cream to stop the burning

Question 39

In the management of patients with a suspected cerebral trauma, which of the following procedures is not generally recommended?

☐ Employ a rapid extrication for all patients
☐ Elevate head of backboard to a 30-degree angle
☐ Provide assisted ventilation if necessary
☐ Contemplate quick transportation

Question 40

Which of the following is not typically observed in the evaluation of muscle strains?

☐ Pronounced muscle weakness
☐ Audible "snap" during muscle tear
☐ Intense localized tenderness
☐ Swelling around the joint

Question 41

Upon arriving at the scene of a single-vehicle collision where a truck skidded off the road and overturned, you find the driver was traveling approximately 40 MPH before encountering an icy patch and losing control. After conducting an initial assessment of the scene, which treatment option would be most suitable for the patient?

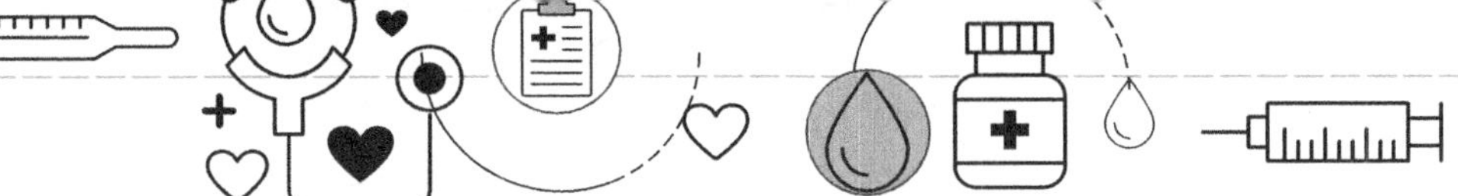

- ☐ Obtain a SAMPLE history and perform a targeted physical examination
- ☐ Measure baseline vital signs and conduct a focused examination based on the chief complaint
- ☐ Conduct a detailed physical assessment to identify life-threatening injuries
- ☐ Initiate a rapid trauma assessment

Question 42

Upon your arrival at the scene of a multi-vehicle collision, accompanied by your colleague Wanda, you find yourselves as the second emergency medical team on-site. Preliminary assessment reveals there are seven individuals involved across two cars, none of which are trapped. In the first vehicle, there is a 42-year-old unconscious pregnant woman, who is 28 weeks along, a 14-year-old female with severe back pain and vocal distress, and a 7-year-old boy with a facial laceration but no other apparent injuries. The second vehicle contains an 86-year-old male, unconscious and leaning against the steering wheel. In the rear seats, there are three teenagers: two on the side of impact experiencing nausea and showing signs of altered mental status, and a third teenage girl, who reports having seizures and vomiting earlier and was en route to the hospital with her grandfather. She was wearing a seatbelt and exhibits no external injuries. Which individuals require immediate medical attention?

- ☐ The girl who had the seizure earlier
- ☐ The 86-year-old man and the pregnant woman
- ☐ The two teenagers with the altered level of consciousness
- ☐ The girl with the back pain

Question 43

Which of the following is not a recommended protocol in the management of rattlesnake envenomation?

- ☐ If feasible, identify the snake
- ☐ Properly position the affected extremity
- ☐ Ensure the patient remains calm
- ☐ Incise the bite site and extract the venom by suction

Question 44

Which type of burn affects both the epidermal and dermal layers, excluding deeper tissues?

- ☐ Partial-thickness burn
- ☐ Double dermis burn
- ☐ Full-thickness burn
- ☐ Baker's burn

Question 45

Which of the following is NOT a symptom of heat-related conditions characterized by elevated skin temperature?

- ☐ unconsciousness
- ☐ accelerated respiration
- ☐ nausea
- ☐ minimal to no sweating

Question 46

A fracture that is only partial and does not extend through the entire bone is termed a _______________ fracture.

- ☐ Oblique
- ☐ Greenstick
- ☐ Transverse
- ☐ Comminuted

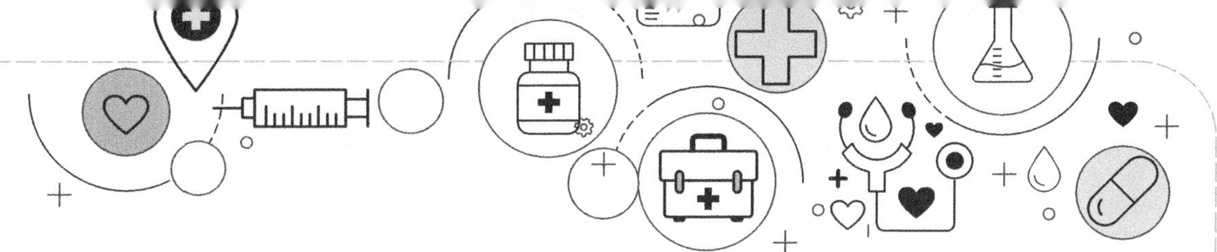

Question 47

Upon arriving at the scene, you find a 35-year-old male lying face down in a bathroom. He is unresponsive, and you proceed to carefully roll him onto his back while maintaining cervical spine stabilization. What should your subsequent action be?

- ☐ Assess the pulse and utilize an AED if needed
- ☐ Employ the AED and perform a SAMPLE history
- ☐ Tap the shoulder and assess for responsiveness
- ☐ Manually secure the airway

Question 48

At 8 a.m., you and your colleague Raymond are dispatched to a multi-vehicle accident on a congested secondary road. Upon your arrival, you observe at least six injured individuals and a chaotic scene with vehicles entangled, obstructing an entire traffic lane, and various fluids accumulating on the ground. You hear cries for help while traffic begins to navigate around the wreckage. Your immediate course of action should be...?

- ☐ Request the fire department, establish a safety perimeter, and aid in maintaining a safe distance for traffic
- ☐ Prioritize triaging the most severely injured and proceed to extricate them based on the severity of their injuries
- ☐ Commence patient extrication while your partner contacts additional ambulance services
- ☐ Notify the patients that legal regulations prevent entry into the accident zone until it has been secured by law enforcement

Question 49

Which actions are performed during a swift trauma evaluation?

- ☐ Palpation
- ☐ Auscultation
- ☐ All of the above
- ☐ Visual Inspection

Question 50

Which of the following most accurately characterizes a partial-thickness burn?

- ☐ A burn that penetrates all skin layers and may impact muscles, bones, or internal organs
- ☐ A burn confined to the outermost layer of the skin
- ☐ A burn covering less than 60% of the body's surface area
- ☐ A burn affecting both the epidermal layer and portions of the dermis

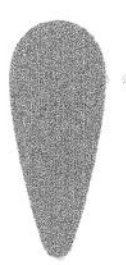

Answers & Explanation
Page 172

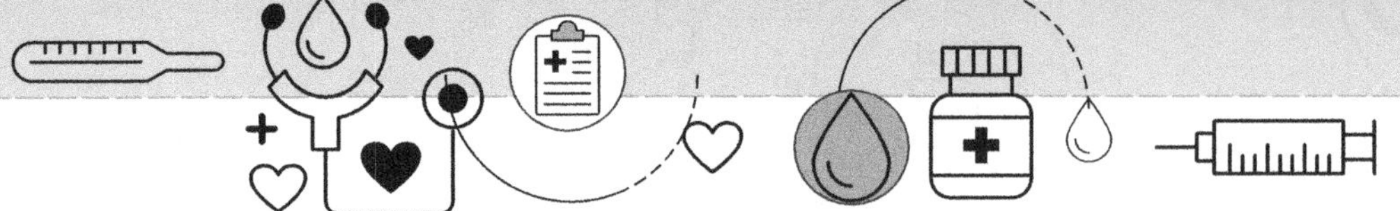

CARDIOLOGY AND RESUSCITATION

Question 1

You and your colleague Grimes receive an emergency call to a location where a stabbing incident has occurred. Two individuals have sustained injuries. One is a woman with a stab wound in the upper right quadrant (URQ) of her abdomen and is exhibiting difficulty in breathing, a pulse rate of 103, and a respiration rate of 35, with shallow breaths. The second patient is a man who has a stab wound in the lower right quadrant (LRQ) and is reporting intense abdominal pain; he has a pulse rate of 48 and a respiration rate of 24. Based on this information, which patient is more likely to present with hypotension (low blood pressure), and what is the rationale behind this conclusion?

- ☐ The male patient, due to the specific type and location of his wound, may be experiencing internal blood loss. Additionally, his pulse rate is notably slow.
- ☐ Neither patient will exhibit hypotension; their blood pressures are more likely to be elevated.
- ☐ The female patient, as her difficulty in breathing could potentially result in lowered blood pressure.
- ☐ The male patient, as a respiration rate of 24 can be associated with low blood pressure.

Question 2

A person exhibiting tachycardia will have which characteristic?

- ☐ A heart rate surpassing 60 bpm
- ☐ Blood pressure falling below 60
- ☐ A heart rate under 60 bpm
- ☐ A heart rate exceeding 100 bpm

Question 3

Levine's sign, characterized by the involuntary clutching of a closed fist to the chest, typically occurs during which condition?

- ☐ Experiencing an acute myocardial infarction
- ☐ Obstructed by a piece of food
- ☐ Undergoing labor
- ☐ Undergoing a transient ischemic attack

Question 4

Identify the option that is not a clinical manifestation of Cardiogenic shock.

- ☐ Cyanotic appearance
- ☐ Dysrhythmic pulse
- ☐ Elevated skin temperature
- ☐ Cool and diaphoretic skin

Question 5

Which of the following can dysrhythmia encompass?

- ☐ Normal cardiac function
- ☐ Either bradycardia or tachycardia
- ☐ Consistent heart rhythms
- ☐ Excessive blood flow

Question 6

The correct size of a blood pressure cuff is essential, particularly in the case of pediatric pa-

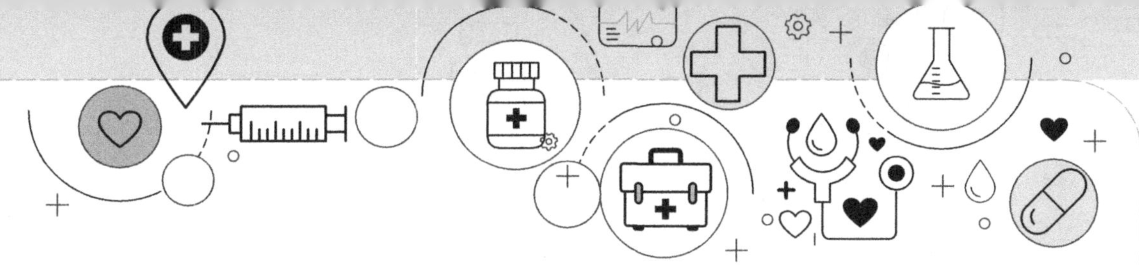

tients. Utilizing a cuff that is excessively small will ______________. Conversely, the use of a cuff that is excessively large will ______________.

- ☐ impede blood flow, affecting the child's circulation / compress the child's arm excessively, causing compartment syndrome
- ☐ provide a falsely lowered measurement / provide a falsely elevated measurement
- ☐ fail to provide an accurate reading due to excessive vessel constriction / fail to provide a reading due to insufficient vessel compression
- ☐ yield a falsely elevated reading / yield a falsely lowered reading

Question 7

Among the subsequent assessment findings and manifestations, which one is unlikely to suggest that a patient has experienced a stroke or transient ischemic attack (TIA)?

- ☐ Headache
- ☐ Bleeding
- ☐ Diplopia
- ☐ Confusion, weakness, or dizziness

Question 8

Whilst navigating through a supermarket, you observe a congregation surrounding an individual lying on the ground. Upon closer inspection, you discover a female, aged 48, who is both pulseless and apneic. What compression rate and depth do you administer?

- ☐ 30:2 / at least 2 inches
- ☐ 30:2 / one third to one half the depth of the chest
- ☐ 30:2 / 1.5 to 2 inches
- ☐ 15:2 / one third to one half the depth of the chest

Question 9

Into which vessel does blood flow upon exiting the left ventricle?

- ☐ Superior Vena Cava
- ☐ Lungs
- ☐ Left atrium
- ☐ Aortic arch

Question 10

What are the three primary etiologies of shock?

- ☐ Injuries, heart incidents, and seizures
- ☐ Inadequate cardiac output, hemorrhage, and vessel dilation
- ☐ Inadequate tissue perfusion, cognitive impairment, and impaired respiratory function
- ☐ Vascular constriction, vascular insufficiency, and respiratory impairment

Question 11

What is the foremost precaution when prescribing aspirin?

- ☐ Coagulation abnormalities
- ☐ Aspirin has no usage precautions
- ☐ Allergic reactions
- ☐ Gastrointestinal upset

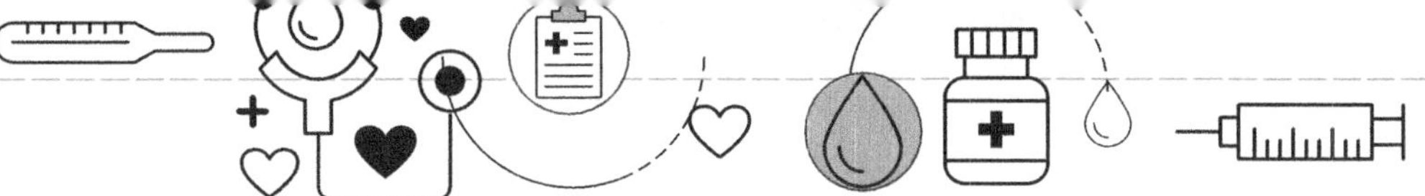

Question 12

In the instance of a cerebral infarction, neural cells that are deprived of adequate oxygenation for a prolonged period will inevitably face necrosis. What is the specific term for these cells?

- ☐ Eschiel cells
- ☐ Nephrotic cells
- ☐ Dead cells
- ☐ Infarcted cells

Question 13

Which chamber of the heart performs the most substantial work?

- ☐ Left atrium
- ☐ Left ventricle
- ☐ Right atrium
- ☐ Right ventricle

Question 14

If an individual is experiencing bradycardia, it indicates they

- ☐ Have a heart rate below 60 beats per minute
- ☐ Have a blood pressure reading of less than 60
- ☐ Have a heart rate exceeding 60 beats per minute
- ☐ Have a heart rate under 100 beats per minute

Question 15

What is the underlying cause of an ischemic stroke?

- ☐ Early-onset atrial contractions
- ☐ Obstruction of cerebral blood flow
- ☐ Rapid transition to an upright position
- ☐ Obstruction in the Inferior vena cava

Question 16

Among the pulses detectable within the vascular network, which one is not recognized?

- ☐ Brachial pulse
- ☐ Radial pulse
- ☐ Anterior pulse
- ☐ Femoral pulse

Question 17

What is the term used for shock resulting from the failure of the heart's pumping capabilities?

- ☐ Hemorrhagic
- ☐ Cardiogenic
- ☐ Hemophilic
- ☐ Psychogenic

Question 18

Identify the response that is not indicative of Hypovolemic Shock:

- ☐ Elevated respiratory rate
- ☐ Rapid, feeble pulse
- ☐ Generalized edema
- ☐ Hypotension

Question 19

Among the following, who should be regarded as a patient requiring immediate medical attention?

- ☐ A 55-year-old woman exhibiting a blood pressure of 178/90
- ☐ A pregnant individual experiencing contractions spaced 15 minutes apart
- ☐ A 24-year-old male with a fractured tibia
- ☐ A 34-year-old man who has sustained multiple bee stings

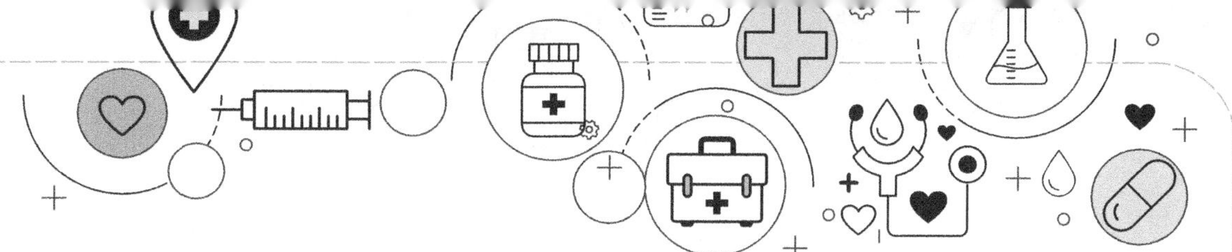

Question 20

Upon examining a 78-year-old female patient, her skin appears cool, moist, and pallid. What would be your diagnosis?

- ☐ Hypoperfusion
- ☐ Hyperglycemia
- ☐ Hyperthermia
- ☐ Vasovagal syncope

Question 21

The initial phase of shock, wherein the physiological mechanisms of the body are capable of coping with the hemorrhage, is termed

- ☐ Reversible shock
- ☐ Irreversible shock
- ☐ Decompensated shock
- ☐ Compensated shock

Question 22

What would be the appropriate sequence of interventions for a 76-year-old woman presenting with a heart rate of 142 beats per minute, accompanied by cyanosis around her lips and nail beds?

- ☐ Employ a bag-valve-mask (BVM) for ventilation and proceed with transportation
- ☐ Persist with assessment to ascertain the cause and contact Advanced Life Support (ALS)
- ☐ Carry out an expedited trauma assessment and transport immediately
- ☐ Continue evaluation during transport and administer high-flow oxygen

Question 23

In the scenario where you are administering CPR alone to a 77-year-old male who has experienced cardiac arrest and is not breathing, what is the best technique to ascertain the effectiveness of your ventilations?

- ☐ Observing the chest for movement up and down
- ☐ Examining the pupils to determine if they are reactive to light
- ☐ Feeling for a carotid pulse while performing compressions
- ☐ Noting if the patient's cheeks inflate with each breath administered

Question 24

In the thorough secondary evaluation, all of the following concerning blood pressure assessment must be considered except:

- ☐ measurement methodologies
- ☐ perfusion correlation
- ☐ arm positioning
- ☐ methods of palpation

Question 25

Shock etiologies are primarily classified into three main types. What are they?

- ☐ Injury, cardiac incident, and seizure
- ☐ Compromised perfusion, altered mental status, and respiratory insufficiency
- ☐ Impaired cardiac function, fluid depletion, and vascular dilation
- ☐ Vascular constriction, inadequate vascular function, and respiratory insufficiency

Question 26

What does the notation 140/P signify?

- ☐ A blood pressure reading of 140 was palpated

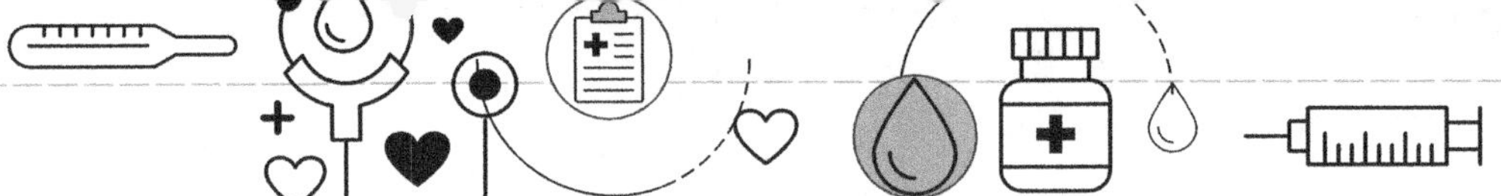

- ☐ A pulse rate of 140 was recorded
- ☐ A respiratory rate of 140 breaths per minute was noted
- ☐ None of the provided options are correct

Question 27

In a SAMPLE history evaluation, what does the letter 'P' signify?

- ☐ Pain
- ☐ Provocation
- ☐ Pallor
- ☐ Pertinent past medical history

Question 28

A patient presents with acute chest discomfort accompanied by diaphoresis and a blood pressure reading of 96/55 mmHg. Among the patient's medications is a prescription for nitroglycerin. After contacting medical control, you receive an order to administer one nitroglycerin tablet sublingually. What would be your course of action?

- ☐ Administer the prescribed nitroglycerin tablet as directed
- ☐ Advise medical control to consult contraindications in the protocol manual for nitroglycerin
- ☐ Re-assess the blood pressure and then administer the nitroglycerin tablet
- ☐ Re-check the patient's blood pressure and seek further guidance

Question 29

A patient presents with nausea and bradycardia. What physiological response is being exhibited?

- ☐ Parasympathetic
- ☐ Sympathetic
- ☐ Vagal
- ☐ Emotional

Question 30

The left atrium and ventricle of the heart ______________ and ______________.

- ☐ propels pulmonary circulation, maintains systemic circulation
- ☐ accepts blood from the lungs, initiates systemic circulation
- ☐ receives systemic circulation, facilitates pulmonary flow
- ☐ receives systemic flow, accepts blood from the lungs

Question 31

In the scope of emergency medical services (EMS), what does the term 'lumen' denote?

- ☐ The internal diameter of a tube
- ☐ The amount of illumination inside an ambulance
- ☐ The circumference of the outer skull
- ☐ The rapid depletion of bodily fluids

Question 32

You are called to assist an elderly male patient who may have had a stroke. Upon arrival, you discover him prone on the floor. He exhibits Decerebrate Rigidity, emits groaning noises, and his eyes fail to react to verbal or painful stimuli. What is his Glasgow Coma Scale (GCS) score?

- ☐ 5
- ☐ 4
- ☐ 6
- ☐ 7

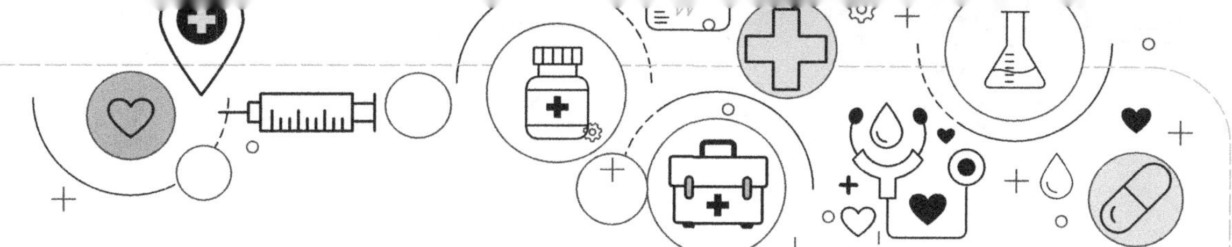

Question 33

Identify the vessel that receives blood ejected from the right ventricle.

- ☐ Pulmonary vein
- ☐ Pulmonary artery
- ☐ Aorta
- ☐ Left ventricle

Question 34

The pulmonary artery originates from the __________ and terminates at the _____________.

- ☐ Right ventricle / lungs
- ☐ Lungs / left ventricle
- ☐ Left atrium / lungs
- ☐ Lungs / right atrium

Question 35

Which part of the heart is often termed the 'workhorse'?

- ☐ Left atrium
- ☐ Left ventricle
- ☐ Right ventricle
- ☐ Right atrium

Question 36

Identify which of the following pediatric patients exhibits bradycardia.

- ☐ An infant with a heart rate of 120 beats per minute
- ☐ A 4-year-old child with a heart rate of 70 beats per minute
- ☐ A 6-year-old child with a heart rate of 100 beats per minute
- ☐ A 12-year-old child with a heart rate of 90 beats per minute

Question 37

Identify the diastolic pressure that fits within the normal parameters for a healthy adult.

- ☐ 55 mm Hg
- ☐ 95 mm Hg
- ☐ 105 mm Hg
- ☐ 125 mm Hg

Question 38

Which of the following situations might indicate that CPR is not warranted?

- ☐ The individual is unresponsive
- ☐ Central cyanosis observed
- ☐ Presence of stiff neck and jaw
- ☐ Absence of pulse and breathing

Question 39

Identify the feature that would not typically be associated with the clinical presentation of Cardiogenic shock.

- ☐ Tissue necrosis
- ☐ Thoracic discomfort
- ☐ Hypotension
- ☐ Heightened nervousness

Question 40

Define perfusion:

- ☐ The delivery of nutrients to the respiratory system
- ☐ The removal of waste from the lymphatic system
- ☐ The elimination of waste from the body's cells
- ☐ The distribution of blood, oxygen, and nutrients to the body's cells

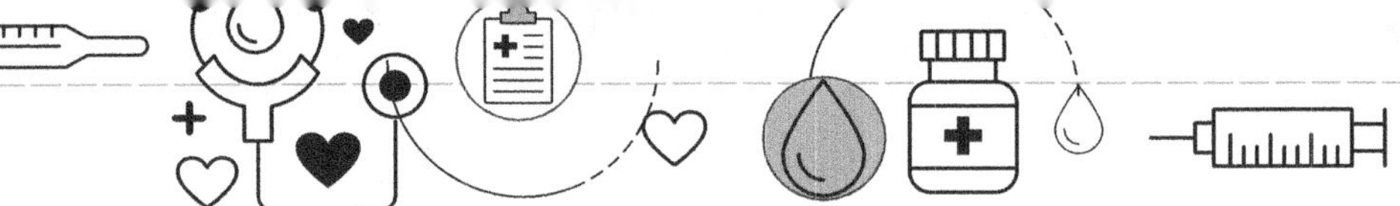

Question 41

The carotid artery transports blood from the ______________ to the ______________.

- ☐ Cardiac region / lower limbs
- ☐ Cardiac region / cranial region
- ☐ Lower limbs / cardiac region
- ☐ Pulmonary region / cardiac region

Question 42

Within what range would one expect the systolic blood pressure of an 8-year-old child to fall?

- ☐ 70 mm Hg
- ☐ Above 80 mm Hg
- ☐ Below 80 mm Hg
- ☐ Above 120 mm Hg

Question 43

Upon arrival at the scene, you encounter four individuals with varying conditions. Which individual should be prioritized for treatment and transport?

- ☐ A 9-year-old child who is alert, breathing at a rate of 26 per minute, with a systolic blood pressure of 68 mm Hg
- ☐ A 24-year-old male suffering from fractures to his collarbone and wrist
- ☐ An 18-year-old individual with a systolic blood pressure of 100 mm Hg
- ☐ A 64-year-old woman experiencing chest pain, with a blood pressure reading of 120/70 and reporting pain at a severity level of 5

Question 44

During a myocardial infarction, aspirin is prescribed primarily to ________________

- ☐ Alleviate headache pain induced by nitroglycerine
- ☐ Break down existing platelet clots
- ☐ Inhibit additional platelet aggregation
- ☐ Relieve muscle-related chest discomfort

Question 45

Identify the option that is not a constituent of the fundamental components to enhance survival outcomes during resuscitation.

- ☐ Timely CPR
- ☐ Timely administration of Aspirin
- ☐ Prompt access
- ☐ Rapid defibrillation

Question 46

Identify the collection that comprises solely of anatomical components of the Circulatory System.

- ☐ Heart, spleen, arteries, and veins
- ☐ Heart, nephritic structures, capillaries, and arterial pathways
- ☐ Heart, pulmonary organs, capillaries, and venous structures.
- ☐ Heart, arterial vessels, capillaries, and venous pathways

Question 47

The primary functions of the respiratory system are to ___________ and ___________.

- ☐ enable oxygen to reach the lungs and bloodstream; expel waste products from the blood and lungs.
- ☐ play a role in lung temperature regulation; assist in the circulatory system maintenance
- ☐ aid in body cooling; contribute to lymphatic system purification

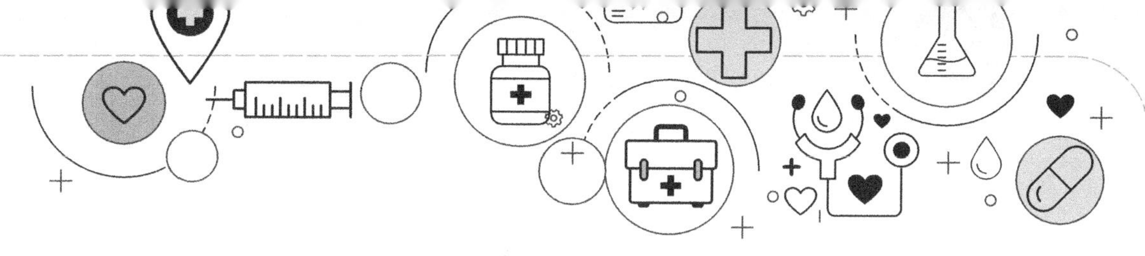

- ☐ introduce waste into the lungs and bloodstream; permit oxygen to exit from the blood and lungs

Question 48

Which anatomical site should be palpated to assess the pulse of an infant?

- ☐ Brachial artery
- ☐ Femoral artery
- ☐ Carotid artery
- ☐ Radial artery

Question 49

A patient exhibits a pulse but lacks respiratory function. Rescue ventilation should be administered ________________.

- ☐ With minimal air to just make the chest elevate.
- ☐ With a volume greater than that used in cardiopulmonary resuscitation.
- ☐ With an air volume of 200 ml except in the case of infants.
- ☐ With an air volume ranging from 500 ml to 800 ml.

Question 50

An alternative term for shock is ______________.

- ☐ Hypoperfusion
- ☐ Hypertension
- ☐ Hypotension
- ☐ Hypoxia

Answers & Explanation
Page 181

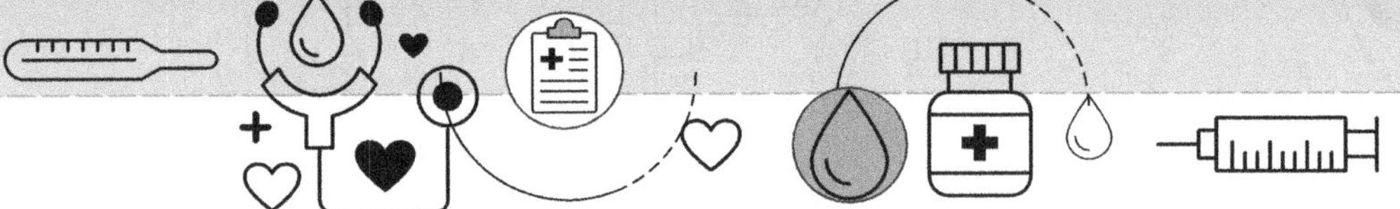

EMS OPERATIONS

Question 1

Are patients entitled to restrict access to their medical documentation?

- ☐ Private
- ☐ From insurance agencies
- ☐ Permanently sealed
- ☐ From judicial entities

Question 2

Interventions are defined as ___________.

- ☐ Applicable to pre-hospital settings
- ☐ Excluded from pre-hospital care
- ☐ Measures taken to resolve an issue
- ☐ An indicator of advanced shock

Question 3

Your emergency medical services team, along with law enforcement, has responded to an incident involving a dilapidated mobile home on the periphery of town. Dispatch has indicated that a 28-year-old male has overdosed on heroin and cocaine. Upon arriving ahead of the county sheriff, you are approached by a distressed teenage girl pleading for assistance for her brother. Assessing the environment and determining it is safe, you enter the mobile home to find bystanders administering CPR to the man. As you begin your evaluation, the man suddenly becomes conscious and attempts to strike you. How should you proceed?

- ☐ Immediately request additional law enforcement support via radio
- ☐ Deliver a forceful punch to subdue him, aiming for the jaw to render him unconscious
- ☐ Enlist the bystanders who were performing CPR to help restrain him on a backboard and gurney so you can administer Narcan
- ☐ Withdraw to the ambulance, maintaining a safe distance from the scene while confirming law enforcement's impending arrival

Question 4

You and your colleague, Obi, have been dispatched to a residence where a 50-year-old male is experiencing respiratory distress. Upon arrival, you observe the patient lying in bed with labored breathing, a respiratory rate of 20, minimal chest expansion, pallor, and a weak pulse. The family informs you that the patient is diagnosed with AIDS. Obi responds by stating, "I apologize, but I do not wish to risk contracting AIDS. I cannot assist," and then exits the premises. What has just transpired?

- ☐ Obi has forsaken his duty to render care to the patient, thereby committing abandonment
- ☐ Obi's actions have inflicted emotional distress on the family, potentially exacerbating the patient's physical condition due to lack of assistance
- ☐ There has been a lapse in communication between you and Obi, eroding the family and patient's confidence in emergency services
- ☐ Obi's assessment prioritizing scene safety is justified, leading to his departure from the unsafe environment

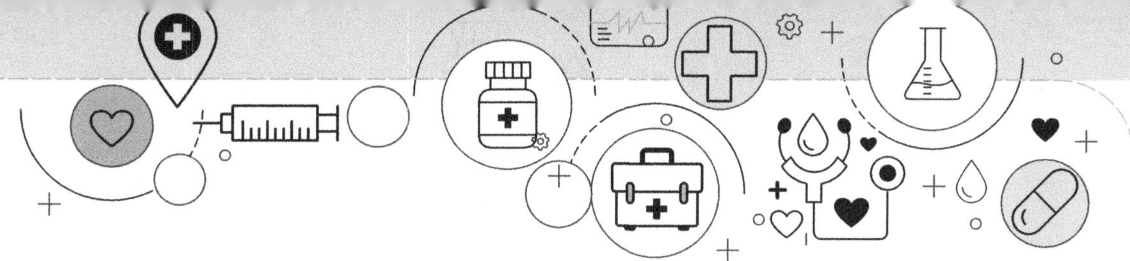

Question 5

In the role of an Emergency Medical Technician, under what circumstances may you be accused of abandonment?

- ☐ Depart from a patient classified as low priority (green) to assist another patient who is in critical condition (red)
- ☐ Leave a patient without ensuring they are transferred to a provider with adequate or superior qualifications
- ☐ Engage in actions that directly result in harm to a patient
- ☐ Fail to evacuate a patient from a burning structure

Question 6

Which of the following actions is NOT a valid method EMTs can use to protect bystanders?

- ☐ Arrest them
- ☐ Evacuate them
- ☐ Keep them away
- ☐ Set up barriers

Question 7

Which of the following is NOT a requisite criterion for establishing negligence on the part of an EMT?

- ☐ An injury must have been sustained by the patient
- ☐ The negligent act or omission must have directly caused the injury
- ☐ The action or inaction must have occurred within the scope of the EMT's duty
- ☐ The patient must provide evidence of their injuries

Question 8

Which of the following elements is NOT relevant when assessing a patient's current medical condition?

- ☐ Include environmental influences
- ☐ Emphasize the current health condition
- ☐ Incorporate personal individual aspects
- ☐ Emphasize patient's historical health background

Question 9

You and your colleague, Zavid, are evaluating a patient who appears to exhibit unusual behavior possibly due to trauma. The patient displays clear signs of altered consciousness and has a conspicuous, bleeding injury on the side of their head. The patient is resistant to your presence and uses profanity towards you. What is the most appropriate course of action?

- ☐ Seek authorization from Medical Control to administer a Sux dart in their neck
- ☐ Instruct your partner to discreetly approach from behind and gently subdue the patient
- ☐ Reach out to medical control and request police aid in handling the patient
- ☐ Reiterate your intention to provide treatment. Should the patient decline, you must withdraw

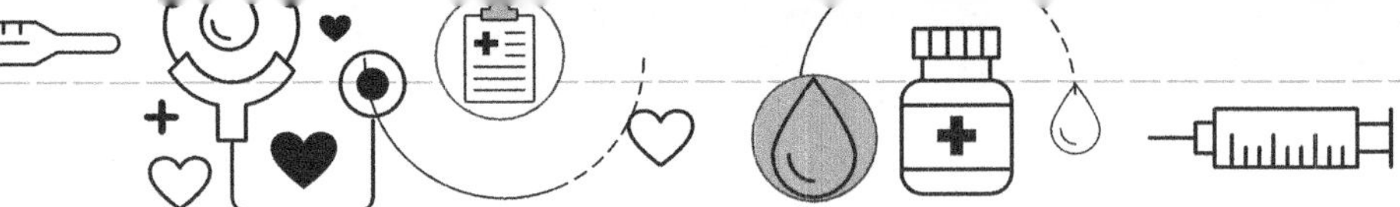

Question 10

In the context of evaluating the cardiovascular system during a secondary assessment, primary attention should initially be directed towards ______________ and ___________.

- ☐ Pulse and perfusion
- ☐ Skin coloration and the presence of erythema
- ☐ Signs of edema and levels of hypertension
- ☐ Indicators of cardiogenic shock and congestive heart failure

Question 11

An individual deemed to be legally competent has the ability to:

- ☐ Decline medical treatment
- ☐ Assume power of attorney over emergency medical services personnel
- ☐ Direct the actions of healthcare providers
- ☐ Experience involuntary loss of bladder control

Question 12

Upon arriving at a retirement facility with your colleague Rodrigo, you observe that numerous staff members and residents are experiencing emesis and vertigo. What should be your primary suspicion?

- ☐ The emergency dispatcher failed to deploy adequate resources
- ☐ A widespread influenza outbreak is occurring
- ☐ A toxic substance may be causing the symptoms
- ☐ Sufficient medical supplies are available for treatment

Question 13

The diagnostic strategy enables the exclusion of life-threatening conditions and subsequently ______________.

- ☐ Conduct a reassessment
- ☐ Address the reported symptoms of the patient
- ☐ Determine the patient's medical condition
- ☐ Transfer the patient to a senior healthcare professional

Question 14

Which of the following is not among the supplementary resources that EMTs call for during hazard mitigation or scene control?

- ☐ Fire department
- ☐ Additional ambulances
- ☐ Law enforcement
- ☐ Health department

Question 15

What is the definition of assault?

- ☐ Inducing fear of harmful physical touch
- ☐ Providing medical treatment without obtaining permission
- ☐ Detaining a willing patient forcefully
- ☐ All of the statements above

Question 16

The appropriate clinical scenarios and symptoms for prescribing a drug are ___________.

- ☐ Unreliable information
- ☐ Potential outcomes for a patient from using the drug
- ☐ Directed by medical authority

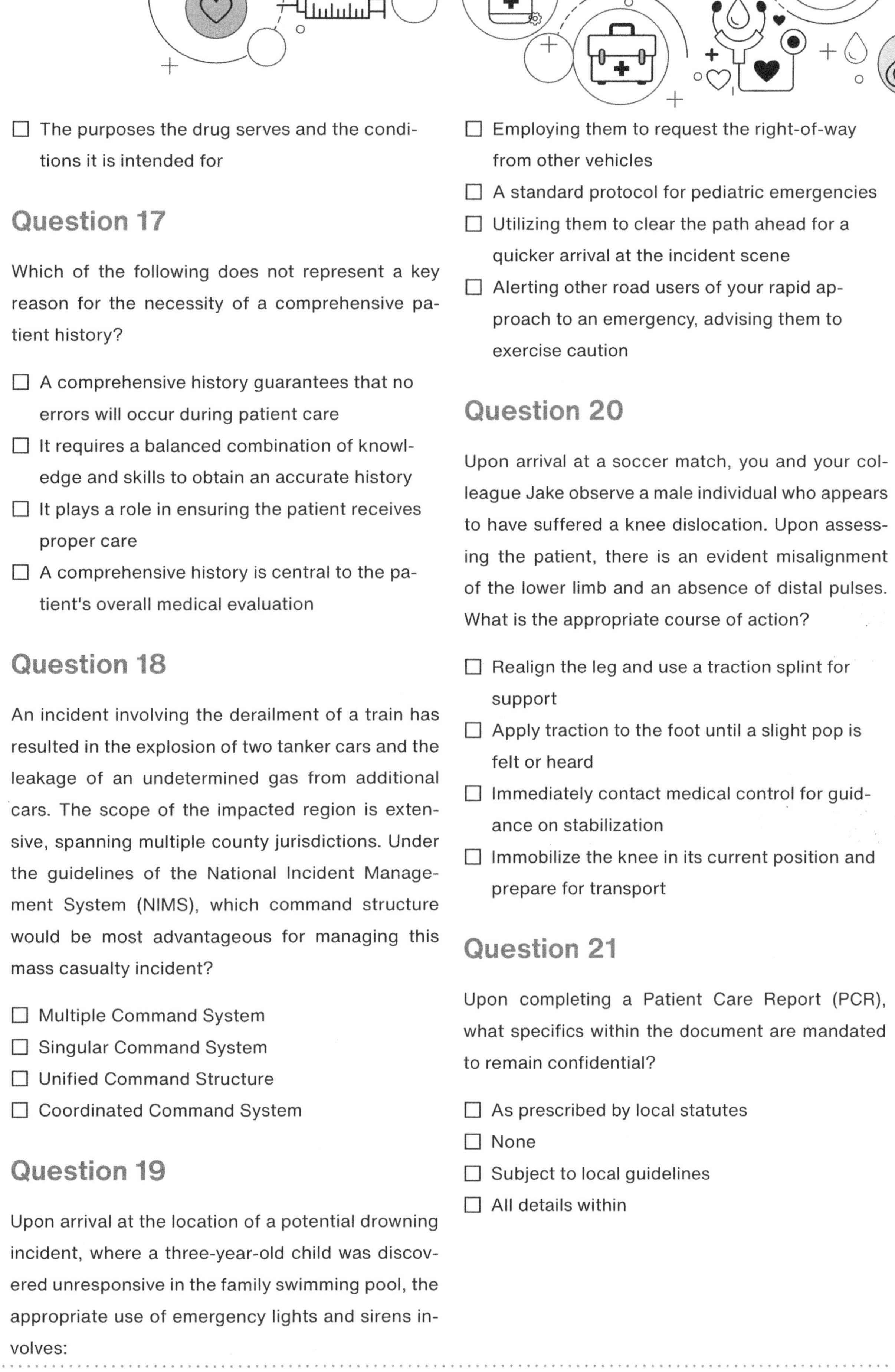

- ☐ The purposes the drug serves and the conditions it is intended for

Question 17

Which of the following does not represent a key reason for the necessity of a comprehensive patient history?

- ☐ A comprehensive history guarantees that no errors will occur during patient care
- ☐ It requires a balanced combination of knowledge and skills to obtain an accurate history
- ☐ It plays a role in ensuring the patient receives proper care
- ☐ A comprehensive history is central to the patient's overall medical evaluation

Question 18

An incident involving the derailment of a train has resulted in the explosion of two tanker cars and the leakage of an undetermined gas from additional cars. The scope of the impacted region is extensive, spanning multiple county jurisdictions. Under the guidelines of the National Incident Management System (NIMS), which command structure would be most advantageous for managing this mass casualty incident?

- ☐ Multiple Command System
- ☐ Singular Command System
- ☐ Unified Command Structure
- ☐ Coordinated Command System

Question 19

Upon arrival at the location of a potential drowning incident, where a three-year-old child was discovered unresponsive in the family swimming pool, the appropriate use of emergency lights and sirens involves:

- ☐ Employing them to request the right-of-way from other vehicles
- ☐ A standard protocol for pediatric emergencies
- ☐ Utilizing them to clear the path ahead for a quicker arrival at the incident scene
- ☐ Alerting other road users of your rapid approach to an emergency, advising them to exercise caution

Question 20

Upon arrival at a soccer match, you and your colleague Jake observe a male individual who appears to have suffered a knee dislocation. Upon assessing the patient, there is an evident misalignment of the lower limb and an absence of distal pulses. What is the appropriate course of action?

- ☐ Realign the leg and use a traction splint for support
- ☐ Apply traction to the foot until a slight pop is felt or heard
- ☐ Immediately contact medical control for guidance on stabilization
- ☐ Immobilize the knee in its current position and prepare for transport

Question 21

Upon completing a Patient Care Report (PCR), what specifics within the document are mandated to remain confidential?

- ☐ As prescribed by local statutes
- ☐ None
- ☐ Subject to local guidelines
- ☐ All details within

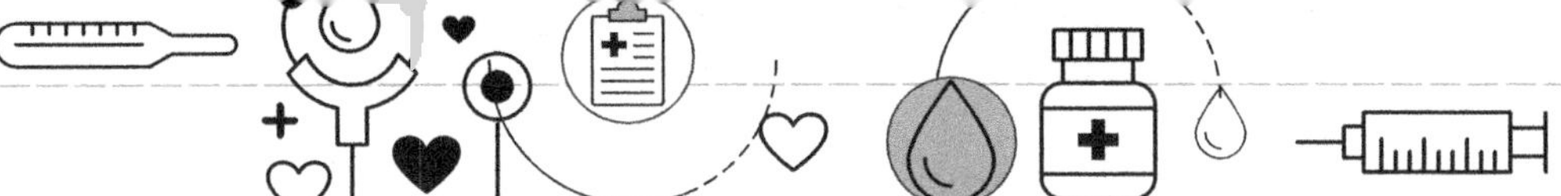

Question 22

An incident involving an overturned tanker truck transporting unidentified chemicals has occurred on the interstate, resulting in the spillage of a luminous liquid from the trailer. Several casualties have been reported and numerous onlookers are experiencing nausea and vomiting. You have been tasked by the Incident Commander to establish a helicopter landing zone. Which of the following areas would be most suitable for this landing zone?

- ☐ A small incline about 80 by 80 feet, positioned uphill and upwind from the danger site.
- ☐ A flat, solid surface situated downhill and no less than 100 meters from the danger site.
- ☐ A level hilltop located at least a mile from the danger site, downwind from any affected area.
- ☐ A sports field immediately beside the danger site that was cleared following reports of vomiting.

Question 23

While returning from a lunch break, you encounter an intersection obstructed by a collision involving two vehicles that are ablaze. What is the most appropriate course of action?

- ☐ Request a Hazmat team's assistance via radio
- ☐ Maintain a safe distance until the situation is under control
- ☐ Assist in extricating the occupants from the vehicles
- ☐ Retrieve the fire extinguisher from the ambulance

Question 24

In the context of a multi-vehicle accident where you have been designated as the Incident Commander's safety officer, your primary duty is:

- ☐ Establishing a "red zone" around the accident site to prevent bystanders and passing vehicles from approaching too closely.
- ☐ Devising the most efficient and secure method of extrication and ensuring that the strategy is clearly communicated to the logistical team.
- ☐ Halting an ongoing extrication when an EMT enters the danger zone of an inactive airbag.
- ☐ Stopping any unauthorized individuals from performing rescue operations during the extrication process.

Question 25

To proficiently steer an ambulance around a bend, the driver must comprehend the appropriate velocity, _______________, and recognize the importance of _____________.

- ☐ The intended final position of the turn / reaching the apex of the turn earlier
- ☐ The current location and planned trajectory / reaching the apex later in the turn
- ☐ The width and estimated length of the curve / initiating the turn earlier
- ☐ The sharpness of the curve / engaging the brakes if the turn is too rapid

Question 26

In the year 1989, the Department of Defense initiated a project aimed at addressing the unique medical needs of law enforcement personnel during tactical missions. What was the designation of this program?

- ☐ CONTOMS
- ☐ TACEMT
- ☐ LEMT
- ☐ EMSTAC

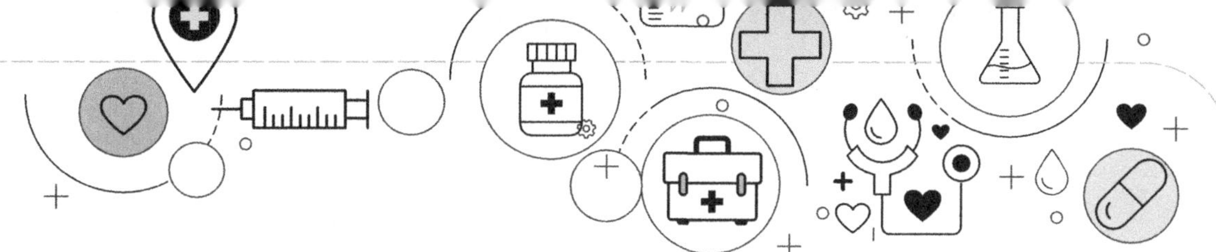

Question 27

In the event that a patient's wallet must be inspected for medical data, it should be done ______________.

- ☐ Privately, away from onlookers, to ensure the patient's confidentiality
- ☐ Visibly, so that others can witness the search
- ☐ Discreetly to avoid drawing attention to the action
- ☐ In a secluded area, such as inside the ambulance, to prevent interruptions

Question 28

Identify the option that does not align with the standard practices for respiratory system evaluation during a secondary medical examination.

- ☐ Assessment of chest shape and symmetry
- ☐ Evaluating respiratory effort
- ☐ Conducting auscultation
- ☐ Refrain from exposing the chest

Question 29

Responding to a call at the county detention center, you are requested to examine an incarcerated individual who recently engaged in a physical altercation. The individual has multiple lacerations and presents with a periorbital hematoma. Upon your attempt to provide assistance, the prisoner adamantly states, 'Leave me alone, I don't need or want your help.' What course of action should you take?

- ☐ Notify the Deputy that you recommend a thorough medical assessment and treatment, and if the detainee refuses care, he should be escorted to the emergency room under law enforcement supervision.
- ☐ Advise the detainee of his right to remain silent and suggest he utilize that right.
- ☐ Have the detainee complete a refusal of treatment form and then depart from the scene.
- ☐ Request the Deputy restrain the detainee to allow you to assess his injuries.

Question 30

What is an advisable procedure for donning latex or vinyl gloves?

- ☐ Wear two layers of gloves for maximum protection
- ☐ Don the gloves in the patient's presence to ensure sterility
- ☐ Put them on during transit to the emergency site
- ☐ Check with the patient for any allergy to latex or vinyl

Question 31

Which of the following elements is inappropriate to be part of a patient's secondary evaluation?

- ☐ Musculoskeletal system
- ☐ Digestive system
- ☐ Neurological system
- ☐ Cardiovascular system

Question 32

Emergency dispatch has reported a motor vehicle accident involving two cars, necessitating the response of both an ambulance and a fire truck. Both vehicles depart the station and head towards the accident site. Upon nearing a heavily trafficked intersection, what safety measures should be observed?

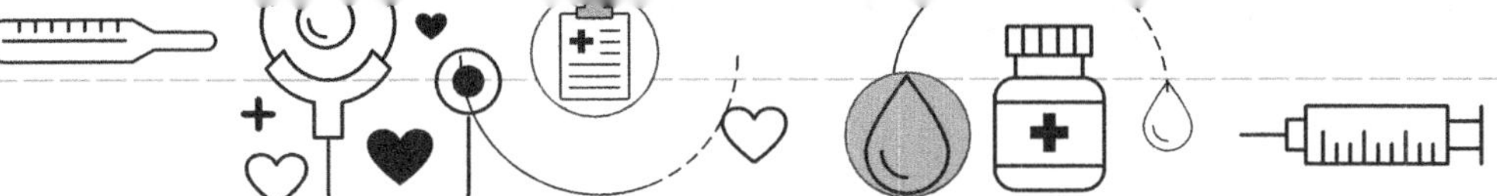

- ☐ Activate a siren with a unique sound distinct from the fire truck's to ensure that drivers are aware of multiple emergency vehicles approaching the intersection
- ☐ Permit the fire truck to navigate the intersection first, as it is more likely to be recognized by drivers than the ambulance
- ☐ Engage all emergency lights and sirens and proceed through the intersection with the understanding that emergency vehicles have priority
- ☐ Reduce the space between the ambulance and the fire truck to facilitate a coordinated and secure passage through the intersection

Question 33

The utilization of Critical Incident Stress Debriefings (CISD) serves to:

- ☐ Assess whether a patient requires Advanced Life Support (ALS) due to critical conditions
- ☐ Evaluate potential misconduct of EMS personnel at an incident
- ☐ Facilitate pre-arrival situational understanding of the incident
- ☐ Aid EMS workers in recuperating after distressing incidents

Question 34

How is a region classified where there is a high level of contamination?

- ☐ Hot zone
- ☐ Green zone
- ☐ Yellow zone
- ☐ Black zone

Question 35

You and your colleague Blaze have been dispatched to an incident involving two individuals who have sustained stab wounds. One patient, a woman, has been stabbed in the upper right quadrant (URQ) and is experiencing respiratory difficulty, with a pulse rate of 103 and shallow respirations at 35 breaths per minute. The other patient, a man, has a stab wound in the lower right quadrant (LRQ), is in significant abdominal pain, and has a pulse of 60 with a respiratory rate of 24. Prior to arriving at the scene, what steps should be taken?

- ☐ Communicate with the police about potential domestic violence and wait across from the scene
- ☐ Prepare the Automated External Defibrillator (AED)
- ☐ Ensure that law enforcement has secured the scene
- ☐ Request law enforcement support and wait at the scene until they arrive

Question 36

Which of the following can be an indicator of child maltreatment?

- ☐ Wounds at different stages of recovery
- ☐ A visibly upset parent
- ☐ An arm injury from a fall
- ☐ A child explaining a ball-related injury

Question 37

In what capacity can a PCR be utilized?

- ☐ Formal legal evidence
- ☐ Informational guide for patient care
- ☐ Essential tool for intubation

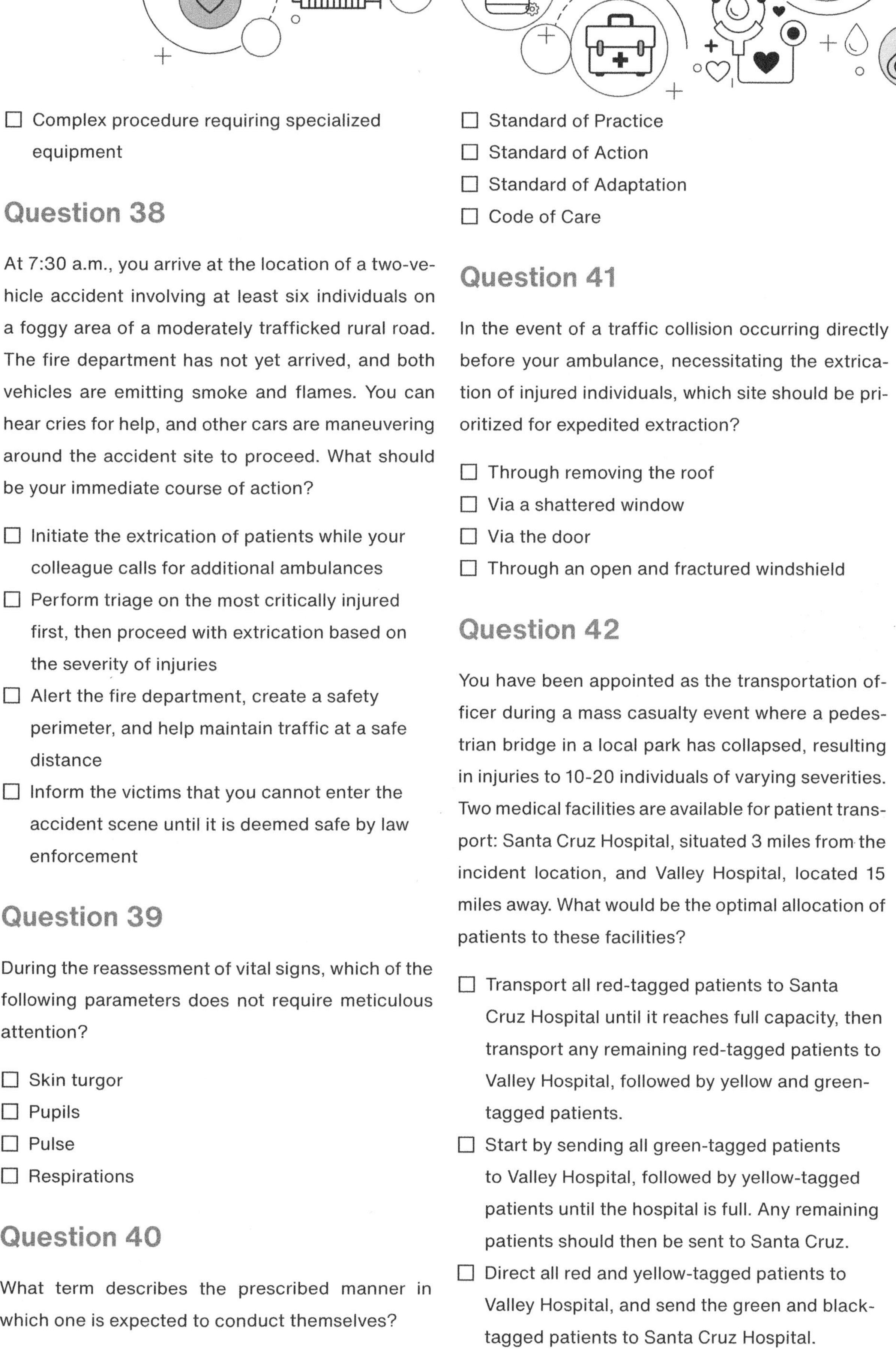

☐ Complex procedure requiring specialized equipment

Question 38

At 7:30 a.m., you arrive at the location of a two-vehicle accident involving at least six individuals on a foggy area of a moderately trafficked rural road. The fire department has not yet arrived, and both vehicles are emitting smoke and flames. You can hear cries for help, and other cars are maneuvering around the accident site to proceed. What should be your immediate course of action?

☐ Initiate the extrication of patients while your colleague calls for additional ambulances
☐ Perform triage on the most critically injured first, then proceed with extrication based on the severity of injuries
☐ Alert the fire department, create a safety perimeter, and help maintain traffic at a safe distance
☐ Inform the victims that you cannot enter the accident scene until it is deemed safe by law enforcement

Question 39

During the reassessment of vital signs, which of the following parameters does not require meticulous attention?

☐ Skin turgor
☐ Pupils
☐ Pulse
☐ Respirations

Question 40

What term describes the prescribed manner in which one is expected to conduct themselves?

☐ Standard of Practice
☐ Standard of Action
☐ Standard of Adaptation
☐ Code of Care

Question 41

In the event of a traffic collision occurring directly before your ambulance, necessitating the extrication of injured individuals, which site should be prioritized for expedited extraction?

☐ Through removing the roof
☐ Via a shattered window
☐ Via the door
☐ Through an open and fractured windshield

Question 42

You have been appointed as the transportation officer during a mass casualty event where a pedestrian bridge in a local park has collapsed, resulting in injuries to 10-20 individuals of varying severities. Two medical facilities are available for patient transport: Santa Cruz Hospital, situated 3 miles from the incident location, and Valley Hospital, located 15 miles away. What would be the optimal allocation of patients to these facilities?

☐ Transport all red-tagged patients to Santa Cruz Hospital until it reaches full capacity, then transport any remaining red-tagged patients to Valley Hospital, followed by yellow and green-tagged patients.
☐ Start by sending all green-tagged patients to Valley Hospital, followed by yellow-tagged patients until the hospital is full. Any remaining patients should then be sent to Santa Cruz.
☐ Direct all red and yellow-tagged patients to Valley Hospital, and send the green and black-tagged patients to Santa Cruz Hospital.

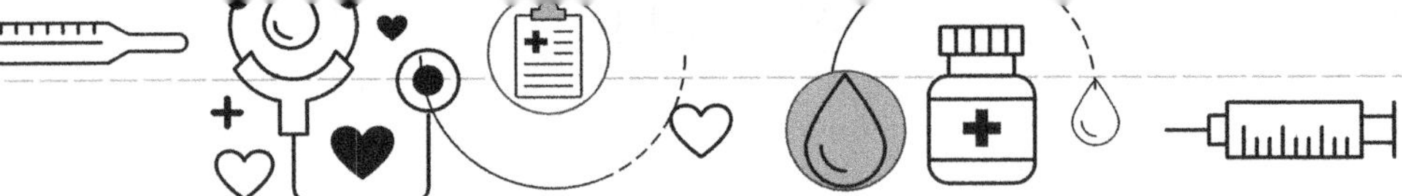

- ☐ Send all green-tagged patients to Valley Hospital after sending all red, yellow, and black-tagged patients to Santa Cruz Hospital.

Question 43

In which context would an expedited evaluation for trauma be conducted?

- ☐ In a hazardous environment
- ☐ At the incident location
- ☐ After the patient has been transported to the ambulance
- ☐ Within a hospital setting

Question 44

What is the recommended course of action if your radio communication extends beyond 30 seconds?

- ☐ Proceed until your message is fully transmitted
- ☐ Request the recipient to contact you via telephone
- ☐ Transmit the message again to ensure it was received
- ☐ Divide into two shorter messages

Question 45

Within the SAMPLE history framework, what does the letter 'S' signify?

- ☐ Severity
- ☐ Significant
- ☐ Signs
- ☐ Superficial

Question 46

Which of the following is not classified as a medication assisted by EMTs:

- ☐ Oxygen
- ☐ Inhaled bronchodilators
- ☐ Epinephrine
- ☐ Nitroglycerin

Question 47

Who is accountable for overseeing the operations of EMS agencies and ensuring EMTs adhere to standards in practice?

- ☐ Agency leaders
- ☐ Transportation department
- ☐ Medical direction
- ☐ Healthcare personnel

Question 48

Which technique is considered optimum for transferring a patient onto a backboard?

- ☐ Four-person lift
- ☐ Four-person log roll
- ☐ Three-person log roll
- ☐ Two-person log roll

Question 49

Within the acronym OPQRST, what does 'R' signify?

- ☐ Rapid breathing very shallow
- ☐ Radial
- ☐ Refraction
- ☐ Radiate

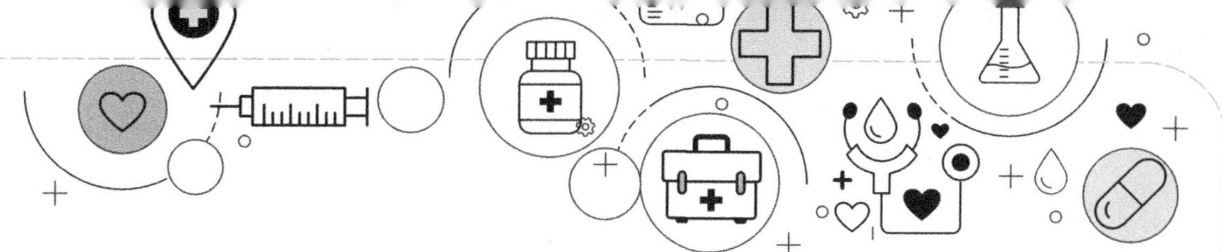

Question 50

For what purpose is the Incident Command System (ICS) implemented?

- ☐ Guarantee the efficient allocation of resources, safety for the public and responders, and the achievement of management objectives during incidents.
- ☐ Set organizational priorities for the National Incident Management System (NIMS) in response to natural disasters, acts of terrorism, or hazardous material incidents.
- ☐ Ensure that responses to mass casualty incidents are timely, coordinated, and effectively managed.
- ☐ Prevent individual agencies from making suboptimal response decisions due to communication failures or resource shortages.

Answers & Explanation
Page 189

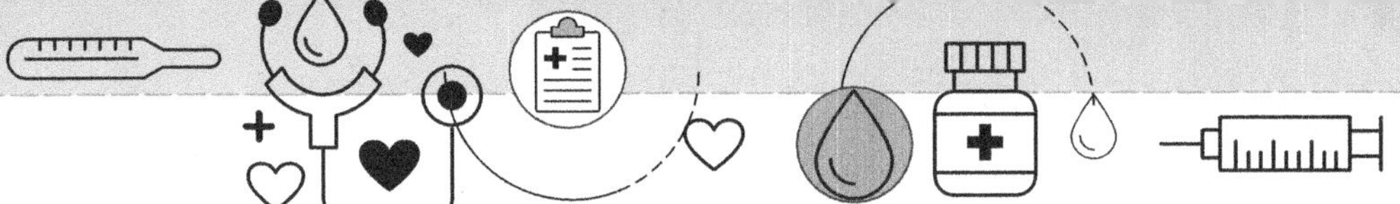

ALS AND ADVANCED QUESTIONS ONLY

Question 1

Which physiological processes are regulated by the autonomic nervous system?

- ☐ Respiratory rhythm
- ☐ Involuntary physiological activities
- ☐ Cardiac pace
- ☐ All aforementioned functions

Question 2

Within the anatomical framework, how would one classify nerves located in the lower extremities?

- ☐ Peripheral
- ☐ Occipital
- ☐ Central
- ☐ Leg nerves

Question 3

The purpose of defibrillation is to ___________.

- ☐ Administer an electric shock to reinitiate cardiac rhythm
- ☐ End critical arrhythmias
- ☐ Cease cardiac activity temporarily
- ☐ Resolve atrial disturbances

Question 4

Identify which items listed below could potentially trigger an allergic response in individuals:

- ☐ Botanical sources
- ☐ Pharmaceutical substances
- ☐ All aforementioned options
- ☐ Seafood, specifically shrimp

Question 5

Dyspnea is most likely to be observed in an individual who is _________.

- ☐ Experiencing respiratory distress
- ☐ Sleeping peacefully
- ☐ Breathing an average of 18 breaths per minute with regularity
- ☐ Younger than 18 years old

Question 6

An acute myocardial infarction (AMI) is commonly referred to as:

- ☐ Cardioverting
- ☐ A heart attack
- ☐ A pneumothorax
- ☐ A hemopneumothorax

Question 7

In the state of shock, the constriction of blood vessels results in the skin becoming _____.

- ☐ Cool
- ☐ Hot
- ☐ Warm
- ☐ Contract

Question 8

Which option listed does not belong to the six principles of accurate and safe medication administration?

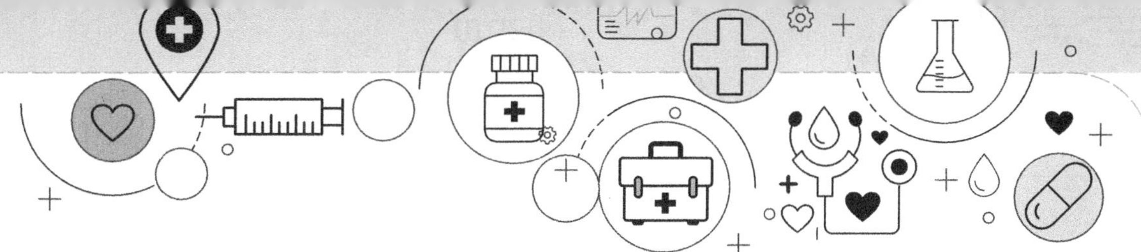

- ☐ Proper documentation
- ☐ Correct patient
- ☐ Injection device
- ☐ Method of administration

Question 9

A breech birth manifests as a/an ________.

- ☐ Arm
- ☐ The infant in a posterior-first position
- ☐ An issue that can be resolved pre-hospitalization
- ☐ None of the provided options

Question 10

What physiological condition might cause extreme thirst in individuals diagnosed with diabetes mellitus?

- ☐ Hyperglycemia
- ☐ Polyuria
- ☐ Hypoglycemia
- ☐ Transport inhibitors

Question 11

Individuals with a tracheostomy may require distinct methods of ventilation compared to those without such an opening. Which of the following statements accurately describes these ventilation methods?

- ☐ Creating a seal over the patient's mouth and nose during ventilation through a stoma, and then unsealing them during passive exhalation, can be an efficacious technique for assisted ventilation
- ☐ A specialized adapter for tracheostomy can be inserted into the stoma or attached to the tracheostomy tube, enabling a bag valve mask to deliver artificial ventilation with 100% oxygen via the BVM port.
- ☐ Using the head tilt chin lift maneuver aids in sustaining an open airway in patients ventilated through a stoma. Placing a rolled towel beneath the neck helps in tracheal positioning.
- ☐ Inserting an Oropharyngeal Airway (OPA) prior to BVM ventilation through a stoma aids in maintaining airway patency when the patient is vomiting. Suctioning to the level of the stoma through the oropharynx can be performed if significant vomitus is present.

Question 12

A 20-year-old male has sustained a back injury at a nearby swimming area. Upon arrival, you and your colleague Missy discover the individual groaning and partially submerged next to a pile of rocks. Eyewitnesses report that he fell approximately 30 feet from a tree he was climbing over the swimming hole. The patient's respiratory rate is 12 breaths per minute, his breathing is extremely shallow with intermittent apnea, his pulse is 72 beats per minute, and his skin is slightly clammy and pale. After securing cervical spine precautions, what would be the most appropriate intervention?

- ☐ Administer high-flow oxygen at 12-15 LPM and conduct a comprehensive physical examination
- ☐ Provide ventilation assistance and raise the

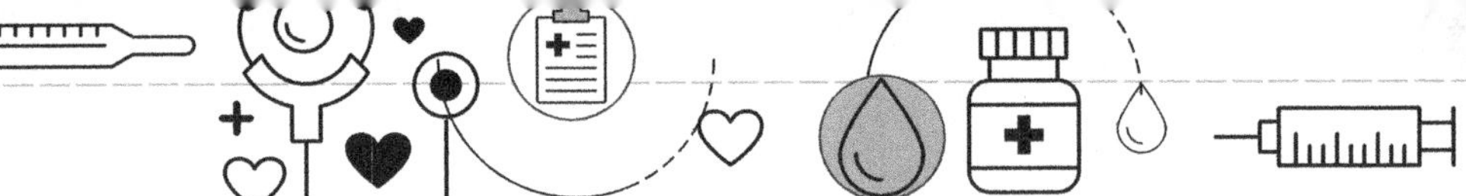

individual's legs

- ☐ Conduct a targeted physical examination for life-threatening injuries followed by transportation
- ☐ Evaluate airway patency, administer high-flow oxygen via non-rebreather mask (NRB), assess circulation, and prepare for transport

Question 13

Your team is summoned to a youth summer camp where a 14-year-old female is experiencing an undetermined illness. According to the camp counselor, the girl began vomiting while playing basketball and now complains of abdominal pain. Upon arrival, you observe the girl seated in the camp office, clutching her stomach. She is significantly overweight, mildly sweating, and her skin is pink and feels normothermic. During the pulse examination, she mentions feeling weak. She is alert and oriented to person, place, and time. What is the most probable diagnosis and which treatment option is most suitable?

- ☐ The girl is experiencing heat stroke and requires immediate cooling with ice. Administer 4 x 81mg salt tablets if she maintains a normal level of consciousness. Provide oxygen through a non-breather mask and ensure airway support during transport.
- ☐ The girl is experiencing heat cramps. She should be given small sips of cool water if she is fully conscious. Move her to a cooler environment and initiate active cooling by misting her with tepid water followed by fanning to promote evaporation. Provide high-flow oxygen, administer intravenous fluids if within your practice scope, and arrange for transport.
- ☐ The girl is experiencing heat exhaustion. She should be relocated to a cooler area and given small sips of cold water if her consciousness is unimpaired. Cool her passively with cold water. Administer high-flow oxygen and a fluid bolus if allowed by protocol. Ensure transport to a hospital for further assessment.
- ☐ The girl has a lower gastrointestinal bleed. Administer high-flow oxygen via a non-rebreather mask and transport her with legs elevated. Manage her for shock and be ready to suction if she vomits or loses consciousness.

Question 14

Following a detonation at a local oil refinery, you have been designated as the triage officer by the Incident Command. What triage color label would be assigned to each of the following cases?

Case 1: a 9-year-old girl with a fractured arm, exhibiting a respiratory rate of 8 breaths per minute.
Case 2: an elderly man with an open fracture of the left thigh bone, showing signs of severe hemorrhagic shock with an absent pulse.
Case 3: an elderly male with a forehead wound and a Glasgow Coma Scale (GCS) score of 8.
Case 4: a 5-year-old boy breathing at a rate of 18 breaths per minute with a minor head injury.

- ☐ Case 1: Red, Case 2: Black, Case 3: Red, Case 4: Green
- ☐ Case 1: Red, Case 2: Black, Case 3: Yellow, Case 4: Yellow
- ☐ Case 1: Yellow, Case 2: Red, Case 3: Black, Case 4: Red
- ☐ Case 1: Red, Case 2: Green, Case 4: Yellow, Case 3: Black

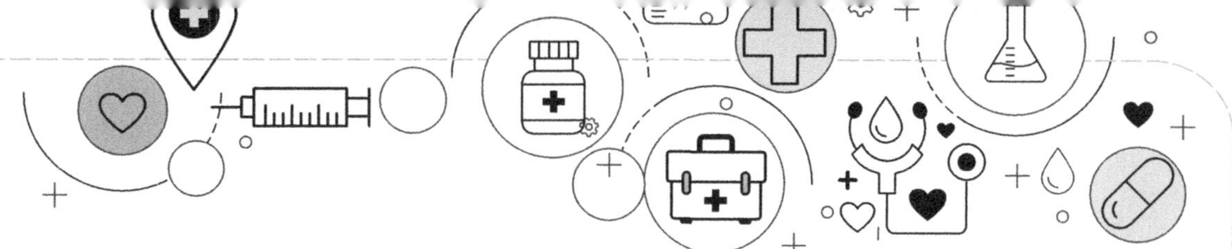

Question 15

Upon your arrival at the location, you encounter a 27-year-old woman experiencing anxiety and respiratory distress. Which question should you prioritize asking?

- ☐ Have you ever experienced panic attacks before?
- ☐ Do you know what today's date is?
- ☐ Could you please tell me your name?
- ☐ When did your difficulty in breathing start?

Question 16

Status asthmaticus is characterized by ___________.

- ☐ An improved likelihood of recovery
- ☐ A potentially fatal scenario
- ☐ The precursor to acute asthma
- ☐ Effective management with standard bronchodilators

Question 17

In what scenario might one observe the manifestation known as Battle's sign in a patient?

- ☐ In the case of rib fractures
- ☐ In the case of a pelvic fracture
- ☐ All aforementioned conditions
- ☐ In the case of skull fractures

Question 18

Through which path does blood travel after being ejected from the left ventricle?

- ☐ Right atrium
- ☐ Lungs
- ☐ Aortic arch
- ☐ Inferior Vena Cava.

Question 19

As the initial Emergency Medical Services unit to arrive at a scene involving multiple casualties, where a crane has collapsed onto an adjacent building from a rooftop, what procedures should you follow in accordance with the Incident Command System (ICS)?

- ☐ Maintain a safe distance and follow the directives of the Incident Commander.
- ☐ Inform dispatch of the necessity for an Incident Commander and initiate patient triage.
- ☐ Report your location to the IC and begin patient triage if the area is deemed secure.
- ☐ Assume the role of Incident Commander until relieved or reassigned by higher authority

Question 20

You arrive at the residence of a 69-year-old male who suddenly experienced dyspnea and dizziness while mowing his lawn. Upon initial evaluation, his integument is erythematous and anhidrotic. His respiratory rate is approximately 22 breaths per minute, and his heart rate stands at 120 beats per minute. His spouse mentions he commenced using Flomax two months ago but is otherwise not on any pharmacological regimen. At that moment, the patient reports a headache. A sphygmomanometric reading reveals his blood pressure to be 100/60 mmHg. What treatment approach is most appropriate for this patient?

- ☐ Transfer him to a cooler setting and disrobe him
- ☐ Expedited transport with limbs elevated and oxygen administered via nasal cannula at 6 LPM
- ☐ Provision of high-flow oxygen through a bag-valve mask (BVM) at 15 LPM

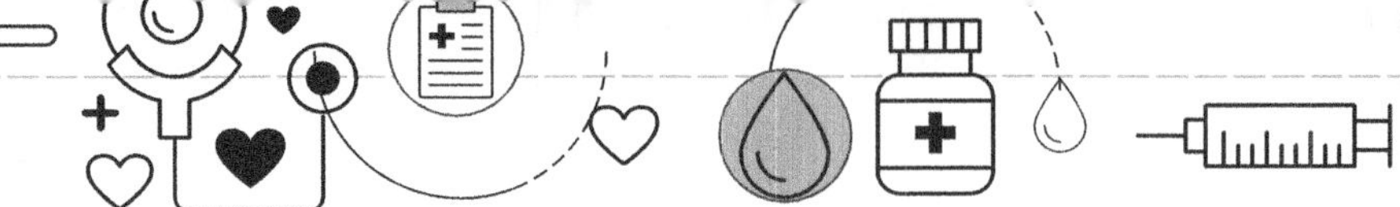

- ☐ Conducting a detailed medical history and physical examination

Question 21

You and your colleague, Stacy, respond to a call at an apartment complex involving a 17-year-old female experiencing abdominal pain. Upon arrival, you observe the patient, who appears pale and is lying on the couch. Her abdomen is visibly distended, and she has a towel on her lap with some blood stains. She is breathing at a rate of 20 breaths per minute, with a pulse rate of 114 beats per minute. The patient denies any trauma and reports a small amount of vaginal bleeding. After administering high-flow oxygen and transferring her to the ambulance, you notice a loop of tissue protruding from her vagina. What condition might this patient be experiencing, and how should she be managed?

- ☐ The patient has preeclampsia with placental abruption. Transport her in a left lateral recumbent position and administer shock treatment. Initiate IV therapy if within the scope of practice.
- ☐ The patient is in labor with a nuchal cord. Transport the patient with her head and torso angled downward while monitoring vital signs en route. Initiate IV therapy within the scope of practice. If the estimated time of arrival is more than 30 minutes, attempt to gently maneuver the cord back into the vagina.
- ☐ The patient is suffering from umbilical cord prolapse. Insert a gloved hand into the vagina to check for cord pulsations, gently lift the baby's head off the cord, and transport the patient in a supine position with elevated hips. Treat for shock and initiate IV therapy according to the scope of practice.
- ☐ The patient has an acute lower gastrointestinal bleed. Transport her in a comfortable position and treat for shock. Establish IV access if within the scope of practice.

Question 22

Shock can be attributed to three primary etiologies. What are they?

- ☐ Inadequate cardiac function, fluid depletion, and vasodilation
- ☐ Trauma, cardiac incident, and seizure
- ☐ Impaired perfusion, altered mental status, and respiratory failure
- ☐ Vascular constriction, impaired vascular function, and respiratory failure

Question 23

During an emergency delivery in the back of an ambulance, you and your partner Jim face a nuchal cord that is too tight to maneuver over the infant's head. Given this situation, what should be your subsequent course of action?

- ☐ Provide support to the infant's head and clear the nose and mouth of any obstructions
- ☐ Clamp the umbilical cord at two points and cut between the clamps
- ☐ Carefully push the infant's head back into the birth canal until the cord is free
- ☐ Stimulate more intense uterine contractions by massaging the uterus, to release the infant

Question 24

During which month of gestation is it most probable for supine hypotensive syndrome to manifest?

- ☐ Third
- ☐ First
- ☐ Sixth

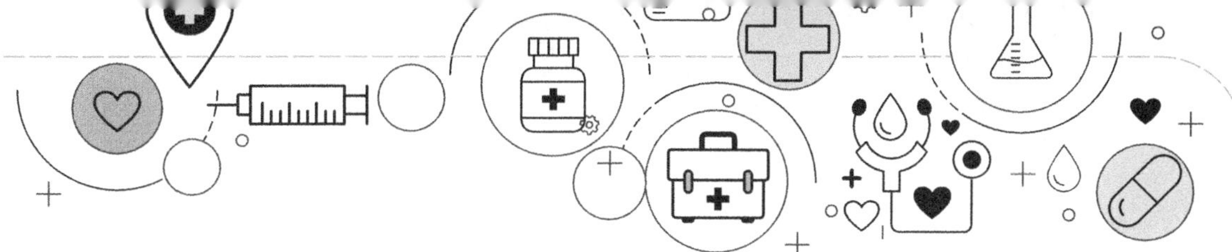

☐ Ninth

Question 25

Upon arrival at a wedding ceremony, you and your colleague Asher encounter a woman who has experienced a syncopal episode. Witnesses report that the incident was triggered by her realization of a dragon tattoo on her daughter's ankle as she proceeded down the aisle. Attendees noted that the woman was gently lowered to the ground, avoiding any traumatic impact. After remaining supine for 10 minutes, she was assisted to an upright position without expressing any discomfort. Despite a pallid appearance, her neurological function appears normal with a Glasgow Coma Scale (GCS) score of 15. What is the most plausible diagnosis for this woman's condition?

☐ Cardiogenic shock
☐ Neurogenic shock
☐ Psychogenic shock
☐ Hemostatic shock

Question 26

You are attending to a 16-year-old female presently in active labor, discovered alone in her automobile. Upon examination, it is evident that the fetal head has already emerged. What action should be taken next in the childbirth process?

☐ Immediately position her in a left lateral recumbent position on a gurney and transport her
☐ Advise her to push and await the delivery of the shoulders
☐ Assess for the presence of a nuchal cord
☐ Administer blow-by oxygen to the neonate and proceed with transportation

Question 27

What term is used to describe the accumulation of air in the cavity between the visceral and parietal pleurae?

☐ Pneumothorax
☐ Pneumatic emphysema
☐ Subcutaneous emphysema
☐ Pleural edema

Question 28

You have been dispatched to a ski resort where a 49-year-old female was discovered after spending the night in an infrequently visited section of the ski area. Upon your arrival, you observe the patient seated, enveloped in a blanket. She exhibits signs of disorientation and is muttering unintelligibly. Her right foot is swathed in towels, and a resort employee reports that it is blistered and significantly swollen. What is the likely diagnosis for this woman, and what would constitute the most appropriate course of treatment?

☐ The patient is hypothermic and has frostbite on her foot. Manage the hypothermia by placing heat packs covered in towels onto the axillary and groin regions. The foot should be loosely covered with a sterile dressing and the patient should be transported to the closest hospital.
☐ The patient has frostbite on her foot and would benefit from the application of heat packs over the towels to facilitate warming. Immediate transport coupled with high-flow oxygen administration is essential.
☐ The patient is hypothermic and should be given small amounts of coffee or tea until her mental status improves. Rub the frostbitten foot to enhance blood circulation and transport her to the nearest healthcare facility.

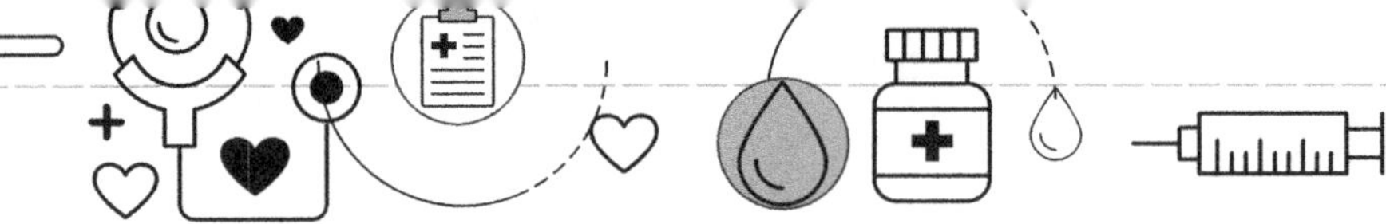

- ☐ The patient has a frostbitten foot and has developed hypoglycemia due to a lack of food since the previous day. Administer oral glucose if her gag reflex is intact. Provide high-flow oxygen using a non-rebreather mask and proceed to the nearest hospital.

Question 29

The term 'cyt-' denotes which of the following?

- ☐ Cell
- ☐ Rib
- ☐ Spine
- ☐ Bladder

Question 30

Upon arriving at the scene, you observe a male approximately in his 60s reclining on the floor of a minimally heated, compact apartment. His lips exhibit a bluish tint and his consciousness level is altered. What is the most plausible diagnosis?

- ☐ Exhibiting bradycardia and tachypnea
- ☐ Displaying diaphoresis and osmotic imbalance
- ☐ Showcasing diaphoresis and multitasking abilities
- ☐ Cyanotic and experiencing hypothermia

Question 31

In pediatric assessments, what is the typical weight range for children aged 2 to 6 years?

- ☐ 15-25 kilograms
- ☐ 15-35 kilograms
- ☐ 64-85 kilograms
- ☐ 35-85 kilograms

Question 32

What is the recommended patient positioning for transportation when managing shock?:

- ☐ Prone with legs elevated
- ☐ Comfortable position
- ☐ Supine with legs elevated
- ☐ Modified Trovestic position

Question 33

Identify an alternative term frequently used for shock:

- ☐ Hypoxia
- ☐ Hypertension
- ☐ Hypoperfusion
- ☐ Hyperperfusion

Question 34

Administering nitroglycerin to a patient during a myocardial infarction will have which primary effect?

- ☐ Cause vasodilation
- ☐ Accelerate cardiac rhythm
- ☐ Induce vasoconstriction
- ☐ Augment cardiac workload

Question 35

What is meconium?

- ☐ Distinctive for its bright red coloration with shades of blue
- ☐ Harmless to the newborn
- ☐ All of the mentioned options
- ☐ An indicator of fetal or maternal distress

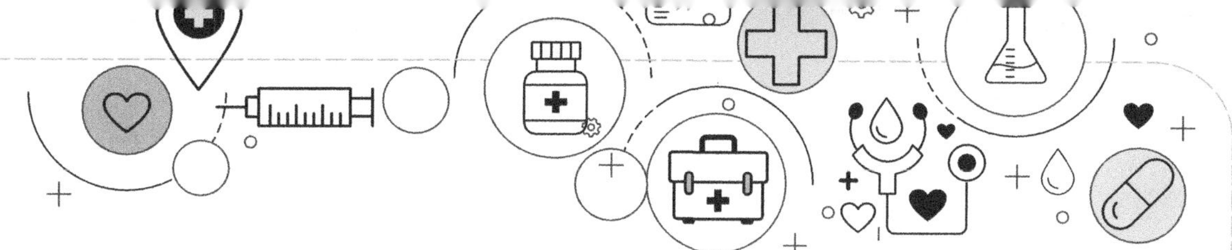

Question 36

What classification of shock is most likely to occur in an individual experiencing a myocardial infarction?

- ☐ Hemorrhagic
- ☐ Cardiogenic
- ☐ Psychogenic
- ☐ Neurogenic

Question 37

Upon arrival at the scene, you and your colleague Rob encounter a woman who is 37 weeks into her pregnancy. She expresses that she feels an imminent need for delivery and requests immediate transportation to the hospital. As Rob monitors her vital signs en route, you begin to evaluate her stage of labor. Notably, she is experiencing vaginal bleeding, leading you to consider the possibility of ____________ or ________________.

- ☐ Multiple gestation such as twins or triplets
- ☐ Preterm labor or umbilical cord prolapse
- ☐ Placenta previa or placental abruption
- ☐ Sustained abdominal trauma

Question 38

During childbirth, if the infant is emerging but the amniotic sac remains intact, what steps should be taken?

- ☐ Proceed with the delivery as usual
- ☐ Carefully break the sac to reveal the baby's head
- ☐ Insert several fingers into the birth canal to rupture the sac
- ☐ Allow the baby's head to naturally push through the sac

Question 39

A distinguishing feature of Cheyne-Stokes respiration is _________.

- ☐ Irregular breathing interspersed with apnea
- ☐ Slow breathing
- ☐ Quick deep breaths
- ☐ Very shallow rapid breathing

Question 40

The gesture known as Levine's sign is indicative of ______________

- ☐ Experiencing a cerebrovascular accident (stroke)
- ☐ Undergoing a myocardial infarction
- ☐ Obstructing their airway with food
- ☐ Being in labor

Question 41

You arrive at Bigrock High School in response to an incident in the chemistry laboratory. A heated test tube has shattered, causing an injury to a student's eye. Upon entering the nurse's office, you observe an 18-year-old male reclined on the examination table, his face partially concealed by a towel. Upon the removal of the towel, it is apparent that fragments of glass are embedded in his facial skin, and he is experiencing ocular bleeding. What is the most appropriate course of action to take?

- ☐ Apply a bandage with moderate pressure to manage the bleeding
- ☐ Extract any visible glass pieces from the eye and apply an occlusive dressing
- ☐ Administer high-flow oxygen and expedite transport
- ☐ Shield the injured eye with a paper cup and secure with a bandage, avoiding pressure

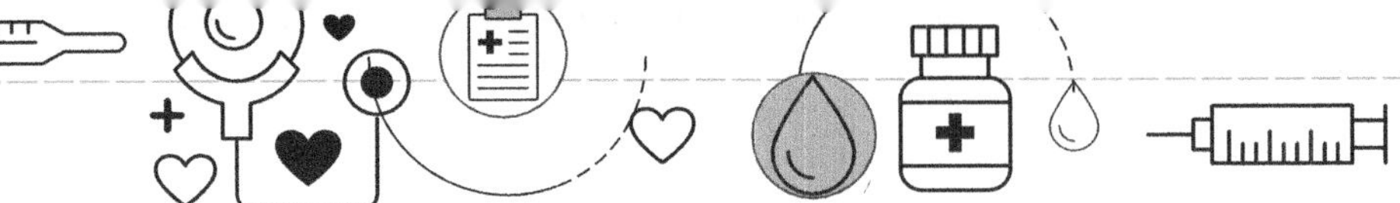

Question 42

Concerning the preservation of a pediatric patient's airway, which of the following statements holds true?

- ☐ It occupies a smaller proportion of the mouth compared to an adult
- ☐ Placing a towel beneath the shoulders assists in aligning the airway
- ☐ A towel under the shoulders should never be used
- ☐ Utilize an oropharyngeal airway sized from the nasal corner to the ear lobe

Question 43

In the event that a patient presents with emesis resembling coffee grounds, which condition would you consider?

- ☐ Esophageal varices
- ☐ Pleuratenial Intestotrophy
- ☐ Gastrointestinal hemorrhage
- ☐ Excessive alcohol consumption

Question 44

What might precipitate cardiogenic shock?

- ☐ Transient Ischemic Attack (TIA)
- ☐ Acute Myocardial Infarction (AMI)
- ☐ An alarming event
- ☐ An electrical accident involving a vehicle

Question 45

How is cardiac output defined?

- ☐ Heart rate multiplied by Stroke rate
- ☐ The total volume of blood expelled by the heart in one minute
- ☐ Product of Cardiac output and Stroke output
- ☐ Product of Stroke volume and Cardiac volume

Question 46

A healthcare provider has instructed you to administer a nitroglycerin spray to a patient via the sublingual route. What method will you employ to deliver the medication?

- ☐ Beneath the tongue
- ☐ Through the skin
- ☐ Through an endotracheal tube
- ☐ Inside the cheek

Question 47

Upon arrival, you and your colleague, Steve, encounter an 85-year-old male seated in a lounge chair, engrossed in smoking a cigar. Initially, his eyes remain shut, but they open when addressed as 'Sir'. He exhibits confusion when questioned about his name but promptly responds by squeezing your hand when requested. What Glasgow Coma Scale (GCS) score would this patient likely receive?

- ☐ 15
- ☐ 13
- ☐ 12
- ☐ 10

Question 48

The organ that adheres to the uterine wall and consists of both maternal and fetal tissues is the ________________.

- ☐ Amniotic
- ☐ Polenta
- ☐ Placenta
- ☐ Cervix

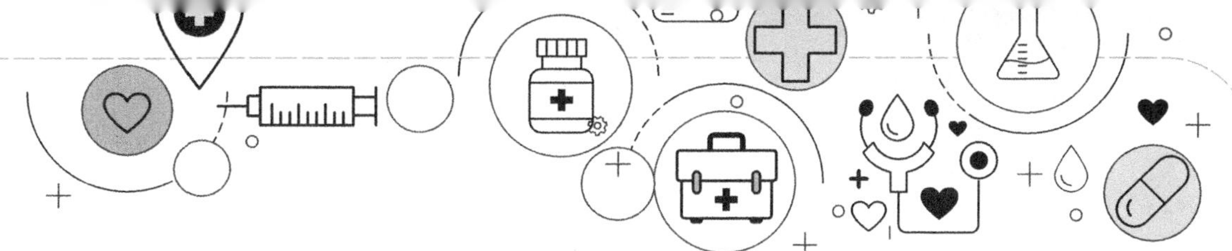

Question 49

At what minimum age is it deemed inappropriate to employ an automatic ventilator?

- ☐ 8
- ☐ 10
- ☐ 12
- ☐ 14

Question 50

Identify the anatomical region referred to as the perineum::

- ☐ The extent of cervical dilation
- ☐ The terminal lumbar vertebra
- ☐ The abdominal lining
- ☐ The area found between the anus and the vaginal opening

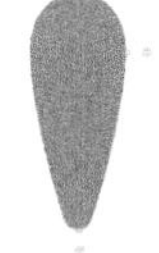

Answers & Explanation
Page 199

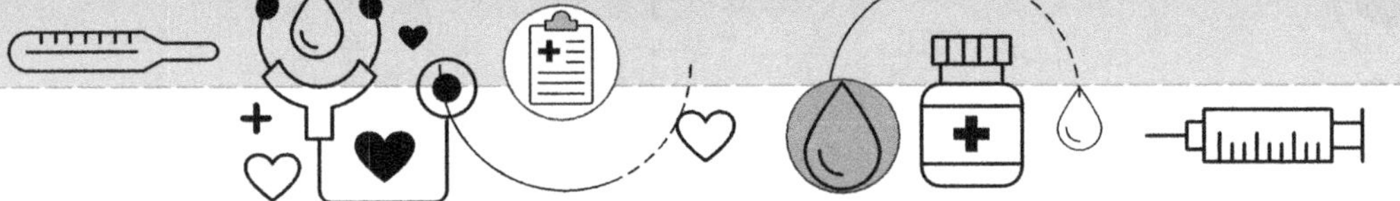

AIRWAY, RESPIRATION AND VENTILATION

Question 1

Upon arrival at a residence to address a 'slip and fall' incident, you and your colleague Bob are informed by an anxious father that his 3-year-old child has tumbled down a staircase of around 20 steps into the basement. The father hands over the unconscious boy, who exhibits shallow, irregular respiration and a pulse rate of 98 beats per minute. After ensuring the child's cervical spine is manually stabilized, you and Bob carefully lay him on the floor. Next, you should:

- ☐ Administer two short rescue breaths, followed by high-flow oxygen via non-rebreather mask, assuming the child's airway is unobstructed.
- ☐ Insert a nasopharyngeal airway and assist breaths at 15-30 per minute while hastening transport.
- ☐ Introduce an oropharyngeal airway and assist breathing with a bag-valve mask, ensuring swift transportation.
- ☐ Initiate CPR with a compression rate of 100 per minute combined with around 5-6 breaths per minute, using a 15:2 compression-to-breath ratio for two rescuers.

Question 2

Identify the upper airway bacterial infection that has the potential to cause severe respiratory distress:

- ☐ Laryngositus
- ☐ Croup
- ☐ Epiglottitis
- ☐ Emphysema

Question 3

A patient exhibits signs indicative of irregular respiratory effort. Which observations would confirm this diagnosis?

- ☐ Abdominal breathing, stridor, retractions, and silent chest
- ☐ Retractions, nasal flaring, abdominal breathing, and sweating
- ☐ Wheezing, nasal flaring, crackles, and sweating
- ☐ Stridor, wheezing, crackles, and silent chest

Question 4

Which of the following does not indicate a proper airway?

- ☐ The individual is fully alert.
- ☐ The individual can speak in complete sentences.
- ☐ The airway is unblocked, allowing air movement to be heard and felt.
- ☐ The vocal sound is normal for the individual.

Question 5

Upon entering a residence, you observe an infant being held by her mother. The child is not crying and appears to be limp in her mother's arms. The infant's complexion appears pale or grayish, and there are no observable efforts of breathing. Which assessment tool is being utilized, and what is the primary action needed to manage this situation?

- ☐ Pediatric Assessment Triangle; Remove the child from the mother, promptly open the air-

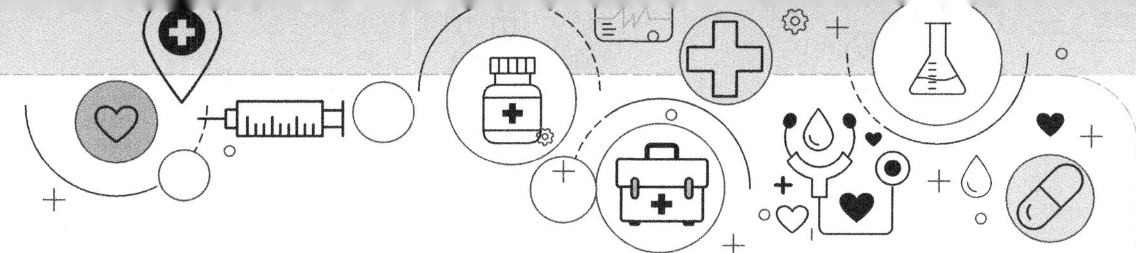

way, and evaluate breathing

- ☐ Rapid Initial Assessment; Collect relevant history from the mother while simultaneously assessing the child's respiratory and circulatory status
- ☐ Rapid Initial Assessment; Direct the mother to lay the child on the floor and begin CPR if there is no evidence of breathing or circulation
- ☐ Pediatric Assessment Triangle; Conduct a swift head-to-toe examination to identify any immediate life-threatening conditions

Question 6

You are dispatched to Medical Park to attend to an individual who has reportedly fallen from his wheelchair. Upon arrival with your colleague Sheila, you observe two bystanders administering CPR on a male who appears to be around 60 years old. What are the recommended rate and depth of chest compressions to perform during CPR in this scenario?

- ☐ 15 compressions to 2 breaths / 2 inches depth
- ☐ 30 compressions to 2 breaths / one third to one half the chest depth
- ☐ 30 compressions to 2 breaths / 2 inches depth
- ☐ 15 compressions to 2 breaths / one third to one half the chest depth

Question 7

All of the following are functions performed by the respiratory system except:

- ☐ Ventilation
- ☐ Respiration
- ☐ Gas exchange between bronchioles and veins
- ☐ Alveolar-capillary gas exchange

Question 8

To what does the term 'bilateral' pertain?

- ☐ Neither side
- ☐ One side
- ☐ All sides
- ☐ Both sides

Question 9

While performing an evaluation of a patient with your colleague Tony, you observe an unusual movement of the thoracic cage during expiration following a blunt force impact to the chest. This aberrant motion suggests what kind of injury?

- ☐ Hemothorax
- ☐ Scapular fracture
- ☐ Flail chest
- ☐ Hemopneumothorax

Question 10

Upon arrival, you and your colleague, Dale, find a female patient exhibiting signs of respiratory distress. She is ambulatory, with her arms elevated, and you can hear wheezing with each inhalation. Witnesses report that she was consuming a hot dog when she began to choke, which occurred approximately 10 minutes ago. What is the most appropriate intervention in this scenario?

- ☐ Administer the Heimlich maneuver
- ☐ Wait for her to lose consciousness and then

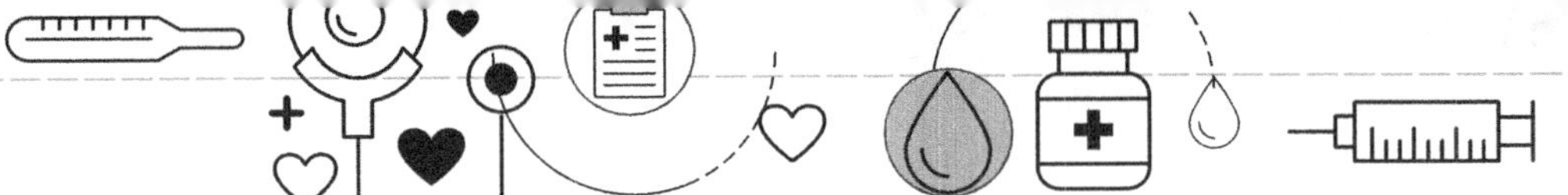

perform chest compressions
- ☐ Motivate her to cough and transport her
- ☐ Encourage her to cough and obtain a PCR signature from a relative

Question 11

According to American Heart Association CPR Guidelines, what is the recommended duration for administering a rescue breath to a pediatric patient?

- ☐ 1 second
- ☐ 5-6 seconds
- ☐ 3-5 seconds
- ☐ 1 minute

Question 12

Upon arriving at a nursing facility, you encounter a 73-year-old male patient with a stoma who is apneic. What is the appropriate intervention?

- ☐ Utilize a Venturi mask for ventilation.
- ☐ Employ a pediatric BVM mask with an adult bag for ventilation.
- ☐ Implement a Nasal Cannula for ventilation.
- ☐ Use a Nasopharyngeal airway to ventilate.

Question 13

Identify which of the following is not recognized as an early indicator of respiratory distress in a 7-year-old female.

- ☐ Head bobbing
- ☐ Intercostal retractions
- ☐ Tachypnea
- ☐ Bluish discoloration of the lips

Question 14

The evaluation of respiratory parameters in anaphylactic patients reveals ____________________ and ________________________.

- ☐ severe respiratory distress and wheezing to diminished lung sounds
- ☐ decreased mental status and wheezing to diminished lung sounds
- ☐ wheezing to diminished lung sounds and increased heart rate
- ☐ rapid pulse and hypotension

Question 15

Cyanosis is frequently indicative of ___________.

- ☐ A yellow tinge in the sclera
- ☐ The presence of hypoxia
- ☐ Restoration of sensation in peripheral areas
- ☐ The patient's condition is improving

Question 16

What is the proportion of oxygen present in the air we inhale?

- ☐ 50%
- ☐ 26%
- ☐ 21%
- ☐ 85%

Question 17

A 61-year-old male patient presents with shortness of breath, without any evidence or history of trauma. Which diagnostic history and physical examination approach would you select for this patient, and what is the most probable diagnosis of his condition?

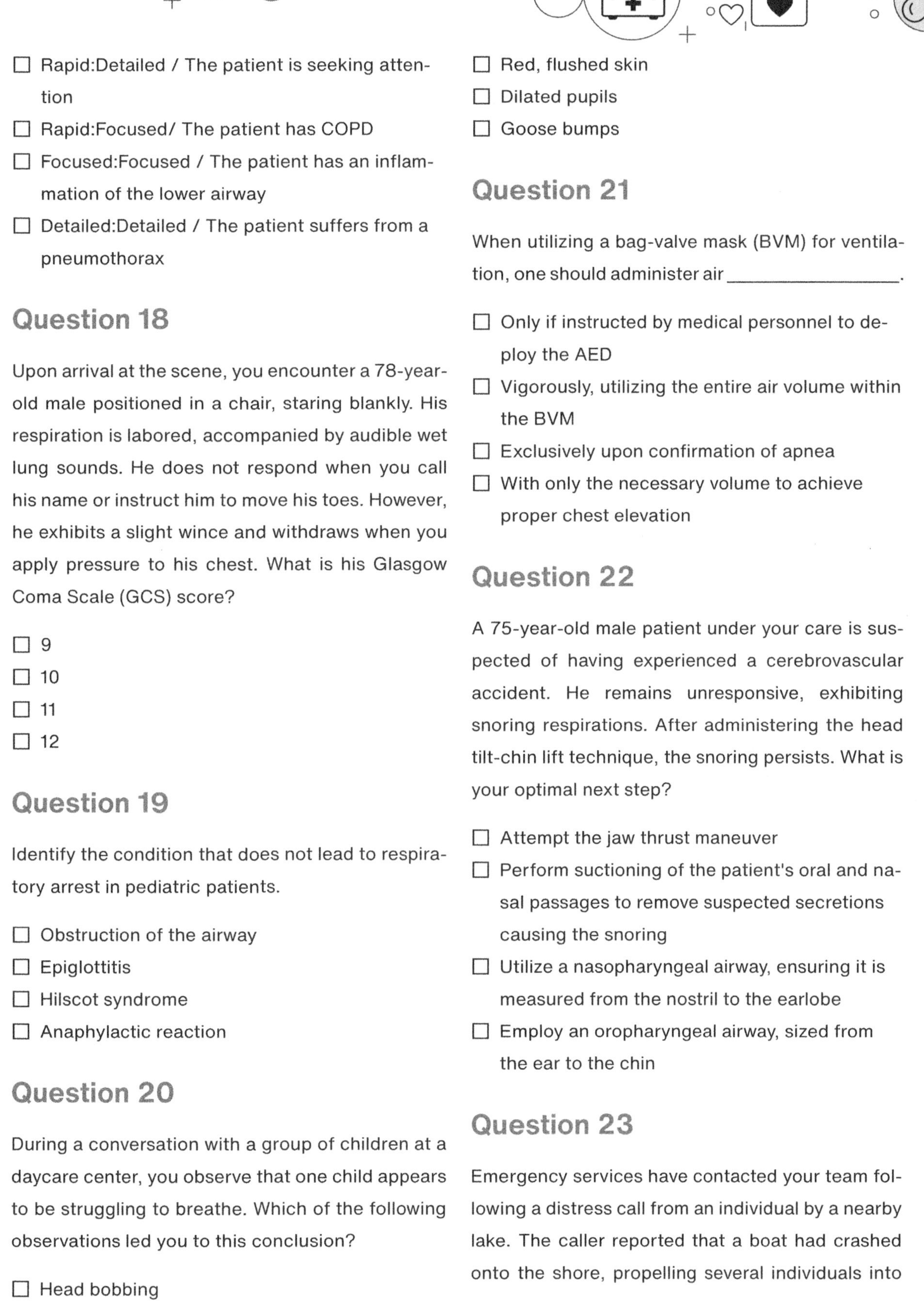

- ☐ Rapid:Detailed / The patient is seeking attention
- ☐ Rapid:Focused/ The patient has COPD
- ☐ Focused:Focused / The patient has an inflammation of the lower airway
- ☐ Detailed:Detailed / The patient suffers from a pneumothorax

Question 18

Upon arrival at the scene, you encounter a 78-year-old male positioned in a chair, staring blankly. His respiration is labored, accompanied by audible wet lung sounds. He does not respond when you call his name or instruct him to move his toes. However, he exhibits a slight wince and withdraws when you apply pressure to his chest. What is his Glasgow Coma Scale (GCS) score?

- ☐ 9
- ☐ 10
- ☐ 11
- ☐ 12

Question 19

Identify the condition that does not lead to respiratory arrest in pediatric patients.

- ☐ Obstruction of the airway
- ☐ Epiglottitis
- ☐ Hilscot syndrome
- ☐ Anaphylactic reaction

Question 20

During a conversation with a group of children at a daycare center, you observe that one child appears to be struggling to breathe. Which of the following observations led you to this conclusion?

- ☐ Head bobbing
- ☐ Red, flushed skin
- ☐ Dilated pupils
- ☐ Goose bumps

Question 21

When utilizing a bag-valve mask (BVM) for ventilation, one should administer air ________________.

- ☐ Only if instructed by medical personnel to deploy the AED
- ☐ Vigorously, utilizing the entire air volume within the BVM
- ☐ Exclusively upon confirmation of apnea
- ☐ With only the necessary volume to achieve proper chest elevation

Question 22

A 75-year-old male patient under your care is suspected of having experienced a cerebrovascular accident. He remains unresponsive, exhibiting snoring respirations. After administering the head tilt-chin lift technique, the snoring persists. What is your optimal next step?

- ☐ Attempt the jaw thrust maneuver
- ☐ Perform suctioning of the patient's oral and nasal passages to remove suspected secretions causing the snoring
- ☐ Utilize a nasopharyngeal airway, ensuring it is measured from the nostril to the earlobe
- ☐ Employ an oropharyngeal airway, sized from the ear to the chin

Question 23

Emergency services have contacted your team following a distress call from an individual by a nearby lake. The caller reported that a boat had crashed onto the shore, propelling several individuals into

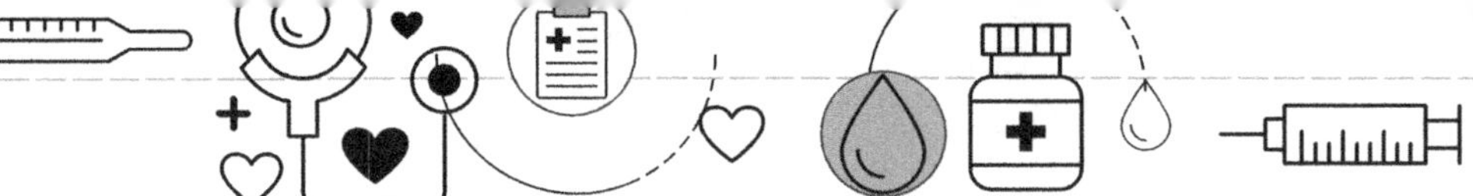

a forested area. Upon arrival, you and your colleague Zeek discover three individuals with minor abrasions performing CPR on a woman in her 30s. They inform you that the patient was thrown into the trees when the boat struck land. Zeek quickly checks for a pulse and finds none at the carotid artery. Both of you initiate CPR. As you prepare to transport the patient to the ambulance, you should provide approximately ____________ per minute using a BVM. During the 30-minute journey, an oral airway adjunct is placed, and a subsequent pulse check indicates the woman now has a strong palpable pulse. What is the appropriate ventilation rate for this patient now? ____________

- ☐ 6 breaths / 10 to 12 breaths per minute
- ☐ 8 to 10 breaths / 10 to 12 breaths per minute
- ☐ 10 to 12 breaths / 12 to 20 breaths per minute
- ☐ 12 to 20 / 12 to 20 breaths per minute

Question 24

You are attending to a 6-year-old girl suffering from an asthma exacerbation. She is having difficulty breathing, and you provide her with oxygen through a non-rebreather mask. Which of the following statements is incorrect in the context of pediatric asthma exacerbations?

- ☐ The child might exhibit signs of cyanosis
- ☐ Pediatric asthma episodes typically resolve without intervention
- ☐ Continuous observation for potential deterioration is essential
- ☐ Administering a bronchodilator via MDI with a spacer is necessary

Question 25

During expiration, what condition is commonly suggested by the abnormal, contradictory excursion of the thoracic cage?

- ☐ Hemopneumothorax
- ☐ Pneumothorax
- ☐ Flail chest
- ☐ Fracture of the clavicle

Question 26

Crackles in the lungs are indicative of:

- ☐ An indication of lower respiratory tract obstruction
- ☐ A symptom directly associated with right-sided heart failure
- ☐ Indicative of an upper respiratory infection and also termed as stridor
- ☐ The noise produced when fractured bone fragments rub together

Question 27

You and your colleague, with whom you have been collaborating for two years, respond to a residence where a female patient reports experiencing chest discomfort and difficulty breathing. She presents with diaphoresis, a heart rate of 110 beats per minute, a respiratory rate of 22 breaths per minute, and a blood pressure of 140/80 mmHg. She denies any prior cardiac or pulmonary conditions. What is the most appropriate course of action?

- ☐ Obtain a sample history and attempt to identify the etiology of her respiratory symptoms
- ☐ Place her in the ambulance and initiate transport as swiftly as possible
- ☐ Contact medical control to seek authorization for administering her spouse's nitroglycerin
- ☐ Conduct an assessment, administer oxygen at a rate of 15 lpm, and proceed with transportation

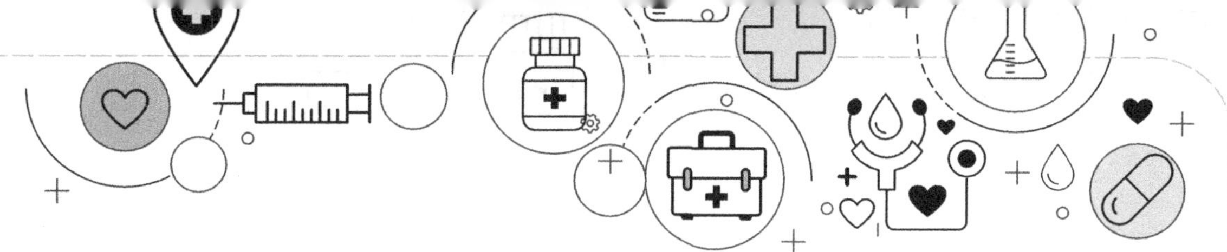

Question 28

The left atrium and ventricle of the cardiac system are responsible for ____________________ and ____________________.

- ☐ receives pulmonary circulation, drives systemic circulation
- ☐ drives pulmonary circulation, drives systemic circulation
- ☐ receives systemic circulation, drives pulmonary circulation
- ☐ receives systemic circulation, receives pulmonary circulation

Question 29

Identify the elements that constitute components of the lower respiratory tract from the options provided:

- ☐ Trachea - alveoli – uvula
- ☐ Trachea - bronchial tree - alveoli
- ☐ Epiglottis - oropharynx - vestibular fold
- ☐ Vocal cords - pharynx - epiglottis

Question 30

After your colleague Gina has used a French tip catheter to clear a patient's airway of vomit, what is the appropriate subsequent action?

- ☐ Discard the catheter in the sharps disposal unit
- ☐ Dispose of the catheter
- ☐ Place an oropharyngeal airway
- ☐ Ready the catheter for future use by rinsing it with sterile water

Question 31

Identify three pathological states frequently associated with an accelerated respiratory rate (tachypnea).

- ☐ Allergic reaction, shock, and CHF
- ☐ Hypoxia, CHF, and shock
- ☐ Fibromyalgia, hypoxia, and ischemia
- ☐ Hypoxia, congestive heart failure, and opiate overdose

Question 32

In pediatric care, certain interventions are necessary to ensure the airway remains unobstructed. Which of the following techniques is deemed appropriate?

- ☐ Employ an oral or nasal airway adjunct
- ☐ Utilize Magill forceps to prevent the child's tongue from obstructing the airway
- ☐ Position a rolled-up towel beneath the child's neck to maintain airway alignment
- ☐ Place the child in the Trendelenburg position with high flow oxygen at 15 liters per minute

Question 33

A report has indicated that a male individual is found unconscious behind a grocery store and is not exhibiting signs of respiration. Upon arrival, you encounter a male sitting solo against a wall with his eyes shut, unresponsive to verbal stimuli. His respiratory rate is 8 irregular breaths per minute, interspersed with episodes of apnea. Adjacent to him lies a small plastic bag containing a white substance. Upon administering a sternal rub, he clutches his chest but remains silent. How would you assess his Glasgow Coma Scale (GCS) score, and what is the most appropriate intervention?

- ☐ GCS score of 6 / Administer high-flow oxygen via Non-Rebreather Mask (NRB) and transport
- ☐ GCS score of 7 / Facilitate ventilation using a

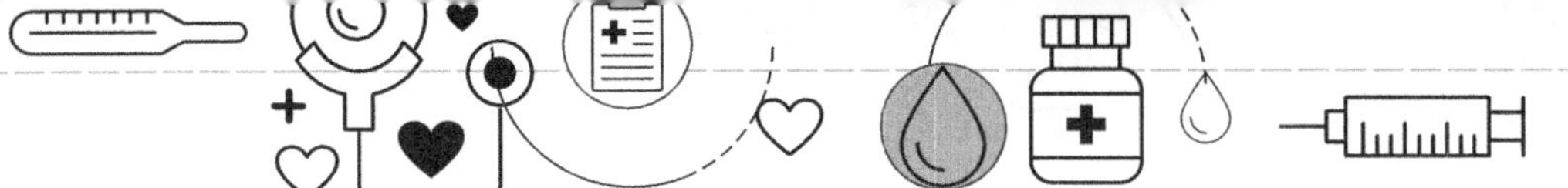

Bag-Valve Mask (BVM)

- ☐ GCS score of 7 / Secure the individual to the gurney due to suspected drug ingestion
- ☐ GCS score of 6 / Insert a nasopharyngeal airway and prepare for suction

Question 34

Upon arrival at the scene where a man is experiencing unexplained respiratory distress, what can you ascertain?

- ☐ It is certain the patient has hit his head
- ☐ It is necessary to call Advanced Life Support
- ☐ It might involve the trachea, epiglottis, or alveoli
- ☐ All of the previous statements are correct

Question 35

Faced with a respiratory failure case, you and your colleague must determine the main objective of providing ventilatory support. What is the primary rationale for this intervention?

- ☐ Providing ventilatory support enhances both oxygenation and ventilation
- ☐ Providing ventilatory support enhances only oxygenation
- ☐ Providing ventilatory support enhances only ventilation
- ☐ Providing ventilatory support enhances only respiration

Question 36

What causes gastric distention in patients undergoing cardiopulmonary resuscitation (CPR)?

- ☐ Utilization of a bag-valve-mask (BVM) that is too small for the patient
- ☐ Excessive air volume during ventilatory support
- ☐ Gastric distention occurs in all patients undergoing CPR
- ☐ Inability of an unconscious patient to properly exhale

Question 37

During a pulmonary examination of a healthy 23-year-old woman, what type of respiratory sounds would you anticipate detecting?

- ☐ Bronchovesicular breath sounds
- ☐ Bronchial breath sounds
- ☐ Vesicular breath sounds
- ☐ Moist breath sounds

Question 38

The initiation of resuscitative efforts should be withheld in cases where unequivocal indications of death are evident. Which of the following is not considered one of these signs?

- ☐ Rigor mortis
- ☐ Decomposition
- ☐ Lividity
- ☐ Lack of cardiac activity

Question 39

What is the primary therapeutic intervention for a patient exposed to noxious gases?

- ☐ Cardiopulmonary Resuscitation (CPR)
- ☐ Thoracentesis
- ☐ Assisted Ventilation
- ☐ Oxygen Therapy

Question 40

A young male, aged 20, has sustained a back injury at a nearby swimming location. Upon arrival,

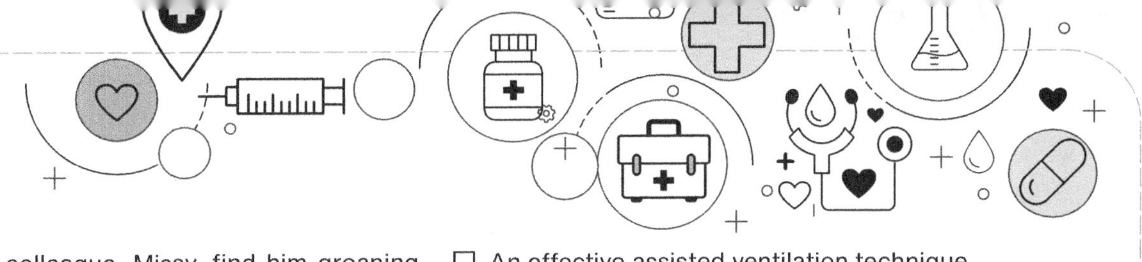

you and your colleague, Missy, find him groaning and partly submerged in water near a rock formation. Bystanders report that he fell approximately 30 feet from a tree he was climbing over the swimming area, landing on the rocks. His breathing rate is 12 breaths per minute, characterized by very shallow breaths with intermittent pauses of apnea. His heart rate is 72 beats per minute, and his skin appears slightly moist and pale. Following the provision of cervical spine stabilization, what should be the next immediate step in managing his condition?

- ☐ Conduct a focused physical examination to look for life-threatening conditions and then initiate transport
- ☐ Administer high-flow oxygen at 12-15 L/min and perform a detailed physical examination
- ☐ Evaluate the airway, administer high-flow oxygen via a non-rebreather mask, assess circulation, and prepare for transport
- ☐ Provide assisted ventilation and elevate his legs

Question 41

Individuals with tracheal stomas require distinct methods of ventilation compared to those without such openings. Which of the following statements regarding these ventilation methods is accurate?

- ☐ A specialized adapter for tracheostomy can be inserted into the stoma or affixed to the tracheostomy tube, allowing a BVM to administer artificial ventilation with 100% oxygen.
- ☐ The head tilt-chin lift technique aids in maintaining airway patency during ventilation through a tracheal stoma. Placing a rolled towel under the neck can ensure proper tracheal alignment.
- ☐ An effective assisted ventilation technique involves sealing the patient's mouth and nose when ventilating through a stoma, and then unsealing them during passive exhalation.
- ☐ Inserting an OPA prior to BVM ventilation through a stoma assists in maintaining airway patency for vomiting patients. Suctioning through the oropharynx to the level of the stoma is permissible if there is significant vomitus.

Question 42

What is a clinical reason for employing a tracheostomy mask?

- ☐ The patient has a tracheal stoma
- ☐ The patient presents symptoms of hypoxia
- ☐ The patient requires a standard oxygen level
- ☐ The patient is experiencing hyperventilation

Question 43

How is the term 'golden hour' best defined?

- ☐ The interval from the moment an injury occurs to when surgery is performed
- ☐ The 60 key assessment points that must be evaluated
- ☐ The duration it takes to react to an emergency call after an injury has happened
- ☐ The final hour of a work shift

Question 44

Identify the procedure that should be avoided in a 9-year-old with a cranial fracture resulting from a horseback riding incident.

- ☐ Examination of limbs
- ☐ Oropharyngeal airway
- ☐ Nasopharyngeal airway
- ☐ Airway evaluation

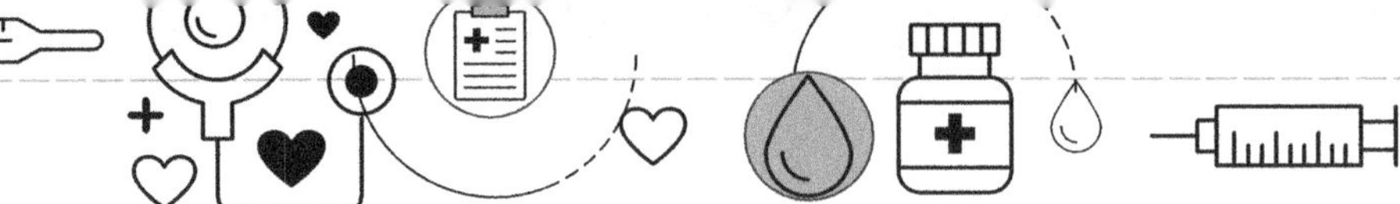

Question 45

An 84-year-old male patient presents with auditory crepitations during lung auscultation, along with reports of chest discomfort and pulmonary congestion. These clinical manifestations may be indicative of which condition?

- ☐ Pulmonary embolism
- ☐ Left ventricular failure
- ☐ Vena cava collapse
- ☐ Right ventricular failure

Question 46

What is a clinical sign that necessitates the suctioning of the upper respiratory tract?

- ☐ A coughing sound observed during a patient's breathing.
- ☐ A snoring sound detected during a patient's breathing.
- ☐ A gurgling noise noted during a patient's respiration.
- ☐ A stridor sound heard during a patient's respiration.

Question 47

What is a key benefit of using supplemental oxygen therapy?

- ☐ Increasing the concentration of oxygen can enhance pulmonary respiration and replace all inert gases
- ☐ Increasing the concentration of oxygen can enhance cellular respiration and replace some inert gases
- ☐ Increasing the concentration of oxygen can enhance cellular respiration and replace all inert gases
- ☐ Increasing the concentration of oxygen can enhance pulmonary respiration and replace some inert gases

Question 48

After attending to a call concerning an unidentified ailment or injury alongside your colleague Aaron, you arrive at an apartment complex and notice a woman lying supine with her eyes closed in the parking lot. Following an assessment ensuring the safety of the environment, what would be the most effective method for obtaining pertinent information about her condition?

- ☐ Manually check her pulse and observe for nasal flaring
- ☐ Locate the individual who made the call and inquire about the situation
- ☐ Immediately initiate ventilation with high-flow oxygen
- ☐ Assess her pulse manually while placing your ear near her mouth and watching the sternum for signs of chest movement

Question 49

Calculate the respiratory minute volume for an individual with a respiratory rate of 20 breaths per minute and a tidal volume of 300 milliliters.

- ☐ 3000 mL/min
- ☐ 4000 mL/min
- ☐ 6000 mL/min
- ☐ 8000 mL/min

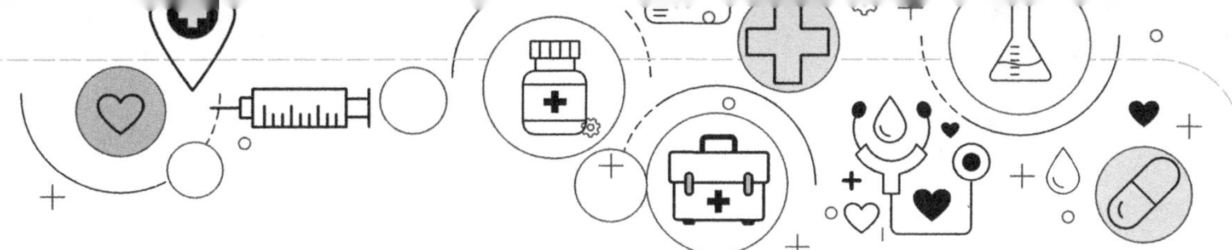

Question 50

You are summoned to a childcare center where a 3-year-old boy has lost consciousness after choking on a plastic toy. Upon arrival, you observe the child in a supine position on the floor while the caregiver is unsuccessfully attempting to administer artificial respirations. 'I am unable to get any air into him!' she exclaims. Upon a swift examination of the oral cavity, a partially visible object deeply embedded near the glottis can be seen. What is the appropriate immediate action to take?

- ☐ Start chest compressions to dislodge the obstruction and periodically check the airway.
- ☐ Flip the child over and administer 5 quick back blows with the head slightly lowered.
- ☐ Insert your fingers into the child's mouth and try to swipe the object out.
- ☐ Initiate abdominal thrusts to dislodge the obstruction and provide ventilation if possible.

Answers & Explanation
Page 209

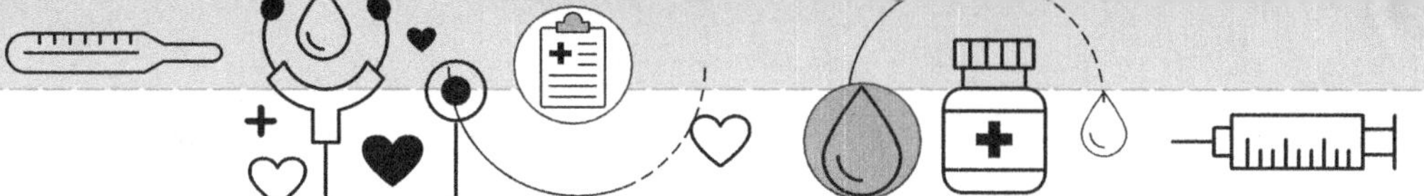

MEDICAL / OBSTETRICS / GYNECOLOGY

Question 1

When a patient experiencing chest pain inquires about the number of chambers in the human heart, how do you respond?

- ☐ There are 5 chambers: the apex, the right and left atria, and the right and left ventricles.
- ☐ There are 4 chambers: the right and left atria, and the right and left ventricles.
- ☐ There are 3 chambers: the mitral, biscuspid, and tricuspid.
- ☐ The heart has no chambers.

Question 2

Encountering an individual lying on their stomach is best described as which position?

- ☐ Prone
- ☐ Fowler
- ☐ Supine
- ☐ Postparty

Question 3

A male motorcyclist involved in a collision with a car displays multiple injuries, including head trauma and several lacerations on his knees and feet. Despite efforts, such as verbal requests and a sternal rub, he does not open his eyes. He mumbles unintelligibly, and his arms and hands are drawn tightly to his chest. He does not respond to instructions to raise his arm. What is his Glasgow Coma Scale (GCS) score?

- ☐ 4
- ☐ 5
- ☐ 6
- ☐ 7

Question 4

In which anatomical structure within the maternal body does embryonic and fetal development occur?

- ☐ Vagina
- ☐ Cervix
- ☐ Placenta
- ☐ Uterus

Question 5

Upon evaluating a stroke patient, you observe the presence of dysarthria. This condition is defined by which of the following symptoms?

- ☐ Slurred speech
- ☐ Difficulty comprehending questions
- ☐ Impairment on the left side of the body
- ☐ Drooping of the face

Question 6

Which of the following accurately characterizes the role of plasma within the human body?

- ☐ It purifies the blood from infections and dead cells
- ☐ It is responsible for transporting carbon dioxide throughout the body
- ☐ It carries cells to different parts of the body
- ☐ It plays the primary role in blood clot formation

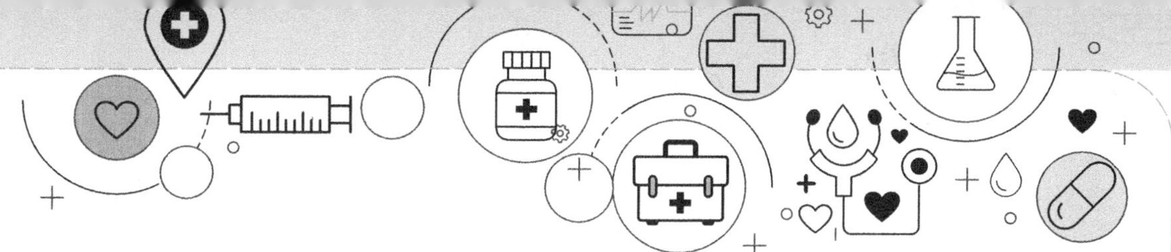

Question 7

Among the following physiological responses, which is regulated by the sympathetic division of the autonomic nervous system?

- ☐ Reduction in pupil size
- ☐ Decreased heart rate and gastrointestinal motility
- ☐ Frequency of breaths
- ☐ Narrowing of blood vessels

Question 8

At which phase of labor is the rupture of the amniotic sac most commonly observed?

- ☐ Initial stage
- ☐ Fourth stage
- ☐ Second stage
- ☐ Third stage

Question 9

Which of the following is not a role of the pancreas?

- ☐ Assists in fat digestion
- ☐ Assists in protein digestion
- ☐ Controls the level of glucose in the bloodstream
- ☐ Controls the level of iron in the bloodstream.

Question 10

Given the rising threat of nerve agent exposure, emergency medical service (EMS) teams must be equipped with appropriate antidote kits. Which of the following options correctly identifies these antidote kits?

- ☐ Mark 1 kits or NAAK
- ☐ Maxkits or Nervadoct kits
- ☐ MOVAK 5 Kits or VOMAK 5 Kits
- ☐ TRAX1 or Vtax kits

Question 11

Upon arriving at a senior care facility, you and your colleague Rodrigo discover that both staff and residents are experiencing vomiting and dizziness. What is the most likely cause?

- ☐ An inadequate number of emergency teams dispatched
- ☐ A widespread flu outbreak
- ☐ An abundance of medical supplies available
- ☐ The presence of a harmful chemical or substance

Question 12

What is an alternative medical term used to describe inadequate blood flow to tissues?

- ☐ Stroke
- ☐ Shock
- ☐ Hypertension
- ☐ Hyperperfusion

Question 13

Upon arrival at a multi-casualty incident with your colleague Lola, which of the following patients should be deemed the highest priority for immediate medical intervention?

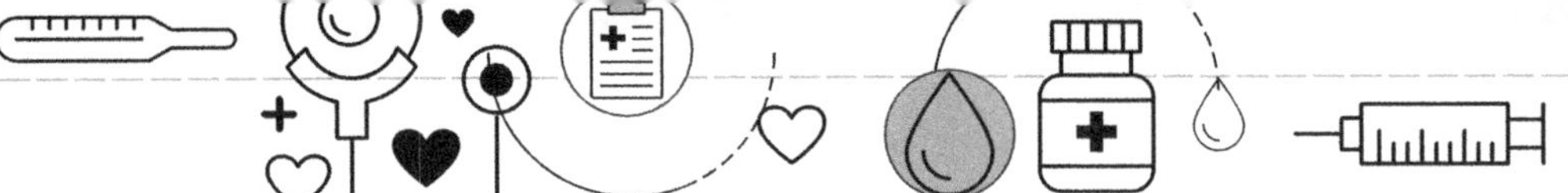

- ☐ A 19-year-old male with an ulna fracture
- ☐ A 29-year-old pregnant woman experiencing contractions every 12 minutes
- ☐ A 24-year-old female who has been stung by a few wasps
- ☐ A 45-year-old woman with a blood pressure of 169/92

Question 14

A severe winter storm has left numerous individuals stranded on a highway for several days. You have been called to assist with the National Guard to provide aid to those suffering from cold exposure. As you gather your supplies, what items should you prioritize and why?

- ☐ Oral glucose; Extended periods without food may result in low blood glucose levels
- ☐ Blankets; Patients encountered will require substantial warming, for which blankets are necessary
- ☐ Drinking water; Dehydration is a highly probable issue
- ☐ Warm IV fluids; To address hypothermia in patients, warm IV fluids will be needed

Question 15

Which clinical manifestations would signify that a patient's condition has escalated from a mild allergic response to anaphylaxis?

- ☐ Experiencing a drop in blood pressure versus an elevation in blood pressure
- ☐ Circulatory shock or severe respiratory distress
- ☐ Having a fast versus a slow heart rate
- ☐ If hives diminish after administering Benadryl

Question 16

What is denoted by the abbreviation 'mmHg'?

- ☐ Millimeters of mercury
- ☐ Millimeters of hydrostat
- ☐ Millimeters of hydrogen
- ☐ Millimeters of pressure

Question 17

What is the term for an infant born with the buttocks presenting first?

- ☐ Cephalic presentation
- ☐ Placental abruption
- ☐ Ryan
- ☐ Breech

Question 18

Syncope can arise from various emergency situations. Which term is commonly used to refer to Syncope?

- ☐ Low blood pressure
- ☐ Emesis
- ☐ Fainting
- ☐ Vomiting

Question 19

What are the primary etiologies of shock?

- ☐ Physical injury, cardiac arrest, and convulsions
- ☐ Inadequate cardiac output, fluid depletion, and excessive vessel dilation
- ☐ Insufficient blood flow, cognitive decline, and compromised respiratory function
- ☐ Vessel constriction, impaired vascular function, and respiratory insufficiency

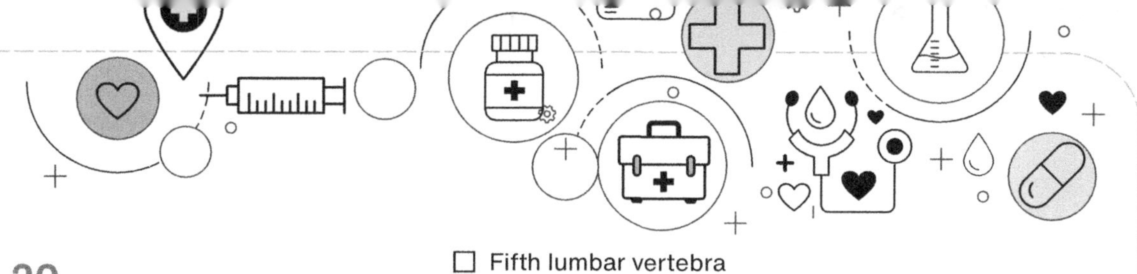

Question 20

What does the term 'Hemiparesis' signify?

- ☐ All of these options
- ☐ Loss of bladder control
- ☐ Presence of blood in urine
- ☐ Unilateral body weakness

Question 21

Upon arriving at the location of an unidentified medical incident with your colleague Abner, what should be your primary focus as you assess the scene?

- ☐ Prescription bottles or items indicating the patient's medical background
- ☐ Potential hazards that could compromise scene safety
- ☐ Signs indicating a physical confrontation
- ☐ An individual who can provide the patient's medical history

Question 22

Regarding the prevalence of seizures in the United States, it is noted to be ________. Emergency Medical Services (EMS) report that approximately _______ of their emergency 911 calls are related to seizures.

- ☐ high, 30%
- ☐ low, 30%
- ☐ low, 10%
- ☐ high, 60%

Question 23

Identify the perineum from the following options.

- ☐ Radius of the cervix when dilated
- ☐ Fifth lumbar vertebra
- ☐ Abdominal lining
- ☐ Region between the anus and vaginal opening

Question 24

Determine the equivalent weight of 150 pounds in kilograms.

- ☐ 67.5 kilograms
- ☐ 90 kilograms
- ☐ 80 kilograms
- ☐ 100 kilograms

Question 25

In the context of the mnemonic OPQRST, what does the letter 'T' represent?

- ☐ Trachea
- ☐ Time
- ☐ Temperature
- ☐ Topography

Question 26

In the context of a detailed ocular examination, upon which of the following should attention not be concentrated?

- ☐ Pigmentation of the pupils
- ☐ Pink, moist conjunctiva
- ☐ Pupil dimensions
- ☐ Light responsiveness

Question 27

In conducting a detailed history of a patient's presenting symptoms, healthcare professionals utilize the acronym OPQRST. What inquiry does the letter 'O' denote?

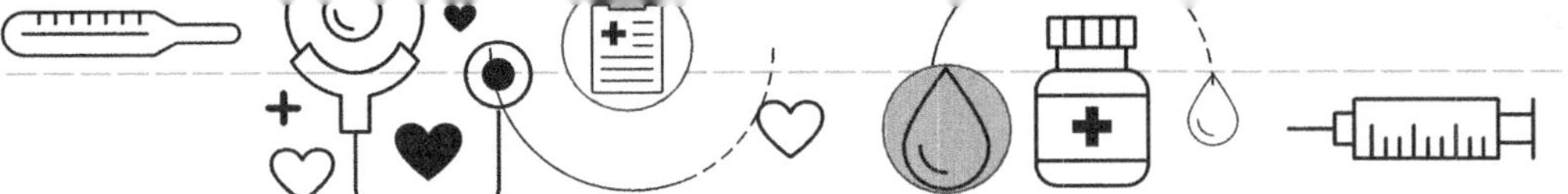

- ☐ Off set
- ☐ When did it start?
- ☐ Have you had Operations?
- ☐ Does it feel Ordinary?

Question 28

In the course of conducting a secondary evaluation of the abdominal region, which of the following should not be closely examined:

- ☐ Rigidity
- ☐ Distention
- ☐ Medical devices
- ☐ Retractions

Question 29

Which of the subsequent factors can induce hypoglycemia?

- ☐ Administering an excessive amount of insulin
- ☐ Insufficient caloric intake
- ☐ All of the mentioned factors
- ☐ Intense physical activity

Question 30

Which of the following symptoms is not characteristic of alcohol withdrawal?

- ☐ Tremors
- ☐ Sweating
- ☐ Pinpoint pupils
- ☐ Hallucinations

Question 31

The temporal characteristics of the immune system's response to an allergenic stimulus can be classified as _______________ and ___________________.

- ☐ slow (exceeding 90 minutes) and rapid (within 90 minutes)
- ☐ slow (over 15 minutes) and rapid (within 15 minutes)
- ☐ slow (more than 30 minutes) and rapid (within 30 minutes)
- ☐ slow (more than 60 minutes) and rapid (within 60 minutes)

Question 32

The most frequent site of an aneurysm is the ___________ and typically presents as ___________________.

- ☐ female population / associated with extreme pain
- ☐ abdominal region / symptomless
- ☐ male population / leading to significant chest discomfort
- ☐ chest cavity / a consequence of an injury

Question 33

The _____________ stage of a seizure, which involves convulsive movements, is the third in sequence.

- ☐ Clonic phase
- ☐ Postictal phase
- ☐ Aura phase
- ☐ Tonic phase

Question 34

How do the primary structural differences between pediatric and adult airways manifest?

- ☐ There are no anatomical differences; children's airways are identical to those of adults.
- ☐ Children's airways are shorter and more compact, facilitating easier visualization of the vocal cords.

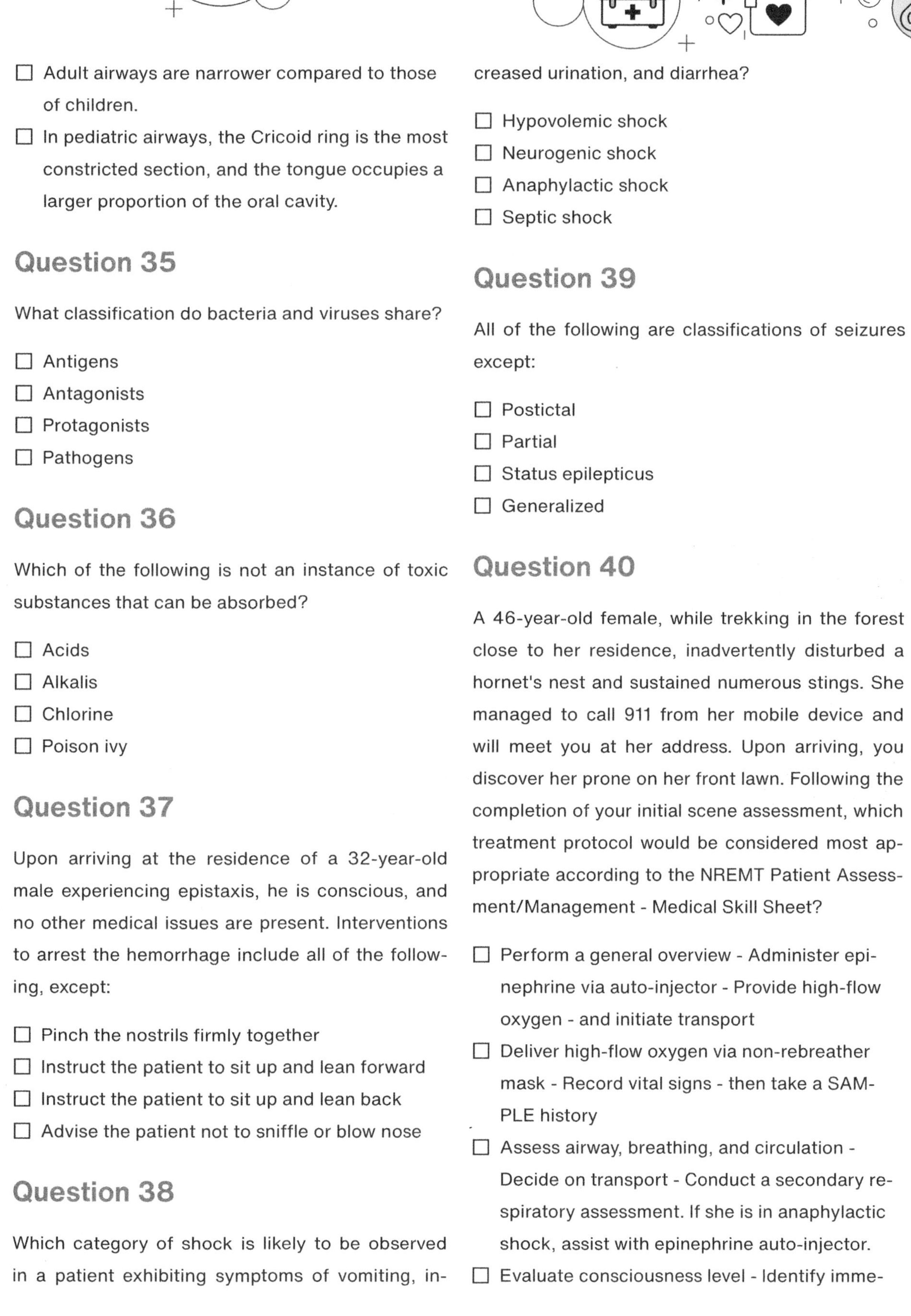

- ☐ Adult airways are narrower compared to those of children.
- ☐ In pediatric airways, the Cricoid ring is the most constricted section, and the tongue occupies a larger proportion of the oral cavity.

Question 35

What classification do bacteria and viruses share?

- ☐ Antigens
- ☐ Antagonists
- ☐ Protagonists
- ☐ Pathogens

Question 36

Which of the following is not an instance of toxic substances that can be absorbed?

- ☐ Acids
- ☐ Alkalis
- ☐ Chlorine
- ☐ Poison ivy

Question 37

Upon arriving at the residence of a 32-year-old male experiencing epistaxis, he is conscious, and no other medical issues are present. Interventions to arrest the hemorrhage include all of the following, except:

- ☐ Pinch the nostrils firmly together
- ☐ Instruct the patient to sit up and lean forward
- ☐ Instruct the patient to sit up and lean back
- ☐ Advise the patient not to sniffle or blow nose

Question 38

Which category of shock is likely to be observed in a patient exhibiting symptoms of vomiting, increased urination, and diarrhea?

- ☐ Hypovolemic shock
- ☐ Neurogenic shock
- ☐ Anaphylactic shock
- ☐ Septic shock

Question 39

All of the following are classifications of seizures except:

- ☐ Postictal
- ☐ Partial
- ☐ Status epilepticus
- ☐ Generalized

Question 40

A 46-year-old female, while trekking in the forest close to her residence, inadvertently disturbed a hornet's nest and sustained numerous stings. She managed to call 911 from her mobile device and will meet you at her address. Upon arriving, you discover her prone on her front lawn. Following the completion of your initial scene assessment, which treatment protocol would be considered most appropriate according to the NREMT Patient Assessment/Management - Medical Skill Sheet?

- ☐ Perform a general overview - Administer epinephrine via auto-injector - Provide high-flow oxygen - and initiate transport
- ☐ Deliver high-flow oxygen via non-rebreather mask - Record vital signs - then take a SAMPLE history
- ☐ Assess airway, breathing, and circulation - Decide on transport - Conduct a secondary respiratory assessment. If she is in anaphylactic shock, assist with epinephrine auto-injector.
- ☐ Evaluate consciousness level - Identify imme-

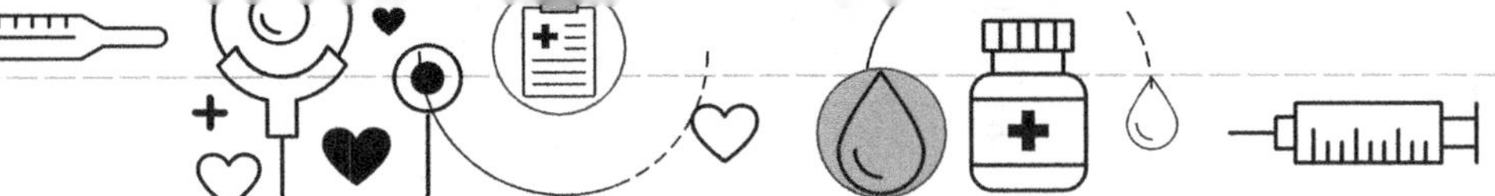

diate threats - Evaluate airway, breathing, and circulation

Question 41

On a warm afternoon in August, you receive an emergency call to attend to a 78-year-old male who has frequently been a patient in your ambulance. The dispatch indicates that his caregiver discovered him lying in an empty bathtub, unable to exit on his own. Upon your arrival, the patient recognizes you and expresses regret for the 911 call, stating that he merely needs assistance to get out of the tub. Observations reveal that his respiratory rate is 20 breaths per minute with normal depth, his skin is slightly flushed, his pulse rate is 118 beats per minute, and his blood pressure reads 138/78. He denies experiencing any pain. What could be the probable cause of his condition and what is the recommended course of action?

- ☐ He has fallen and likely injured himself, which has resulted in his inability to exit the bathtub independently. Utilize cervical spine precautions and a Ked-sled to transfer him to a backboard.
- ☐ He is experiencing hypothermia. Cover him with a blanket and help him out of the bathtub. Apply heat packs to his underarms and groin area, provide high-flow oxygen, and transport him to the nearest hospital for further evaluation.
- ☐ The only issue is his physical inability to leave the bathtub. Assist him out of the tub and reassess his vital signs.
- ☐ He is suffering from heat exhaustion and dehydration. Assist him out of the bathtub and into a cool, air-conditioned environment. Provide small sips of water and administer high-flow oxygen. Transport him if he consents.

Question 42

You are attending to a 46-year-old male individual diagnosed with Type 1 diabetes mellitus. Emergency services were contacted by his partner, who discovered him in a fetal position on the bathroom floor, with a towel positioned beneath his head upon her return home from work. There are no apparent signs of physical injury. The patient is non-responsive, but his respiratory rate is stable at 16 breaths per minute, with adequate depth. His partner reports having a phone conversation with him earlier in the day, during which he appeared to be in good health. What is the most plausible reason for this individual's altered level of consciousness?

- ☐ He administered his insulin dose but did not consume food, resulting in hypoglycemia.
- ☐ He consumed an excessive amount of sugar, leading to hyperglycemia.
- ☐ He neglected his insulin regimen, causing hypoglycemia.
- ☐ He is experiencing a diabetic coma due to excessive insulin production by the pancreas.

Question 43

Upon responding with your colleague Wanda to a multi-vehicle collision, you are the second ambulance to reach the site. Your primary assessment reveals seven individuals involved across two vehicles, and extrication is unnecessary for any. In the first vehicle, you find a 42-year-old pregnant woman at 28 weeks gestation who is unconscious, a distressed 14-year-old girl reporting back pain, and a 7-year-old boy with a facial laceration but otherwise uninjured. The second vehicle contains an 86-year-old male driver slumped over the steering wheel and three teenagers in the back seat. The two teens on the impact side exhibit nausea and al-

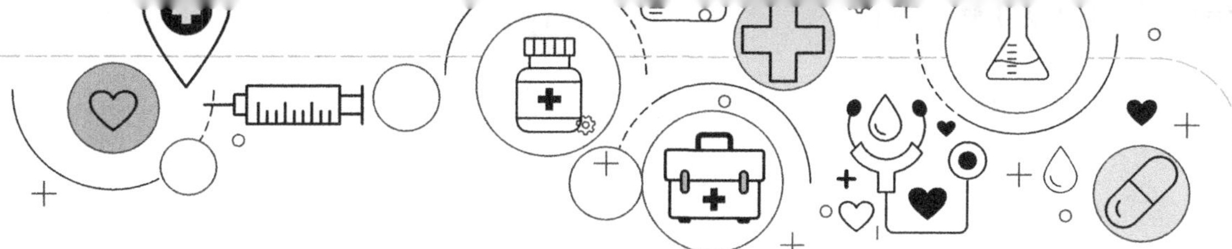

tered consciousness levels. The third teenager, a girl in the back seat, mentions she experienced seizures and vomiting earlier and her grandfather was driving her to the hospital; she shows no signs of injury and was wearing a seatbelt. Whom should your medical team prioritize for immediate attention?

- ☐ The girl who experienced seizures earlier
- ☐ The two teenagers with altered consciousness
- ☐ The girl reporting back pain
- ☐ The 86-year-old male and the pregnant woman

Question 44

You are summoned to the Shadypines elder care facility to attend to an octogenarian male exhibiting altered consciousness and tachycardia. Upon arrival, a nurse is measuring his blood pressure, which registers at 98/62 mmHg. The patient is diaphoretic, tremulous, and febrile. The nurse informs you that he has diabetes mellitus and was recently discharged from the hospital following a surgery for diverticulitis two days prior. Despite multiple attempts to rouse him by calling his name, he fails to open his eyes. The only verbal response he provides when questioned is the repetition of the name "Katherine." He is unresponsive to commands to move his extremities but withdraws his hand to his chest and moans when subjected to a sternal rub. What is this patient's Glasgow Coma Scale (GCS) score, and what is the most probable diagnosis for his condition?

- ☐ GCS of 8/ He has congestive heart failure
- ☐ GCS of 9/ He is in septic shock
- ☐ GCS of 6/ He is having an allergic reaction to antibiotics
- ☐ GCS of 7/ He is in insulin shock

Question 45

Given no additional context, assess the condition of the following pediatric patient: A 12-month-old male presenting with a heart rate of 110 bpm, a respiratory rate of 30 per minute, and a systolic blood pressure of 90 mmHg.

- ☐ Healthy
- ☐ Unwell
- ☐ Critical
- ☐ Fair

Question 46

How is 'behavior' most accurately characterized?

- ☐ An individual's reaction to occurrences that disrupt daily activities.
- ☐ The thoughts an individual has regarding their surroundings.
- ☐ Any activity performed by a person that deviates from their usual routine.
- ☐ Observable responses by an individual to their environment, including their actions.

Question 47

The phenomenon where a blood clot dislodges and migrates to another part of the circulatory system is known as ______________.

- ☐ Thrombus
- ☐ Aneurysm
- ☐ Embolism
- ☐ Clot

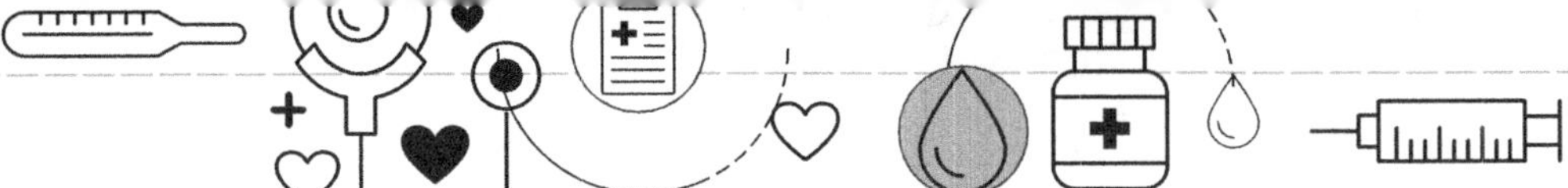

Question 48

All of the following are recognized long-term consequences of chronic alcohol consumption, except:

- ☐ Infertility
- ☐ Hepatitis
- ☐ Seizures
- ☐ Elevated risk for breast cancer

Question 49

In the context of a diabetic crisis, the preference for administering glucose over sucrose is due to what reason?

- ☐ Complex sugars expedite cellular activation processes
- ☐ Glucose, being a monosaccharide, is metabolized more rapidly
- ☐ Sucrose, being a monosaccharide, is required, while the body needs polysaccharides
- ☐ Monosaccharides have a slower rate of absorption in the body

Question 50

Define the term Hyperglycemia.

- ☐ A medical condition characterized by elevated blood glucose levels beyond the normal range.
- ☐ A medical condition where blood glucose levels remain within normal parameters.
- ☐ A medical condition involving blood glucose levels that are close to normal.
- ☐ A medical condition marked by blood glucose levels that are below the normal range.

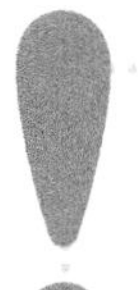

Answers & Explanation
Page 220

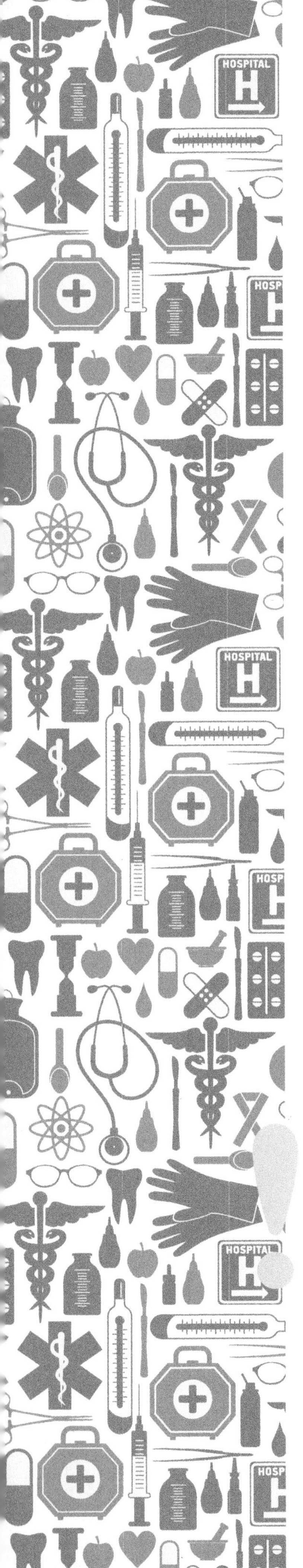

Dear Reader,

We understand that preparing for the NREMT exam can feel like a challenging task, and that's why we want to provide you with additional tools to support your journey toward success.

As a valued customer, you have exclusive access to our advanced e-learning platform, "Learnik," designed to enhance your study experience and offer targeted resources to help you excel in the NREMT exam. By scanning the QR code below, you'll unlock a wealth of supplementary learning resources directly related to the topics covered in this book.

On Learnik, you'll find a variety of interactive features to optimize your preparation:

Scenario-Based Quizzes: The platform generates personalized quizzes based on real-life scenarios and the content of the book you've purchased. These quizzes are designed to reinforce your understanding of key concepts and skills essential for the NREMT exam and help you track your progress.

But there's more! Learnik also offers a wide range of bonus content to enrich your learning experience:

Audiobooks: Study on the go with our professionally narrated audiobooks, allowing you to learn during your commute or downtime.

Flashcards: An effective tool for quickly memorizing essential medical terminology, procedures, and guidelines. Our flashcards are structured to present critical facts in a clear and concise format.

These resources are designed to complement your study routine, making your preparation more comprehensive and efficient. They are available exclusively to our valued customers like you, helping to maximize your chances of success in the NREMT exam.

So why wait? Scan the QR code below and embark on your learning journey with Learnik. It's the perfect way to elevate your NREMT exam preparation. We're here to support you every step of the way as you work toward your goals.

Thank you for choosing our educational materials, and we wish you all the best in your NREMT exam preparation!

For any issues, feel free to contact us at *info@learnik.com*

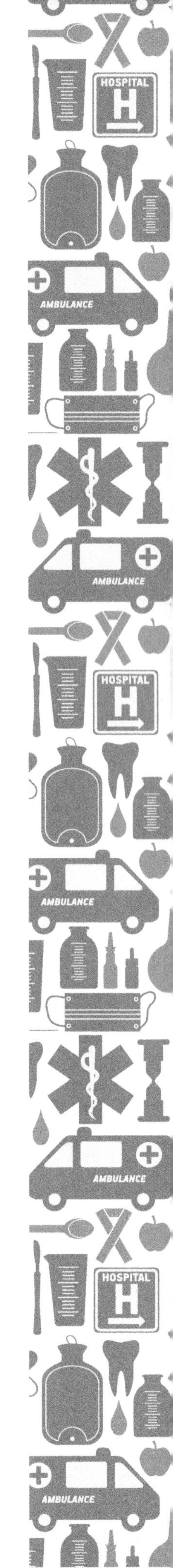

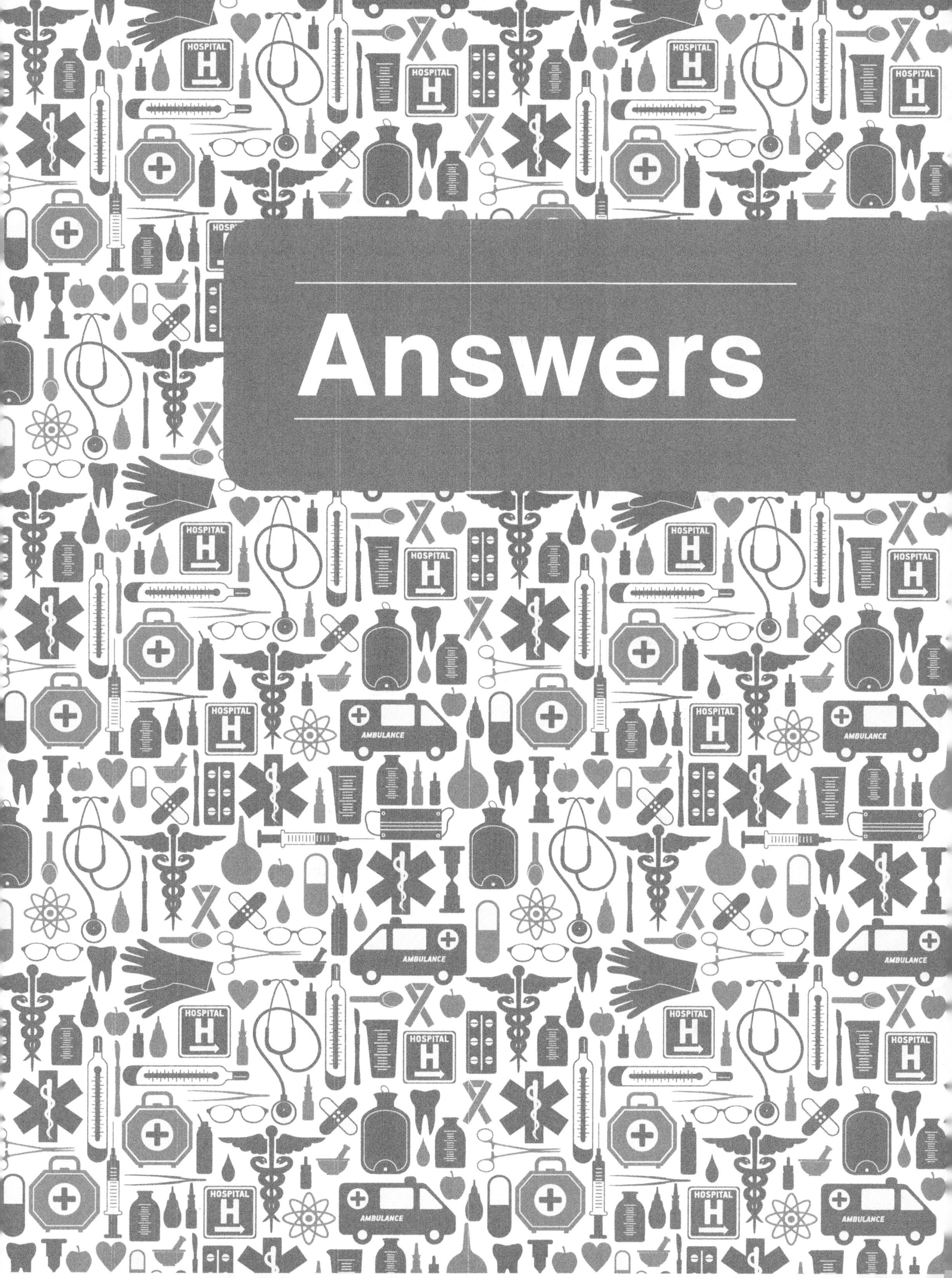

Answers

TRAUMA

Question 1

A male patient in his 20s presents with an open fracture on the lateral aspect of his lower leg. Which bone is most probably fractured?

☐ **Fibula**

Explanation: The fibula, being the thinner and smaller bone located on the outer side of the lower leg, is the most likely to be fractured in this scenario.

Question 2

Which position is optimal for a patient experiencing shock?

☐ **Supine with legs elevated**

Explanation: Elevating the legs while lying flat supine is generally recommended to facilitate venous return to the heart.

Question 3

In the context of using a traction splinting apparatus, complete the following statement: Fasten the splint's support straps around the limb and disengage the ____________ once the ________________ is achieved.

☐ **Manual traction / mechanical traction**

Explanation: After applying the mechanical traction, it is appropriate to let go of the manual stabilization of the limb.

Question 4

An extensive physical assessment ought to be performed ________________.

☐ **Subsequent to executing vital emergency interventions**

Explanation: A comprehensive physical examination should commence only once immediate threats to life have been addressed.

Question 5

Which of the following options does not categorize a mechanism of injury associated with penetrating trauma based on velocity?

☐ **Vital velocity**

Explanation: Penetrating trauma is typically classified into high, medium, and low velocity categories, where velocity denotes the rate of speed.

Question 6

In the context of the AVPU scale utilized to evaluate a patient's consciousness, what does the letter 'V' denote?

☐ **Responsive to verbal stimuli**

Explanation: Alert - Verbal - Pain - Unresponsive (Unconscious).

Question 7

In the context of performing an initial evaluation on a patient with a substantial mechanism of injury (MOI), which option listed below is not pertinent to evaluating their respiratory function?

☐ **Conduct a quick neurological assessment**

Explanation: The initial evaluation for respiratory function in a patient with a significant MOI should encompass the following: Evaluating ventilation, inspecting the thorax and neck, auscultating breath sounds, and delivering high-flow oxygen.

Question 8

The prefix 'cost-' denotes which anatomical structure?

☐ **Ribcage**

Explanation: The prefix 'cost-' is associated with the ribcage.

Question 9

In which of the following scenarios is it necessary to don gloves, a gown, mask, and protective eyewear?

☐ **Arterial bleeding control**

Explanation: Managing arterial bleeding, where blood spurts, necessitates full protective gear.

Question 10

In which part of the human body can the radius be found?

☐ **Adjacent to the thumb in the arm**

Explanation: The radius is a bone situated on the lateral side of the forearm, adjacent to the thumb.

Question 11

Initial shock is known as ____; in contrast, advanced shock is referred to as _____.

☐ **Compensated / decompensated**

Explanation: In the initial stages of shock, the body successfully compensates for its effects. However, as the condition progresses beyond the body's compensatory mechanisms, it transitions into advanced or decompensated shock.

Question 12

Which of the following actions are advisable when managing traumatic vaginal bleeding?

☐ **Insert gloved fingers into the vagina**

Explanation: Essential steps in handling vaginal bleeding due to trauma include checking for pregnancy, using a sterile absorbent pad, and identifying the cause of the injury. Inserting fingers or other objects into the vaginal area should be avoided.

Question 13

Thermal health conditions are classified into which two primary categories?

☐ **'cold-related'; 'heat-related'**

Explanation: Thermal health conditions are generally categorized into 'cold-related' and 'heat-related' illnesses.

Question 14

Individuals exhibiting discrepant pupil sizes are likely to have what condition?

☐ **Could be a normal variant**

Explanation: Anisocoria is a phenomenon observed in 2 to 4 percent of the population, characterized by naturally unequal pupil sizes.

Question 15

In the study of trauma kinematics, all of the following represent types of blunt trauma collisions except:

☐ **Organs impacting external to the body**

Explanation: In Trauma Kinematics, blunt trauma collisions encompass: a vehicle hitting another object, the patient impacting a part of the vehicle, and internal organs impacting each other within the body.

Question 16

What is your initial assessment of the patient?

☐ **An evaluation that helps determine the severity of the patient's condition**

Explanation: This comprises observing the patient's physical state, surroundings, and primary complaint, aiding in evaluating the urgency of the situation.

Question 17

In the acronym DCAPBTLS, to what does the letter 'S' refer?

☐ **Swelling**

Explanation: This acronym denotes: Deformity, contusions, abrasions, penetrations (punctures), burns, tenderness, lacerations, and swelling.

Question 18

Under what circumstances would you extract a foreign object embedded in the cheek?

☐ **It poses a threat to the airway**

Explanation: AThe necessity to remove the object arises if it compromises the airway.

Question 19

What is the most recommended position for transporting a patient experiencing shock?

☐ **Lying flat with legs raised**

Explanation: Positioning the patient supine with elevated legs is beneficial to facilitate the return of blood to the heart.

Question 20

In the AVPU scale utilized to evaluate a patient's responsiveness, what does the letter 'P' denote?

☐ **Pain**

Explanation: The AVPU scale consists of: Alert, Verbal, Pain, and Unconscious (unresponsive).

Question 21

In the context of the SAMPLE acronym in medical history taking, the query "Have you previously experienced any cardiac issues?" corresponds to which letter?

☐ **P**

Explanation: PAST medical history.

Question 22

Which of the following does not describe a typical injury mechanism in orthopedic trauma?

☐ **Torsional force**

Explanation: In orthopedic trauma, mechanisms of injury include: Direct impact can fracture the bone at the site of the blow. Indirect force results in damage away from the impact site. It is imperative to consider associated injuries and determine the point of contact and the mechanism of injury (MOI). A twisting force is frequently observed in knee injuries.

Question 23

Identify the option that does not belong to the upper limb anatomy.

☐ **Patella**

Explanation: The patella, known as the kneecap, is a component of the lower limbs. Conversely, the other options are elements of the upper limbs: the radius and ulna constitute the forearm's bones, and the humerus forms the upper arm structure.

Question 24

Upon arriving at a mass casualty incident along with your colleague Jermain, you initiate treatment for a severe arterial hemorrhage on a woman who had been ejected from a vehicle. As you provide her with a trauma dressing to hold and ask her to apply pressure, you hear an infant crying nearby. You proceed to investigate the source of the distressing sound coming from the car. What actions have you taken?

☐ **Abandoned the patient**

Explanation: Abandoning a patient refers to the act of leaving them without ensuring the same or a superior level of medical care continues in your stead. The Good Samaritan Law does not offer protections in cases of negligence, abandonment, or any situation where the patient's best interests are compromised.

Question 25

Which of the following is not a factor to consider in cases of electrical emergencies?

☐ **Lightning rarely leads to cardiac arrest**

Explanation: Critical factors in electrical emergencies encompass: superficial skin injuries that do not reflect the severity of burns, the presence of both entrance and exit wounds, the potential for cardiac arrest precipitated by electrical exposure, and the occurrence of cardiac arrest due to lightning strikes.

Question 26

During exposure to cold environments, which of the following does NOT contribute to an increased risk of cold-related injuries?

☐ **Reduction in local blood circulation**

Explanation: Factors such as the individual's clothing, age, duration of exposure, consumption of alcohol or other substances, level of physical activity, and pre-existing medical conditions or injuries are known to influence the risk of sustaining a cold injury.

Question 27

You respond to a situation involving a postal service vehicle that has lost control on a dirt track and overturned. Eyewitnesses have indicated that the vehicle ignited, and the postal worker is outside attempting to recover scattered mail. Upon your arrival, the fire brigade has just extinguished the flames, and the driver is observing the smoldering debris from a distance. Your immediate course of action should be:

☐ **Implement cervical spine stabilization using a standing backboard**

Explanation: Considering the high-impact incident involving a vehicular rollover, it is prudent to implement cervical spine immobilization using a standing backboard procedure. The driver may appear ambulatory due to adrenaline, which can conceal significant injuries; thus, they may still be susceptible to cervical or spinal damage.

Question 28

In the context of the SAMPLE assessment, the observation of a patient's pallor is classified as ________.

☐ **A sign**

Explanation: A sign is something that can be objectively observed, whereas a symptom is reported by the patient.

Question 29

What is a common consequence of a scalp laceration?

☐ **Severe bleeding**

Explanation: Scalp wounds are known to bleed significantly due to the extensive network of blood vessels in the area.

Question 30

Which response alternative does not fall under the distinctive anatomical, physiological, and pathophysiological considerations for injured elderly patients?

☐ **Brain enlargement heightening the risk of cerebral hemorrhaging after head trauma**

Explanation: Distinctive considerations for the anatomy, physiology, and pathophysiology of injured elderly patients include: Alterations in pulmonary, cardiovascular, neurological, and musculoskeletal systems render older individuals more prone to trauma; circulatory changes result in an inability to sustain normal vital signs during hemorrhage, with blood pressure decreasing more rapidly; the increased prevalence of multiple medications may impact assessments, notably vital signs and blood clotting processes; brain atrophy increases the likelihood of intracerebral hemorrhage following head trauma; skeletal modifications, such as curvature of the upper spine, may necessitate additional padding during spinal immobilization; diminished strength, sensory deficits, and chronic medical conditions heighten the risk of falls.

Question 31

Your colleague proposes that the patient may have sustained a zygomatic fracture. This would imply injury to which region of the body?

☐ **Facial area**

Explanation: The zygoma refers to the cheekbone, thus indicating facial trauma.

Question 32

You and your colleague have been dispatched to an ATV incident. Upon arrival, you find a 60-year-old male lying adjacent to the roadway. He reports that he lost control of the four-wheeler, resulting in it overturning multiple times. Which of the following options represents the MOST accurate procedural sequence?

☐ **BSI - Direct assistant to maintain manual head immobilization - Assess circulation, motor, and sensory functions - Apply cervical collar**

Explanation: Despite the NREMT discontinuing the evaluation of longboard spinal immobilization skills for candidates, it remains a critical procedure when required. Always begin with Body Substance Isolation (BSI) precautions before any patient contact. Ensure the application or direction of manual spinal stabilization, maintaining the head and neck in a neutral alignment. Additionally, check Circulation, Sensory, and Motor functions before applying a cervical collar to establish a baseline reference.

Question 33

The term 'evisceration' refers to which of the following conditions?

☐ **An internal organ extending through a bodily opening**

Explanation: Evisceration occurs when an internal organ exits through an opening in the body, typically due to a wound.

Question 34

You and your colleague Mary have been dispatched to a motor vehicle accident involving a single car and a moose. What should be your initial priority?

☐ **Ensure the scene is safe**

Explanation: Ensuring a safe environment should be the foremost concern. Eliminate any potential hazards beforehand.

Question 35

What does the letter 'R' signify in the OPQRST acronym?

☐ **Radiate**

Explanation: Radiate refers to whether the pain extends to other areas of the body, such as how heart attack pain can spread to the shoulder.

Question 36

In the mnemonic DCAPBTLS, to what does the letter 'P' refer?

☐ **Penetrations**

Explanation: DCAPBTLS is an acronym for Deformities, Contusions, Abrasions, Penetrations (or Punctures), Burns, Tenderness, Lacerations, Swelling.

Question 37

Upon arriving at the scene where an individual has been involved in a vehicular collision, you note significant damage to the front of the car. The individual is positioned upright in the driver's seat, reporting pain in the back and chest, which limits their ability to breathe deeply. What is the appropriate method to extricate this individual from the vehicle?

☐ **Employ a KED or similar device and then secure the patient to a spine board**

Explanation: The recommended technique involves utilizing a KED (Kendrick Extrication Device) or a similar apparatus to stabilize the patient while seated, followed by transferring them onto a spine board to ensure safe removal.

Question 38

Which of the following is NOT typically part of the standard protocol for burn treatment?

☐ **Apply cream to stop the burning**

Explanation: Common procedures in the management of burns include: halting the burning process, securing the airway, using dry, sterile, non-adherent dressings, removing jewelry and clothing, administering treatment for shock, preventing hypothermia, and ensuring transfer to an appropriate medical facility. It is critical to note that children and the elderly are more vulnerable and have increased mortality rates due to burns, and one should also be vigilant for potential signs of abuse.

Question 39

In the management of patients with a suspected cerebral trauma, which of the following procedures is not generally recommended?

☐ **Employ a rapid extrication for all patients**

Explanation: The management of individuals with suspected brain injuries typically includes: Ensuring a patent airway if the patient is unable to do so autonomously, the administration of supplemental oxygen, assisting ventilation when necessary, controlling external hemorrhage, elevating the head of the backboard by 30 degrees, rapidly transporting the patient, providing psychological support, and maintaining thorough communication and accurate documentation.

Question 40

Which of the following is not typically observed in the evaluation of muscle strains?

☐ **Swelling around the joint**

Explanation: Diagnostic indicators for muscle strains generally encompass: An audible "snap" at the moment of muscle rupture, pronounced muscle weakness, acute onset of sharp pain, and intense localized tenderness.

Question 41

Upon arriving at the scene of a single-vehicle collision where a truck skidded off the road and overturned, you find the driver was traveling approximately 40 MPH before encountering an icy patch and losing control. After conducting an initial assessment of the scene, which treatment option would be most suitable for the patient?

☐ **Initiate a rapid trauma assessment**

Explanation: Given the significant mechanism of injury from the vehicle rolling at 40 MPH, a rapid trauma assessment should be prioritized. This rapid evaluation is crucial to identifying and addressing any immediate life-threatening conditions.

Question 42

Upon your arrival at the scene of a multi-vehicle collision, accompanied by your colleague Wanda, you find yourselves as the second emergency medical team on-site. Preliminary assessment reveals there are seven individuals involved across two cars, none of which are trapped. In the first vehicle, there is a 42-year-old unconscious pregnant woman, who is 28 weeks along, a 14-year-old female with severe back pain and vocal distress, and a 7-year-old boy with a facial laceration but no other apparent injuries. The second vehicle contains an 86-year-old male, unconscious and leaning against the steering wheel. In the rear seats, there are three teenagers: two on the side of impact experiencing nausea and showing signs of altered mental status, and a third teenage girl, who reports having seizures and vomiting earlier and was en route to the hospital with her grandfather. She was wearing a seatbelt and exhibits no external injuries. Which individuals require immediate medical attention?

☐ **The 86-year-old man and the pregnant woman**

Explanation: Immediate medical intervention is warranted for individuals presenting with the lowest levels of responsiveness, notably the unconscious elderly man and the unconscious pregnant woman.

Question 43

Which of the following is not a recommended protocol in the management of rattlesnake envenomation?

☐ **Incise the bite site and extract the venom by suction**

Explanation: The management of rattlesnake envenomation involves several key steps, including: documenting the time of the bite for proper transport, ensuring slow venous return, maintaining the patient's calmness, immobilizing the affected limb, appropriately positioning the extremity, cleansing the bite area with soap and water, and identifying the snake if feasible.

Question 44

Which type of burn affects both the epidermal and dermal layers, excluding deeper tissues?

☐ **Partial-thickness burn**

Explanation: A superficial burn solely impacts the epidermis, whereas a secondary or partial-thickness burn involves both the epidermis and dermis.

Question 45

Which of the following is NOT a symptom of heat-related conditions characterized by elevated skin temperature?

☐ **nausea**

Explanation: Heat-related conditions, particularly those with elevated skin temperature, are often identified by symptoms such as minimal to no sweating—although, in cases of exertion-induced heat stroke, sweating may still occur; unconsciousness; accelerated respiration; an increased heart rate; and convulsions.

Question 46

A fracture that is only partial and does not extend through the entire bone is termed a _____ fracture.

☐ **Greenstick**

Explanation: A greenstick fracture involves an incomplete break partially through the bone's shaft, possibly resulting in significant bending, and is most common in children. An oblique fracture runs diagonally across the bone. A transverse fracture cuts across the bone horizontally. In a comminuted fracture, the bone is shattered or crushed into multiple fragments.

Question 47

Upon arriving at the scene, you find a 35-year-old male lying face down in a bathroom. He is unresponsive, and you proceed to carefully roll him onto his back while maintaining cervical spine stabilization. What should your subsequent action be?

☐ **Tap the shoulder and assess for responsiveness**

Explanation: In alignment with the NREMT medical and trauma protocols, the next priority is to evaluate the patient's responsiveness using the AVPU scale prior to airway management.

Question 48

At 8 a.m., you and your colleague Raymond are dispatched to a multi-vehicle accident on a congested secondary road. Upon your arrival, you observe at least six injured individuals and a chaotic scene with vehicles entangled, obstructing an entire traffic lane, and various fluids accumulating on the ground. You hear cries for help while traffic begins to navigate around the wreckage. Your immediate course of action should be...?

☐ **Request the fire department, establish a safety perimeter, and aid in maintaining a safe distance for traffic**

Explanation: Ensuring scene safety is paramount in this situation. The most critical action to take initially is to prevent the accident scene from escalating. This involves assisting with managing traffic and the crowd until emergency services arrive. Only then should medical care be administered in a secure environment.

Question 49

Which actions are performed during a swift trauma evaluation?

☐ **All of the above**

Explanation: These actions are methods employed to ascertain the presence of a medical or traumatic crisis.

Question 50

Which of the following most accurately characterizes a partial-thickness burn?

☐ **A burn affecting both the epidermal layer and portions of the dermis**

Explanation: A partial-thickness (second-degree) burn affects both the epidermis and the upper dermis without causing damage to the subcutaneous layer. The affected area typically appears moist, with a mottled red or white appearance and the presence of blisters. Such burns are noted for causing significant pain.

CARDIOLOGY AND RESUSCITATION

Question 1

You and your colleague Grimes receive an emergency call to a location where a stabbing incident has occurred. Two individuals have sustained injuries. One is a woman with a stab wound in the upper right quadrant (URQ) of her abdomen and is exhibiting difficulty in breathing, a pulse rate of 103, and a respiration rate of 35, with shallow breaths. The second patient is a man who has a stab wound in the lower right quadrant (LRQ) and is reporting intense abdominal pain; he has a pulse rate of 48 and a respiration rate of 24. Based on this information, which patient is more likely to present with hypotension (low blood pressure), and what is the rationale behind this conclusion?

☐ **The male patient, due to the specific type and location of his wound, may be experiencing internal blood loss. Additionally, his pulse rate is notably slow.**

Explanation: The male patient with a pulse rate of 48 and a lower right quadrant stab wound suggests the possibility of internal hemorrhaging, which can lead to decreased blood pressure.

Question 2

A person exhibiting tachycardia will have which characteristic?

☐ **A heart rate exceeding 100 bpm**

Explanation: A heart rate below 60 bpm is categorized as bradycardia, while a rate exceeding 100 bpm qualifies as tachycardia.

Question 3

Levine's sign, characterized by the involuntary clutching of a closed fist to the chest, typically occurs during which condition?

☐ **Experiencing an acute myocardial infarction**

Explanation: Levine's sign involves the gripping of a closed fist against the chest, often indicative of an acute myocardial infarction (AMI).

Question 4

Identify the option that is not a clinical manifestation of Cardiogenic shock.

☐ **Elevated skin temperature**

Explanation: Cardiogenic shock is characterized by a spectrum of clinical signs and symptoms: chest discomfort; dysrhythmic pulse; diminished pulse strength; hypotension; cyanosis observable on lips and beneath the nails; skin that is cool and moist; heightened anxiety; crackles in lung auscultation; and pulmonary edema.

Question 5

Which of the following can dysrhythmia encompass?

☐ **Either bradycardia or tachycardia**

Explanation: Alterations in cardiac rhythm may result in the heart operating at an accelerated or decelerated rate, or displaying irregular patterns.

Question 6

The correct size of a blood pressure cuff is essential, particularly in the case of pediatric patients. Utilizing a cuff that is excessively small will ______. Conversely, the use of a cuff that is excessively large will ________.

☐ **yield a falsely elevated reading / yield a**

falsely lowered reading

Explanation: Employing a cuff that is too small results in an inaccurately elevated blood pressure reading, while using a cuff that is too large leads to an inaccurately low reading.

Question 7

Among the subsequent assessment findings and manifestations, which one is unlikely to suggest that a patient has experienced a stroke or transient ischemic attack (TIA)?

☐ **Bleeding**

Explanation: Common findings and symptoms indicative of a stroke or TIA include: confusion, dizziness, weakness; alterations in consciousness; combative behavior, uncooperativeness, or restlessness; facial drooping, difficulty swallowing, tongue deviation; diplopia or blurred vision; speech difficulties or aphasia; reduced or absent motor function in one or more limbs; headache; sensory deficits in one or more limbs or other body parts; and coma.

Question 8

Whilst navigating through a supermarket, you observe a congregation surrounding an individual lying on the ground. Upon closer inspection, you discover a female, aged 48, who is both pulseless and apneic. What compression rate and depth do you administer?

☐ **30:2 / at least 2 inches**

Explanation: According to the guidelines set forth by the American Heart Association (AHA) for adult CPR, a compression-to-ventilation ratio of 30:2 must be employed. Furthermore, compressions should reach a minimum depth of 2 inches.

Question 9

Into which vessel does blood flow upon exiting the left ventricle?

☐ **Aortic arch**

Explanation: Upon departing from the left ventricle, the blood is conveyed into the aortic arch.

Question 10

What are the three primary etiologies of shock?

☐ **Inadequate cardiac output, hemorrhage, and vessel dilation**

Explanation: Shock primarily arises due to inadequate cardiac performance, significant hemorrhage or fluid depletion, and abnormal dilation of blood vessels.

Question 11

What is the foremost precaution when prescribing aspirin?

☐ **Coagulation abnormalities**

Explanation: The principal concern associated with aspirin use involves the risk of bleeding disorders, particularly within the gastrointestinal tract.

Question 12

In the instance of a cerebral infarction, neural cells that are deprived of adequate oxygenation for a prolonged period will inevitably face necrosis. What is the specific term for these cells?

☐ **Infarcted cells**

Explanation: Cells that have succumbed to necrosis due to prolonged oxygen deprivation are referred to as infarcted.

Question 13

Which chamber of the heart performs the most substantial work?

☐ **Left ventricle**

Explanation: The left ventricle is tasked with propelling blood into the aorta and subsequently throughout the entire body, frequently earning it the title of the heart's powerhouse.

Question 14

If an individual is experiencing bradycardia, it indicates they

☐ **Have a heart rate below 60 beats per minute**

Explanation: A heart rate under 60 beats per minute is classified as bradycardia.

Question 15

What is the underlying cause of an ischemic stroke?

☐ **Obstruction of cerebral blood flow**

Explanation: An ischemic stroke occurs due to an interruption in the cerebral blood supply, leading to a deficiency in oxygen delivery to brain tissues.

Question 16

Among the pulses detectable within the vascular network, which one is not recognized?

☐ **Anterior pulse**

Explanation: The known pulses within the vascular system include the carotid, femoral, radial, brachial, temporal, apical, and popliteal pulses.

Question 17

What is the term used for shock resulting from the failure of the heart's pumping capabilities?

☐ **Cardiogenic**

Explanation: Shock caused by significant blood loss is referred to as hemorrhagic shock. When the heart's function fails, it is termed cardiogenic shock. Psychogenic shock occurs due to intense emotional distress or fright.

Question 18

Identify the response that is not indicative of Hypovolemic Shock:

☐ **Generalized edema**

Explanation: Hypovolemic shock manifests with the following clinical features: a rapid, feeble pulse; hypotension; altered mental status; cyanosis observable at the lips and under the nails; cool and moist skin; and an elevated respiratory rate.

Question 19

Among the following, who should be regarded as a patient requiring immediate medical attention?

☐ **A 55-year-old woman exhibiting a blood pressure of 178/90**

Explanation: A blood pressure reading of 178/90 signifies a state of hypertensive crisis, thus prioritizing that patient. The others, while potentially becoming urgent cases depending on their progress, do not present as the highest priority based on the current information provided.

Question 20

Upon examining a 78-year-old female patient, her skin appears cool, moist, and pallid. What would be your diagnosis?

☐ **Vasovagal syncope**

Explanation: Cool and pallid skin may indicate insufficient oxygenation or reduced perfusion to the tissues.

Question 21

The initial phase of shock, wherein the physiological mechanisms of the body are capable of coping with the hemorrhage, is termed

☐ **Compensated shock**

Explanation: The initial phase of shock, wherein the physiological mechanisms of the body are capable of coping with the hemorrhage, is termed compensated shock. During compensated shock, the individual's systolic blood pressure remains above 90, ensuring sufficient tissue perfusion.

Question 22

What would be the appropriate sequence of interventions for a 76-year-old woman presenting with a heart rate of 142 beats per minute, accompanied by cyanosis around her lips and nail beds?

☐ **Continue evaluation during transport and administer high-flow oxygen**

Explanation: In such critical scenarios, the immediate administration of oxygen is paramount. This should be done while swiftly transporting the patient to the hospital.

Question 23

In the scenario where you are administering CPR alone to a 77-year-old male who has experienced cardiac arrest and is not breathing, what is the best technique to ascertain the effectiveness of your ventilations?

☐ **Observing the chest for movement up and down**

Explanation: Observing the elevation and depression of the patient's chest provides the most dependable indication of effective ventilations during both solo and dual rescuer CPR.

Question 24

In the thorough secondary evaluation, all of the following concerning blood pressure assessment must be considered except:

☐ **methods of palpation**

Explanation: Within the framework of a secondary assessment, pertinent elements of blood pressure monitoring encompass: the size of the equipment, appropriate cuff placement, patient positioning, arm positioning, measurement methodologies, and how it correlates with perfusion.

Question 25

Shock etiologies are primarily classified into three main types. What are they?

☐ **Impaired cardiac function, fluid depletion, and vascular dilation**

Explanation: The fundamental etiologies of shock include impaired cardiac performance, loss of circulatory fluid, and vascular dilation.

Question 26

What does the notation 140/P signify?

☐ **A blood pressure reading of 140 was palpated**

Explanation: This notation is employed when documenting blood pressure measurement using the palpation technique.

Question 27

In a SAMPLE history evaluation, what does the letter 'P' signify?

☐ **Pertinent past medical history**

Explanation: Understanding previous medical encounters is frequently crucial in clinical assessments.

Question 28

A patient presents with acute chest discomfort accompanied by diaphoresis and a blood pressure reading of 96/55 mmHg. Among the patient's medications is a prescription for nitroglycerin. After contacting medical control, you receive an order to administer one nitroglycerin tablet sublingually. What would be your course of action?

☐ **Re-check the patient's blood pressure and seek further guidance**

Explanation: Administering nitroglycerin to a patient with a systolic blood pressure lower than 100 mmHg can significantly reduce blood pressure, potentially leading to dangerous hypotension and is generally contraindicated. Consideration must also be given to the responsibility and liability implicated in choosing to deviate from the given order.

Question 29

A patient presents with nausea and bradycardia. What physiological response is being exhibited?

☐ **Parasympathetic**

Explanation: The parasympathetic nervous system is implicated in reducing heart rate and increasing gastrointestinal activity.

Question 30

The left atrium and ventricle of the heart ___________and _________.

☐ **accepts blood from the lungs, initiates systemic circulation**

Explanation: The left portion of the heart is responsible for accepting oxygenated blood from the pulmonary veins and establishing systemic circulation.

Question 31

In the scope of emergency medical services (EMS), what does the term 'lumen' denote?

☐ **The internal diameter of a tube**

Explanation: Within EMS terminology, 'lumen' pertains to the internal diameter of medical tubing, such as endotracheal (ET) tubes, needles, or nasopharyngeal airways. It can also refer to the diameter of a blood vessel.

Question 32

You are called to assist an elderly male patient who may have had a stroke. Upon arrival, you discover him prone on the floor. He exhibits Decerebrate Rigidity, emits groaning noises, and his eyes fail to react to verbal or painful stimuli. What is his Glasgow Coma Scale (GCS) score?

☐ **4**

Explanation: Decerebrate Rigidity corresponds to an abnormal extension score of 2, vocalizing only groans equates to a verbal response score of 2, and the lack of eye response to stimuli results in a score of 1.

Question 33

Identify the vessel that receives blood ejected from the right ventricle.

☐ **Pulmonary artery**

Explanation: The right ventricle pumps blood into the pulmonary artery, which transports the blood to the lungs for oxygenation. Once oxygenated, the blood returns to the heart through the pulmonary vein.

Question 34

The pulmonary artery originates from the _______ and terminates at the _________.

☐ **Right ventricle / lungs**

Explanation: This vessel transports deoxygenated blood from the right ventricle to the lungs for oxygenation. Subsequently, the oxygen-rich blood travels to the left atrium.

Question 35

Which part of the heart is often termed the 'workhorse'?

☐ **Left ventricle**

Explanation: The left ventricular chamber is chiefly accountable for propelling blood into the aorta and thereafter to the body's systemic circulation. It is colloquially known as the 'workhorse.'

Question 36

Identify which of the following pediatric patients exhibits bradycardia.

☐ **A 4-year-old child with a heart rate of 70 beats per minute**

Explanation: In the context of pediatric patients who are unwell or injured, bradycardia is defined as a heart rate below 80 beats per minute for children and below 100 beats per minute for infants.

Question 37

Identify the diastolic pressure that fits within the normal parameters for a healthy adult.

☐ **55 mm Hg**

Explanation: The norms for diastolic pressure can differ by source. According to the American Heart Association, a pressure below 80 mm Hg is considered normal. Emergency Medical Services (EMS) literature lists normal ranges from 50-90 mm Hg or 60-89 mm Hg. The National Health Service (NHS) cites an average blood pressure reading of 120/80 mm Hg. This query asks for the most appropriate value, noting that the other options do not fall within any recognized standards.

Question 38

Which of the following situations might indicate that CPR is not warranted?

☐ **Presence of stiff neck and jaw**

Explanation: The presence of a stiff neck and jaw may suggest rigor mortis, a state during which CPR would not be performed if the individual is also without a pulse and not breathing. It is important to confirm rigor mortis in at least two joints. The remaining options all suggest potential conditions under which CPR may be required.

Question 39

Identify the feature that would not typically be associated with the clinical presentation of Cardiogenic shock.

☐ **Tissue necrosis**

Explanation: The clinical manifestations of Cardiogenic shock encompass the following: thoracic discomfort; arrhythmic heartbeat; diminished pulse strength; hypotension; cyanotic discoloration (notably of the lips and subungual regions); skin that is cool and diaphoretic; heightened nervousness; audible crackles in the lungs; and fluid accumulation in the pulmonary system.

Question 40

Define perfusion:

☐ **The distribution of blood, oxygen, and nutrients to the body's cells**

Explanation: Perfusion refers to the distribution of blood, oxygen, and essential nutrients to the cells of the body. Inadequate perfusion can lead to cellular death.

Question 41

The carotid artery transports blood from the __________ to the __________.

☐ **Cardiac region / cranial region**

Explanation: In a medical emergency where an individual is unresponsive, the carotid artery, located in the cervical region, serves as an essential site for pulse assessment. This artery facilitates the passage of blood from the cardiac muscle to the cerebral regions.

Question 42

Within what range would one expect the systolic blood pressure of an 8-year-old child to fall?

☐ **Above 80 mm Hg**

Explanation: A systolic blood pressure between 80 and 120 mm Hg is typical for children of this age group.

Question 43

Upon arrival at the scene, you encounter four individuals with varying conditions. Which individual should be prioritized for treatment and transport?

☐ **A 9-year-old child who is alert, breathing at a rate of 26 per minute, with a systolic blood pressure of 68 mm Hg**

Explanation: Understanding that a pediatric patient exhibiting a systolic blood pressure below 70 mm Hg is in a critical state, is crucial to this determination.

Question 44

During a myocardial infarction, aspirin is prescribed primarily to __________

☐ **Inhibit additional platelet aggregation**

Explanation: Aspirin functions to inhibit further platelet aggregation, but it does not have the capacity to break up existing clots.

Question 45

Identify the option that is not a constituent of the fundamental components to enhance survival outcomes during resuscitation.

☐ **Timely administration of Aspirin**

Explanation: Key components to enhance survival outcomes during resuscitation comprise: Prompt access, timely cardiopulmonary resuscitation (CPR), rapid defibrillation, and swift advanced medical care.

Question 46

Identify the collection that comprises solely of anatomical components of the Circulatory System.

☐ **Heart, arterial vessels, capillaries, and venous pathways**

Explanation: Components that constitute the Circulatory System are as follows: Heart, Blood Vessels (which include arteries, veins, and capillaries), together with Blood.

Question 47

The primary functions of the respiratory system are to __________ and __________.

☐ **enable oxygen to reach the lungs and bloodstream; expel waste products from the blood and lungs.**

Explanation: The respiratory system facilitates the ingress of oxygen into the pulmonary system and bloodstream, while also enabling the expulsion of waste gases from the bloodstream and lungs.

Question 48

Which anatomical site should be palpated to assess the pulse of an infant?

☐ **Brachial artery**

Explanation: When examining an infant, the brachial artery located in the arm should be utilized for pulse assessment.

Question 49

A patient exhibits a pulse but lacks respiratory function. Rescue ventilation should be administered ______________.

☐ **With minimal air to just make the chest elevate.**

Explanation: Each rescue breath ought to be sufficient to cause observable elevation of the chest.

Question 50

An alternative term for shock is ____________.

☐ **Hypotension**

Explanation: Shock is synonymous with hypotension, a condition defined by abnormally low blood pressure, derived from 'hypo' meaning 'under' or 'below' and 'tension' referring to vascular pressure.

EMS OPERATIONS

Question 1

Are patients entitled to restrict access to their medical documentation?

☐ **Private**

Explanation: Patients possess the right to ensure the confidentiality of their medical records.

Question 2

Interventions are defined as ____________.

☐ **Measures taken to resolve an issue**

Explanation: Interventions encompass items such as cervical collars, airway management tools, splinting devices, and medications like morphine.

Question 3

Your emergency medical services team, along with law enforcement, has responded to an incident involving a dilapidated mobile home on the periphery of town. Dispatch has indicated that a 28-year-old male has overdosed on heroin and cocaine. Upon arriving ahead of the county sheriff, you are approached by a distressed teenage girl pleading for assistance for her brother. Assessing the environment and determining it is safe, you enter the mobile home to find bystanders administering CPR to the man. As you begin your evaluation, the man suddenly becomes conscious and attempts to strike you. How should you proceed?

☐ **Withdraw to the ambulance, maintaining a safe distance from the scene while confirming law enforcement's impending arrival**

Explanation: While the impulse to respond physically to a combative patient is understandable, it is generally discouraged and should only be considered as a last resort for self-defense. It is not advisable to solicit the help of bystanders in restraining the patient. Your primary duty is to ensure your own safety. Although immediate radio communication for law enforcement support might seem prudent, it is redundant as they are already en route. Moreover, if the individual has already displayed aggression, calling the police might escalate his agitation further.

Question 4

You and your colleague, Obi, have been dispatched to a residence where a 50-year-old male is experiencing respiratory distress. Upon arrival, you observe the patient lying in bed with labored breathing, a respiratory rate of 20, minimal chest expansion, pallor, and a weak pulse. The family informs you that the patient is diagnosed with AIDS. Obi responds by stating, "I apologize, but I do not wish to risk contracting AIDS. I cannot assist," and then exits the premises. What has just transpired?

☐ **Obi has forsaken his duty to render care to the patient, thereby committing abandonment**

Explanation: Refusal to provide care to this patient constitutes abandonment, regardless of Obi's concerns about infectious risk. This action may also breach the Americans with Disabilities Act and could be considered negligent if additional criteria are fulfilled. Obi's statement did not result in communication failure. While the family and patient may be dissatisfied with Obi's behavior, it is overly presumptive to claim that he has undermined their trust in emergency medical services. Furthermore, evaluating potential psychological harm to the family on-scene is unlikely.

Question 5

In the role of an Emergency Medical Technician, under what circumstances may you be accused of abandonment?

☐ **Leave a patient without ensuring they are transferred to a provider with adequate or superior qualifications**

Explanation: Once patient care has been initiated, you are required to sustain it, unless you arrange for a handover to another provider with equivalent or superior qualifications.

Question 6

Which of the following actions is NOT a valid method EMTs can use to protect bystanders?

☐ **Arrest them**

Explanation: EMTs can ensure bystander safety by: evacuating them from the area, keeping them away from the scene, or setting up barriers. EMTs do not possess the legal authority to carry out arrests.

Question 7

Which of the following is NOT a requisite criterion for establishing negligence on the part of an EMT?

☐ **The patient must provide evidence of their injuries**

Explanation: The necessity for a patient to prove their injuries does not constitute one of the four essential criteria for establishing negligence. The missing criterion is that the EMT's act or omission must fall below the accepted standard of care.

Question 8

Which of the following elements is NOT relevant when assessing a patient's current medical condition?

☐ **Emphasize patient's historical health background**

Explanation: The assessment of a patient's current medical condition emphasizes the present health state, includes environmental factors, and incorporates various individual aspects.

Question 9

You and your colleague, Zavid, are evaluating a patient who appears to exhibit unusual behavior possibly due to trauma. The patient displays clear signs of altered consciousness and has a conspicuous, bleeding injury on the side of their head. The patient is resistant to your presence and uses profanity towards you. What is the most appropriate course of action?

☐ **Reach out to medical control and request police aid in handling the patient**

Explanation: If it is suspected that the patient's irrational behavior stems from the injury and they pose a potential danger to themselves or others, it is advisable to contact medical control and seek police assistance to ensure the patient receives proper medical care. While the idea of a Sux dart sounds appealing, such a solution doesn't exist yet, so alternative measures must be considered.

Question 10

In the context of evaluating the cardiovascular system during a secondary assessment, primary attention should initially be directed towards

______________ and ____________.

☐ **Pulse and perfusion**

Explanation: In the context of evaluating the cardiovascular system during a secondary assessment, primary attention should initially be directed towards PULSE and PERFUSION.

Question 11

An individual deemed to be legally competent has the ability to:

☐ **Decline medical treatment**

Explanation: A person who possesses sufficient cognitive abilities retains the right to decline medical interventions provided that they have the capacity to make informed decisions. Legal competency is determined exclusively by judicial authorities. Your role entails assessing the individual's capacity for making informed decisions.

Question 12

Upon arriving at a retirement facility with your colleague Rodrigo, you observe that numerous staff members and residents are experiencing emesis and vertigo. What should be your primary suspicion?

☐ **A toxic substance may be causing the symptoms**

Explanation: The presentation of similar symptoms among multiple individuals frequently indicates the presence of an environmental emergency, necessitating thorough investigation prior to entering the affected area.

Question 13

The diagnostic strategy enables the exclusion of life-threatening conditions and subsequently ______________.

☐ **Address the reported symptoms of the patient**

Explanation: Post-diagnosis, attention should be focused on addressing the patient's reported issues. There is no requirement to diagnose anew, reassess, or delegate the patient to another healthcare professional.

Question 14

Which of the following is not among the supplementary resources that EMTs call for during hazard mitigation or scene control?

☐ **Health department**

Explanation: EMTs typically request additional resources such as more ambulances, the fire department, and law enforcement to assist with hazard mitigation and scene management.

Question 15

What is the definition of assault?

☐ **Inducing fear of harmful physical touch**

Explanation: Assault pertains to actions that induce apprehension of harmful or offensive physical contact. In contrast, actual physical contact with an individual without their consent or against their will constitutes battery.

Question 16

The appropriate clinical scenarios and symptoms for prescribing a drug are ___________.

☐ **The purposes the drug serves and the conditions it is intended for**

Explanation: Indications for a medication refer to the specific clinical scenarios and symptoms that justify its prescribing.

Question 17

Which of the following does not represent a key reason for the necessity of a comprehensive patient history?

☐ **A comprehensive history guarantees that no errors will occur during patient care**

Explanation: The critical aspects highlighting the necessity of a comprehensive patient history are: Serving as the main element in the patient's overall medical assessment, the requirement of a blend of expertise and knowledge to accurately gather the history, and its role in guaranteeing the patient receives appropriate care.

Question 18

An incident involving the derailment of a train has resulted in the explosion of two tanker cars and the leakage of an undetermined gas from additional cars. The scope of the impacted region is extensive, spanning multiple county jurisdictions. Under the guidelines of the National Incident Management System (NIMS), which command structure would be most advantageous for managing this mass casualty incident?

☐ **Unified Command Structure**

Explanation: A Unified Command Structure permits the integration of various agencies such as Emergency Medical Services (EMS), Fire Departments, Police, Municipal Authorities, County Commissioners, among others.

Question 19

Upon arrival at the location of a potential drowning incident, where a three-year-old child was discovered unresponsive in the family swimming pool, the appropriate use of emergency lights and sirens involves:

☐ **Employing them to request the right-of-way from other vehicles**

Explanation: Sound devices are intended to request the right-of-way from other motorists and should not be used to forcefully clear traffic. It is advisable to be well-versed with the regulations pertaining to emergency light and siren usage in your jurisdiction.

Question 20

Upon arrival at a soccer match, you and your colleague Jake observe a male individual who appears to have suffered a knee dislocation. Upon assessing the patient, there is an evident misalignment of the lower limb and an absence of distal pulses. What is the appropriate course of action?

☐ **Immediately contact medical control for guidance on stabilization**

Explanation: If distal pulses are absent, it is crucial to consult with medical control to determine the next steps, unless a field reduction procedure is within your authorized scope of practice as a paramedic. Splinting the affected limb might be required, but transporting the patient as a low-priority case would be improper.

Question 21

Upon completing a Patient Care Report (PCR), what specifics within the document are mandated to remain confidential?

☐ **All details within**

Explanation: All personal data within a Patient Care Report must be treated as confidential. Disclosure of such information to unauthorized individuals contravenes HIPAA regulations.

Question 22

An incident involving an overturned tanker truck transporting unidentified chemicals has occurred on the interstate, resulting in the spillage of a luminous liquid from the trailer. Several casualties have been reported and numerous onlookers are experiencing nausea and vomiting. You have been tasked by the Incident Commander to establish a helicopter landing zone. Which of the following areas would be most suitable for this landing zone?

☐ **A small incline about 80 by 80 feet, positioned uphill and upwind from the danger site.**

Explanation: It is critical to opt for a site that is both higher in elevation and upwind from the hazardous site. Moreover, the location should not be in an area that has been evacuated due to symptoms of vomiting.

Question 23

While returning from a lunch break, you encounter an intersection obstructed by a collision involving two vehicles that are ablaze. What is the most appropriate course of action?

☐ **Maintain a safe distance until the situation is under control**

Explanation: The optimal response is to remain at a safe distance until the hazardous situation has been managed. Approaching the unsafe area is not advisable. Although summoning Hazmat personnel and using the ambulance's fire extinguisher are possible steps, they do not constitute the best immediate action.

Question 24

In the context of a multi-vehicle accident where you have been designated as the Incident Commander's safety officer, your primary duty is:

☐ **Halting an ongoing extrication when an EMT enters the danger zone of an inactive airbag.**

Explanation: As the Safety Officer, your role involves overseeing the scene's activities and alerting the Incident Commander to any potential hazards. Additionally, it is crucial to halt any procedures that pose an immediate danger to the health or safety of the response team or bystanders.

Question 25

To proficiently steer an ambulance around a bend, the driver must comprehend the appropriate velocity, ______________________, and recognize the importance of ______________________.

☐ **The current location and planned trajectory / reaching the apex later in the turn**

Explanation: When negotiating a curve, it is advantageous to hit the apex later in the turn, as this helps the vehicle stay within the traffic lane. Early apexing tends to push the vehicle to the outside edge of the lane as it exits the curve.

Question 26

In the year 1989, the Department of Defense initiated a project aimed at addressing the unique medical needs of law enforcement personnel during tactical missions. What was the designation of this program?

☐ **CONTOMS**

Explanation: The program known as CONTOMS assists tactical Emergency Medical Technicians (EMTs) in aiding law enforcement. CONTOMS stands for Counter Narcotics and Terrorism Operational Medical Support.

Question 27

In the event that a patient's wallet must be inspected for medical data, it should be done ___________.

☐ **Visibly, so that others can witness the search**

Explanation: Conducting this search in the presence of others is prudent to mitigate any potential allegations of theft.

Question 28

Identify the option that does not align with the standard practices for respiratory system evaluation during a secondary medical examination.

☐ **Refrain from exposing the chest**

Explanation: Components of a respiratory system evaluation during a secondary assessment include: exposing the chest as warranted by the environment, assessing chest configuration and symmetry, evaluating respiratory effort, and performing auscultation.

Question 29

Responding to a call at the county detention center, you are requested to examine an incarcerated individual who recently engaged in a physical altercation. The individual has multiple lacerations and presents with a periorbital hematoma. Upon your attempt to provide assistance, the prisoner adamantly states, 'Leave me alone, I don't need or want your help.' What course of action should you take?

☐ **Notify the Deputy that you recommend a thorough medical assessment and treatment, and if the detainee refuses care, he should be escorted to the emergency room under law enforcement supervision.**

Explanation: Your preliminary observation reveals that the detainee has sustained injuries necessitating a comprehensive examination and potentially urgent medical intervention. The observable wounds may suggest a closed head trauma or possibly internal damage corresponding to the lacerations. Under the jurisdiction of law enforcement, the detainee can be transported involuntarily for further medical evaluation.

Question 30

What is an advisable procedure for donning latex or vinyl gloves?

☐ **Put them on during transit to the emergency site**

Explanation: Wearing gloves en route to an emergency can expedite response times in critical situations.

Question 31

Which of the following elements is inappropriate to be part of a patient's secondary evaluation?

☐ **Digestive system**

Explanation: A comprehensive secondary evaluation of a patient must encompass the following elements: General inspection, respiratory examination, cardiovascular examination, neurological assessment, musculoskeletal check, and evaluation of all anatomical areas.

Question 32

Emergency dispatch has reported a motor vehicle accident involving two cars, necessitating the response of both an ambulance and a fire truck. Both vehicles depart the station and head towards the accident site. Upon nearing a heavily trafficked intersection, what safety measures should be observed?

☐ **Activate a siren with a unique sound distinct from the fire truck's to ensure that drivers are aware of multiple emergency vehicles approaching the intersection**

Explanation: The optimal recommendation is to employ a siren with a distinct sound that differs from the one used by the fire truck. This is because drivers typically expect only one emergency vehicle and can be better alerted to the presence of multiple vehicles if the siren sounds are different.

Question 33

The utilization of Critical Incident Stress Debriefings (CISD) serves to:

☐ **Aid EMS workers in recuperating after distressing incidents**

Explanation: CISD is implemented to assist Emergency Medical Services (EMS) workers in expediting their recovery post exposure to critical incidents and emotionally taxing situations.

Question 34

How is a region classified where there is a high level of contamination?

☐ **Hot zone**

Explanation: A highly contaminated region is termed as the hot zone.

Question 35

You and your colleague Blaze have been dispatched to an incident involving two individuals who have sustained stab wounds. One patient, a woman, has been stabbed in the upper right quadrant (URQ) and is experiencing respiratory difficulty, with a pulse rate of 103 and shallow respirations at 35 breaths per minute. The other patient, a man, has a stab wound in the lower right quadrant (LRQ), is in significant abdominal pain, and has a pulse of 60 with a respiratory rate of 24. Prior to arriving at the scene, what steps should be taken?

☐ **Ensure that law enforcement has secured the scene**

Explanation: Do not proceed to the scene until it has been deemed safe. The mere presence of law enforcement does not guarantee safety. Await explicit confirmation from authorities before attending to victims at a crime scene.

Question 36

Which of the following can be an indicator of child maltreatment?

☐ **Wounds at different stages of recovery**

Explanation: Observing wounds or bruises at various healing stages in a child is sometimes indicative of maltreatment. The presence of an irate parent does not necessarily imply maltreatment, and the other responses reflect common occurrences among children.

Question 37

In what capacity can a PCR be utilized?

☐ **Formal legal evidence**

Explanation: Prehospital Care Reports are admissible as evidence in legal proceedings.

Question 38

At 7:30 a.m., you arrive at the location of a two-vehicle accident involving at least six individuals on a foggy area of a moderately trafficked rural road. The fire department has not yet arrived, and both vehicles are emitting smoke and flames. You can hear cries for help, and other cars are maneuvering around the accident site to proceed. What should be your immediate course of action?

☐ **Alert the fire department, create a safety perimeter, and help maintain traffic at a safe distance**

Explanation: The primary concern in this scenario is ensuring scene safety. The most effective way to assist is by managing traffic and crowd control to prevent the situation from worsening, thereby allowing emergency personnel to operate safely when they arrive and enabling you to provide medical care in a secure environment.

Question 39

During the reassessment of vital signs, which of the following parameters does not require meticulous attention?

☐ **Skin turgor**

Explanation: In the process of reassessing vital parameters, it is essential to closely monitor respirations, pulse, blood pressure, and pupils. Skin turgor, however, is not a primary consideration in this context.

Question 40

What term describes the prescribed manner in which one is expected to conduct themselves?

☐ **Code of Care**

Explanation: The notion of a 'Standard of care' dictates the expected conduct and responsibilities one owes to others.

Question 41

In the event of a traffic collision occurring directly before your ambulance, necessitating the extrication of injured individuals, which site should be prioritized for expedited extraction?

☐ **Via the door**

Explanation: Before opting to use specialized extrication tools, like the Jaws of Life, it is imperative to inspect all doors. Frequently, a door might be operable, allowing for the safe and efficient removal of the casualty.

Question 42

You have been appointed as the transportation officer during a mass casualty event where a pedestrian bridge in a local park has collapsed, resulting in injuries to 10-20 individuals of varying severities. Two medical facilities are available for patient transport: Santa Cruz Hospital, situated 3 miles from the incident location, and Valley Hospital, located 15 miles away. What would be the optimal allocation of patients to these facilities?

☐ **Transport all red-tagged patients to Santa Cruz Hospital until it reaches full capacity, then transport any remaining red-tagged patients to Valley Hospital, followed by yellow and green-tagged patients.**

Explanation: The most effective strategy is to transport the most critically injured individuals (red-tagged) to the nearest medical center, while sending patients with lesser injuries (yellow and green-tagged) to the farther hospital. This may be adjusted depending on the need for specialized care, such as sending a yellow-tagged pediatric patient to a pediatric center even if it is not the closest facility.

Question 43

In which context would an expedited evaluation for trauma be conducted?

☐ **At the incident location**

Explanation: An expedited trauma evaluation is executed on-site to identify any immediate threats to life.

Question 44

What is the recommended course of action if your radio communication extends beyond 30 seconds?

☐ **Divide into two shorter messages**

Explanation: Dividing extensive communications into shorter segments can help to avoid repeating lengthy messages.

Question 45

Within the SAMPLE history framework, what does the letter 'S' signify?

☐ **Signs**

Explanation: The correct answer is 'Signs or symptoms.'

Question 46

Which of the following is not classified as a medication assisted by EMTs:

☐ **Oxygen**

Explanation: Medications such as epinephrine, nitroglycerin, and inhaled bronchodilators are within the EMT-assisted category. Conversely, Oxygen administration is performed directly by EMTs.

Question 47

Who is accountable for overseeing the operations of EMS agencies and ensuring EMTs adhere to standards in practice?

☐ **Medical direction**

Explanation: The overarching responsibility for supervision is attributed to medical direction.

Question 48

Which technique is considered optimum for transferring a patient onto a backboard?

☐ **Four-person log roll**

Explanation: Utilizing the four-person log roll is the advocated procedure for appropriately transferring a patient onto a backboard.

Question 49

Within the acronym OPQRST, what does 'R' signify?

☐ **Radiate**

Explanation: 'R' stands for the concept of radiation, which asks if the pain extends to other areas of the body, such as experiencing shoulder pain during a myocardial infarction.

Question 50

For what purpose is the Incident Command System (ICS) implemented?

☐ **Guarantee the efficient allocation of resources, safety for the public and responders, and the achievement of management objectives during incidents.**

Explanation: The main objective of the Incident Command System is to create a systematic, safe, and effectively managed incident environment. It is adaptable for both minor incidents involving a single unit and large-scale situations requiring numerous resources and multi-agency collaboration.

ALS AND ADVANCED QUESTIONS ONLY

Question 1

Which physiological processes are regulated by the autonomic nervous system?

☐ **All aforementioned functions**

Explanation: The autonomic nervous system governs all the listed functions.

Question 2

Within the anatomical framework, how would one classify nerves located in the lower extremities?

☐ **Peripheral**

Explanation: Peripheral nerves encompass all nerves outside the central nervous system, including the spinal column and brain.

Question 3

The purpose of defibrillation is to ____________.

☐ **End critical arrhythmias**

Explanation: Defibrillation aims to restore normal ventricular rhythms.

Question 4

Identify which items listed below could potentially trigger an allergic response in individuals:

☐ **All aforementioned options**

Explanation: It is important to note that other factors, such as insect bites and various consumables, can also induce allergic reactions.

Question 5

Dyspnea is most likely to be observed in an individual who is _________.

☐ **Experiencing respiratory distress**

Explanation: Dyspnea refers to a condition characterized by shortness of breath or difficulty in breathing.

Question 6

An acute myocardial infarction (AMI) is commonly referred to as:

☐ **A heart attack**

Explanation: The formal term for a heart attack.

Question 7

In the state of shock, the constriction of blood vessels results in the skin becoming ______.

☐ **Cool**

Explanation: The skin experiences a decrease in temperature during shock.

Question 8

Which option listed does not belong to the six principles of accurate and safe medication administration?

☐ **Injection device**

Explanation: The six principles include: patient, medication, dosage, method of administration, timing, and proper documentation.

Question 9

A breech birth manifests as a/an ________.

☐ **The infant in a posterior-first position**

Explanation: In breech deliveries, the infant presents with a posterior-first position. Immediate transportation to a medical facility is critical.

Question 10

What physiological condition might cause extreme thirst in individuals diagnosed with diabetes mellitus?

☐ **Polyuria**

Explanation: Excessive urination, as the body endeavors to expel surplus glucose, induces significant thirst in the individual.

Question 11

Individuals with a tracheostomy may require distinct methods of ventilation compared to those without such an opening. Which of the following statements accurately describes these ventilation methods?

☐ **Creating a seal over the patient's mouth and nose during ventilation through a stoma, and then unsealing them during passive exhalation, can be an efficacious technique for assisted ventilation**

Explanation: A tracheostomy or stoma is a permanent aperture situated at the base or midline of the trachea. When ventilating through a stoma, maneuvers such as head tilt or jaw thrust are ineffective, as they only shift the tongue away from the pharynx situated above the tracheostomy site. There is no unique adapter necessary for tracheostomies; the adapter part of a standard BVM suffices. Moreover, the BVM cannot be directly connected to the stoma and instead requires a seal formed by a child or infant mask if no tube is present. An OPA provides limited benefit for patients ventilated through a tracheostomy and should be removed if the patient is vomiting, with suctioning performed only up to the base of the tongue.

Question 12

A 20-year-old male has sustained a back injury at a nearby swimming area. Upon arrival, you and your colleague Missy discover the individual groaning and partially submerged next to a pile of rocks. Eyewitnesses report that he fell approximately 30 feet from a tree he was climbing over the swimming hole. The patient's respiratory rate is 12 breaths per minute, his breathing is extremely shallow with intermittent apnea, his pulse is 72 beats per minute, and his skin is slightly clammy and pale. After securing cervical spine precautions, what would be the most appropriate intervention?

☐ **Provide ventilation assistance and raise the individual's legs**

Explanation: This individual requires ventilatory assistance due to inadequate respiratory rate and depth. Treatment should also include slight elevation of the legs to manage shock, as well as the use of blankets and potentially heat packs to maintain body temperature.

Question 13

Your team is summoned to a youth summer camp where a 14-year-old female is experiencing an undetermined illness. According to the camp counselor, the girl began vomiting while playing basketball and now complains of abdominal pain. Upon arrival, you observe the girl seated in the camp office, clutching her stomach. She is significantly overweight, mildly sweating, and her skin is pink and feels normothermic. During the pulse examination, she mentions feeling weak. She is alert and oriented to person, place, and time. What is the most probable diagnosis and which treatment option is most suitable?

☐ **The girl is experiencing heat cramps. She should be given small sips of cool water if she is fully conscious. Move her to a cooler environment and initiate active cooling by misting her with tepid water followed by fanning to promote evaporation. Provide high-flow oxygen, administer intravenous fluids if within your practice scope, and arrange for transport.**

Explanation: Heat cramps manifest with symptoms such as vomiting, sweating, abdominal pain, and weakness. In contrast, heat exhaustion typically presents with pale skin and excessive sweating due to more severe salt and fluid depletion. When treating heat cramps, only room-temperature water should be given orally, as cold water can exacerbate nausea. For heat exhaustion, oral intake is not recommended, and cooling should be achieved using tepid water to avoid sudden vasoconstriction and shivering. Given the absence of altered level of consciousness and hyperthermia, heat stroke is unlikely in this case.

Question 14

Following a detonation at a local oil refinery, you have been designated as the triage officer by the Incident Command. What triage color label would be assigned to each of the following cases?

Case 1: a 9-year-old girl with a fractured arm, exhibiting a respiratory rate of 8 breaths per minute.

Case 2: an elderly man with an open fracture of the left thigh bone, showing signs of severe hemorrhagic shock with an absent pulse.

Case 3: an elderly male with a forehead wound and a Glasgow Coma Scale (GCS) score of 8.

Case 4: a 5-year-old boy breathing at a rate of 18 breaths per minute with a minor head injury.

☐ **Case 1: Red, Case 2: Black, Case 3: Red, Case 4: Green**

Explanation: Due to her slow breathing rate, the first patient should be classified as priority 1 or given a red tag. The second patient, lacking a pulse and in severe shock, would be given a black tag, indicating a likely fatal prognosis. The third patient, with a significantly reduced level of consciousness, also requires a red tag. The fourth patient, presenting only with a minor head trauma and stable respiratory rate, would be labeled with a green tag.

Question 15

Upon your arrival at the location, you encounter a 27-year-old woman experiencing anxiety and respiratory distress. Which question should you prioritize asking?

☐ **Could you please tell me your name?**

Explanation: In the execution of a patient evaluation, immediately following the scene size-up, the initial phase is the primary assessment. This begins with forming an overall impression, followed by evaluating the level of consciousness, ensuring the airway is clear, evaluating breathing and circulation, and pinpointing life-threatening conditions throughout this process. While all the suggested questions are relevant at various stages of the assessment, the optimal initial inquiry is to ascertain the patient's name. This vital information establishes the identity of the individual you are engaging with and facilitates assessing the patient's general state based on their reaction, which subsequently aids in evaluating the airway status. This initial interaction is foundational for the remainder of the assessment. Commence by introducing yourself and inquiring about the patient's name. The subsequent questions are integral during the detailed history-taking phase of the assessment.

Question 16

Status asthmaticus is characterized by ___________

☐ **A potentially fatal scenario**

Explanation: Status asthmaticus refers to a critical asthma episode that is extended in duration, severe in intensity, and unresponsive to conventional bronchodilator treatment.

Question 17

In what scenario might one observe the manifestation known as Battle's sign in a patient?

☐ **In the case of skull fractures**

Explanation: Battle's sign, often characterized by bruising behind the ear, may indicate the presence of fractures in the skull.

Question 18

Through which path does blood travel after being ejected from the left ventricle?

☐ **Aortic arch**

Explanation: Upon ejection from the left ventricle, blood enters the aorta followed by the systemic circulation via the aortic arch.

Question 19

As the initial Emergency Medical Services unit to arrive at a scene involving multiple casualties, where a crane has collapsed onto an adjacent building from a rooftop, what procedures should you follow in accordance with the Incident Command System (ICS)?

☐ **Assume the role of Incident Commander until relieved or reassigned by higher authority**

Explanation: Upon arriving at the scene as the initial EMS responder, you should communicate with dispatch to establish yourself as the Incident Commander (IC) until advised otherwise. When additional responders arrive, responsibilities may be reallocated to roles such as triage, transportation, treatment, or logistics.

Question 20

You arrive at the residence of a 69-year-old male who suddenly experienced dyspnea and dizziness while mowing his lawn. Upon initial evaluation, his integument is erythematous and anhidrotic. His respiratory rate is approximately 22 breaths per minute, and his heart rate stands at 120 beats per minute. His spouse mentions he commenced using Flomax two months ago but is otherwise not on any pharmacological regimen. At that moment, the patient reports a headache. A sphygmomanometric reading reveals his blood pressure to be 100/60 mmHg. What treatment approach is most appropriate for this patient?

☐ **Transfer him to a cooler setting and disrobe him**

Explanation: The patient exhibits clinical manifestations of hyperthermia or heat stroke. Tachycardia and tachypnea are compensatory responses to hypotension likely induced by dehydration. Immediate intervention should involve relocating the patient to a cooler environment, administering intravenous fluids, and employing both active and passive cooling techniques. High-flow oxygen delivered via a non-rebreather mask (NRB) should be incorporated into the management plan.

Question 21

You and your colleague, Stacy, respond to a call at an apartment complex involving a 17-year-old female experiencing abdominal pain. Upon arrival, you observe the patient, who appears pale and is lying on the couch. Her abdomen is visibly distended, and she has a towel on her lap with some blood stains. She is breathing at a rate of 20 breaths per minute, with a pulse rate of 114 beats per minute. The patient denies any trauma and reports a small amount of vaginal bleeding. After administering high-flow oxygen and transferring her to the ambulance, you notice a loop of tissue protruding from her vagina. What condition might this patient be experiencing, and how should she be managed?

☐ **The patient is suffering from umbilical cord prolapse. Insert a gloved hand into the vagina to check for cord pulsations, gently lift the baby's head off the cord, and transport the patient in a supine position with elevated hips. Treat for shock and initiate IV therapy according to the scope of practice.**

Explanation: The patient is likely in labor and experiencing umbilical cord prolapse. This condition occurs when a loop of the umbilical cord emerges from the vagina before any part of the baby, risking compression between the baby's head and the mother's pelvis, which can impede blood flow to the baby. If the cord is pulsing, it indicates circulation is still present. Do not attempt to push the cord back into the vagina. Cover the exposed cord with a sterile, warm, and moist towel.

Question 22

Shock can be attributed to three primary etiologies. What are they?

☐ **Inadequate cardiac function, fluid depletion, and vasodilation**

Explanation: The fundamental etiologies of shock include inadequate cardiac function, hemorrhage or fluid depletion, and vasodilation.

Question 23

During an emergency delivery in the back of an ambulance, you and your partner Jim face a nuchal cord that is too tight to maneuver over the infant's head. Given this situation, what should be your subsequent course of action?

☐ **Clamp the umbilical cord at two points and cut between the clamps**

Explanation: Ensuring the baby's airway is unobstructed should be the top priority. Properly severing the cord would be the most prudent action at this juncture.

Question 24

During which month of gestation is it most probable for supine hypotensive syndrome to manifest?

☐ **Ninth**

Explanation: In the later stages of pregnancy, the fetus' weight can exert pressure on the inferior vena cava when the woman lies on her back, potentially leading to decreased and lower blood pressure.

Question 25

Upon arrival at a wedding ceremony, you and your

colleague Asher encounter a woman who has experienced a syncopal episode. Witnesses report that the incident was triggered by her realization of a dragon tattoo on her daughter's ankle as she proceeded down the aisle. Attendees noted that the woman was gently lowered to the ground, avoiding any traumatic impact. After remaining supine for 10 minutes, she was assisted to an upright position without expressing any discomfort. Despite a pallid appearance, her neurological function appears normal with a Glasgow Coma Scale (GCS) score of 15. What is the most plausible diagnosis for this woman's condition?

☐ **Psychogenic shock**

Explanation: Individuals experiencing psychogenic shock typically show improvement in circulation and perfusion after a brief period in the supine position.

Question 26

You are attending to a 16-year-old female presently in active labor, discovered alone in her automobile. Upon examination, it is evident that the fetal head has already emerged. What action should be taken next in the childbirth process?

☐ **Assess for the presence of a nuchal cord**

Explanation: After the fetal head presents, it is crucial to assess for the presence of a nuchal cord. If a nuchal cord is detected, one should attempt to gently maneuver it over the infant's head by inserting a finger between the neck and the umbilical cord. Should the cord be too constricted, it must be clamped in two places and severed. A loose cord can be easily repositioned over the baby's head. Generally, cutting the umbilical cord is deferred until after the entire delivery and once the cord ceases pulsation, which can take up to 30 minutes and is typically not necessary in pre-hospital settings.

Question 27

What term is used to describe the accumulation of air in the cavity between the visceral and parietal pleurae?

☐ **Pneumothorax**

Explanation: Air can infiltrate the space separating the visceral and parietal pleurae either from the lung tissue or due to an external chest injury, resulting in a condition known as pneumothorax.

Question 28

You have been dispatched to a ski resort where a 49-year-old female was discovered after spending the night in an infrequently visited section of the ski area. Upon your arrival, you observe the patient seated, enveloped in a blanket. She exhibits signs of disorientation and is muttering unintelligibly. Her right foot is swathed in towels, and a resort employee reports that it is blistered and significantly swollen. What is the likely diagnosis for this woman, and what would constitute the most appropriate course of treatment?

☐ **The patient has frostbite on her foot and would benefit from the application of heat packs over the towels to facilitate warming. Immediate transport coupled with high-flow oxygen administration is essential.**

Explanation: In cases where a patient presents with frostbite on an extremity coupled with hypothermia, the initial focus should be on addressing the hypothermia. This involves warming the core body areas using heat packs. Rewarming frostbitten extremities should be avoided in the field setting to prevent further damage. Methods such as physically rubbing the frostbitten area could exacerbate the condition. Stimulants like coffee and tea are not advisable. If the patient's mental state is stable, warm, non-stimulating fluids are permissible.

Question 29

The term 'cyt-' denotes which of the following?

☐ **Cell**

Explanation: 'Cyt-' is derived from the Greek word for 'cell'.

Question 30

Upon arriving at the scene, you observe a male approximately in his 60s reclining on the floor of a minimally heated, compact apartment. His lips exhibit a bluish tint and his consciousness level is altered. What is the most plausible diagnosis?

☐ **Cyanotic and experiencing hypothermia**

Explanation: The term 'cyanotic' pertains to the bluish coloration resulting from oxygen-deprived blood evident beneath the skin. Given the cold environment of the apartment, the most appropriate answer is the first one.

Question 31

In pediatric assessments, what is the typical weight range for children aged 2 to 6 years?

☐ **15-25 kilograms**

Explanation: Children within the age range of 2 to 6 years generally have an estimated weight between 15 and 25 kilograms.

Question 32

What is the recommended patient positioning for transportation when managing shock?

☐ **Supine with legs elevated**

Explanation: A supine position with elevated legs is advantageous as it facilitates the return of venous blood to the heart.

Question 33

Identify an alternative term frequently used for shock:

☐ **Hypoperfusion**

Explanation: Shock is synonymous with hypotension, derived from 'hypo-' meaning below average, and 'tension' referring to vascular pressure.

Question 34

Administering nitroglycerin to a patient during a myocardial infarction will have which primary effect?

☐ **Cause vasodilation**

Explanation: Nitroglycerin primarily induces vasodilation, which alleviates the heart's burden by reducing venous return and myocardial oxygen demand.

Question 35

What is meconium?

☐ **An indicator of fetal or maternal distress**

Explanation: Meconium refers to the first excretion from a fetus, which poses a potential risk to fetal respiratory well-being.

Question 36

What classification of shock is most likely to occur in an individual experiencing a myocardial infarction?

☐ **Cardiogenic**

Explanation: Shock caused by the loss of blood is termed hemorrhagic. Cardiogenic shock results from the failure of the heart to function properly as a pump. Psychogenic shock arises from an emotional shock or fright.

Question 37

Upon arrival at the scene, you and your colleague Rob encounter a woman who is 37 weeks into her pregnancy. She expresses that she feels an imminent need for delivery and requests immediate transportation to the hospital. As Rob monitors her vital signs en route, you begin to evaluate her stage of labor. Notably, she is experiencing vaginal bleeding, leading you to consider the possibility of ______________ or __________________.

☐ **Placenta previa or placental abruption**

Explanation: Placental abruption occurs when the placenta detaches prematurely from the uterine wall. Placenta previa involves the placenta positioning itself over the cervix, thus obstructing the birth canal ahead of the baby. Optimal management involves positioning the patient on her left side to avert supine hypotension.

Question 38

During childbirth, if the infant is emerging but the amniotic sac remains intact, what steps should be taken?

☐ **Carefully break the sac to reveal the baby's head**

Explanation: TIf the baby's head starts to appear while the amniotic sac is still unbroken, you should facilitate the breaking of the sac. There is no need for inserting fingers into the birth canal.

Question 39

A distinguishing feature of Cheyne-Stokes respiration is __________.

☐ **Irregular breathing interspersed with apnea**

Explanation: Cheyne-Stokes respiration often appears in individuals suffering from head trauma and is defined by an irregular breathing pattern characterized by alternating episodes of rapid breathing and apnea.

Question 40

The gesture known as Levine's sign is indicative of

____

☐ **Undergoing a myocardial infarction**

Explanation: Levine's sign refers to a person grasping their chest with a clenched fist placed over the sternum; it is often indicative of an Acute Myocardial Infarction (AMI).

Question 41

You arrive at Bigrock High School in response to an incident in the chemistry laboratory. A heated test tube has shattered, causing an injury to a student's eye. Upon entering the nurse's office, you observe an 18-year-old male reclined on the examination table, his face partially concealed by a towel. Upon the removal of the towel, it is apparent that fragments of glass are embedded in his facial skin, and he is experiencing ocular bleeding. What is the most appropriate course of action to take?

☐ **Shield the injured eye with a paper cup and secure with a bandage, avoiding pressure**

Explanation: Eye injuries are potentially severe and the priority is to prevent exacerbation of the injury. It is crucial to avoid applying pressure to eye injuries and refraining from removing glass unless it is mandated by protocol or is life-threatening. Administering high-flow oxygen and rapidly transporting the patient, while important, do not directly address the management of the eye injury. The optimal course of action is to shield the injured eye with protection for hospital transportation. Additionally, covering the unaffected eye is advisable.

Question 42

Concerning the preservation of a pediatric patient's airway, which of the following statements holds true?

☐ **Placing a towel beneath the shoulders assists in aligning the airway**

Explanation: Positioning a towel beneath the shoulders of a child is critical for proper alignment, aiding in ventilation and maintaining a clear airway.

Question 43

YIn the event that a patient presents with emesis resembling coffee grounds, which condition would you consider?

☐ **Gastrointestinal hemorrhage**

Explanation: The presence of vomit resembling coffee grounds serves as an indicator of gastrointestinal hemorrhage. Esophageal varices typically present with bright red blood. The remaining alternatives are fictitious.

Question 44

What might precipitate cardiogenic shock?

☐ **Acute Myocardial Infarction (AMI)**

Explanation: The prefix 'cardio' refers to the heart, suggesting that myocardial infarction is the cause. Conversely, shock induced by a sudden emotional disturbance is classified as psychogenic.

Question 45

How is cardiac output defined?

☐ **The total volume of blood expelled by the heart in one minute**

Explanation: Cardiac output refers to the total volume of blood that the heart propels through the circulatory system every minute. It is calculated by multiplying the heart rate by the stroke volume.

Question 46

A healthcare provider has instructed you to administer a nitroglycerin spray to a patient via the sublingual route. What method will you employ to deliver the medication?

☐ **Beneath the tongue**

Explanation: The term sublingual denotes placement beneath the tongue.

Question 47

Upon arrival, you and your colleague, Steve, encounter an 85-year-old male seated in a lounge chair, engrossed in smoking a cigar. Initially, his eyes remain shut, but they open when addressed as 'Sir'. He exhibits confusion when questioned about his name but promptly responds by squeezing your hand when requested. What Glasgow Coma Scale (GCS) score would this patient likely receive?

☐ **13**

Explanation: The patient receives a score of 3 for eye-opening in response to verbal stimuli, a score of 6 for following the command to squeeze your hand, and a score of 4 for producing a confused verbal response, totaling a GCS score of 13.

Question 48

YThe organ that adheres to the uterine wall and consists of both maternal and fetal tissues is the ________________.

☐ **Placenta**

Explanation: The placenta is instrumental in the transference of essential nutrients and some waste products—including substances like nicotine and alcohol—from mother to fetus.

Question 49

At what minimum age is it deemed inappropriate to employ an automatic ventilator?

☐ **8**

Explanation: It is advised against utilizing an automatic ventilator for pediatric patients younger than 8 years old due to a heightened risk of injury.

Question 50

Identify the anatomical region referred to as the perineum:

☐ **The area found between the anus and the vaginal opening**

Explanation: The perineum is the external region situated between the anus and the vagina

AIRWAY, RESPIRATION AND VENTILATION

Question 1

Upon arrival at a residence to address a 'slip and fall' incident, you and your colleague Bob are informed by an anxious father that his 3-year-old child has tumbled down a staircase of around 20 steps into the basement. The father hands over the unconscious boy, who exhibits shallow, irregular respiration and a pulse rate of 98 beats per minute. After ensuring the child's cervical spine is manually stabilized, you and Bob carefully lay him on the floor. Next, you should:

☐ **Introduce an oropharyngeal airway and assist breathing with a bag-valve mask, ensuring swift transportation.**

Explanation: Applying a nasopharyngeal airway is contraindicated in cases of potential head injury due to the risk of escalating intracranial pressure or causing further damage.

Question 2

Identify the upper airway bacterial infection that has the potential to cause severe respiratory distress:

☐ **Epiglottitis**

Explanation: Epiglottitis is frequently induced by a bacterial invasion affecting the epiglottis and adjacent tissues. Symptoms often include drooling, anxiety, cyanosis, and shallow breathing. Inspiratory stridor may also be present. Without timely and proper medical intervention, epiglottitis can swiftly lead to airway obstruction and fatality. In contrast, Croup is primarily an infection below the vocal cords usually caused by a parainfluenza virus, though other viral and bacterial agents can also be responsible.

Question 3

A patient exhibits signs indicative of irregular respiratory effort. Which observations would confirm this diagnosis?

☐ **Retractions, nasal flaring, abdominal breathing, and sweating**

Explanation: Indicators of irregular respiratory effort encompass retractions, nasal flaring, abdominal breathing, and sweating. On the other hand, sounds such as wheezing, crackles, and a silent chest denote lung abnormalities but do not specifically diagnose abnormal respiratory effort.

Question 4

Which of the following does not indicate a proper airway?

☐ **The individual is fully alert.**

Explanation: Characteristics of a proper airway include: an open airway with detectable airflow, the patient speaking in complete sentences, and the patient's voice sounding normal.

Question 5

Upon entering a residence, you observe an infant being held by her mother. The child is not crying and appears to be limp in her mother's arms. The infant's complexion appears pale or grayish, and there are no observable efforts of breathing. Which assessment tool is being utilized, and what is the primary action needed to manage this situation?

☐ **Pediatric Assessment Triangle; Remove the child from the mother, promptly open the airway, and evaluate breathing**

Explanation: The Pediatric Assessment Triangle is a quick visual assessment tool that evaluates the child's appearance, respiratory effort, and skin circulation. It is essential to immediately ensure the airway is open and assess the patient's breathing in a scenario where apnea is suspected.

Question 6

You are dispatched to Medical Park to attend to an individual who has reportedly fallen from his wheelchair. Upon arrival with your colleague Sheila, you observe two bystanders administering CPR on a male who appears to be around 60 years old. What are the recommended rate and depth of chest compressions to perform during CPR in this scenario?

☐ **30 compressions to 2 breaths / 2 inches depth**

Explanation: According to the American Heart Association (AHA) Guidelines for Cardiopulmonary Resuscitation (CPR), adults should receive chest compressions at a ratio of 30 compressions to 2 breaths. The recommended depth of compressions is approximately 2 inches. This scenario also highlights the reality that the specifics of a situation can differ from initial dispatch information, emphasizing the need for readiness to adapt to evolving situations.

Question 7

All of the following are functions performed by the respiratory system except:

☐ **Gas exchange between bronchioles and veins**

Explanation: The respiratory system's roles encompass ventilation, respiration, gas exchange between alveoli and capillaries, and serving as a buffer.

Question 8

To what does the term 'bilateral' pertain?

☐ **Both sides**

Explanation: The prefix 'bi-' denotes two or both.

Question 9

While performing an evaluation of a patient with your colleague Tony, you observe an unusual movement of the thoracic cage during expiration following a blunt force impact to the chest. This aberrant motion suggests what kind of injury?

☐ **Flail chest**

Explanation: A condition known as flail chest is characterized by a segment of the ribcage becoming detached, leading the affected part to move in opposition to the rest of the chest. This rare condition results from significant blunt chest trauma.

Question 10

Upon arrival, you and your colleague, Dale, find a female patient exhibiting signs of respiratory distress. She is ambulatory, with her arms elevated, and you can hear wheezing with each inhalation. Witnesses report that she was consuming a hot dog when she began to choke, which occurred approximately 10 minutes ago. What is the most appropriate intervention in this scenario?

☐ **Motivate her to cough and transport her**

Explanation: It is crucial to avoid performing the Heimlich maneuver unless there is a total obstruction of the airway. The optimal response in this case is to motivate the patient to continue coughing and arrange for immediate transportation to a medical facility.

Question 11

According to American Heart Association CPR Guidelines, what is the recommended duration for administering a rescue breath to a pediatric patient?

☐ **1 second**

Explanation: The guidelines advise that a rescue breath should be delivered within a 1-second time frame.

Question 12

Upon arriving at a nursing facility, you encounter a 73-year-old male patient with a stoma who is apneic. What is the appropriate intervention?

☐ **Employ a pediatric BVM mask with an adult bag for ventilation.**

Explanation: Individuals with tracheal stomas necessitate ventilation directly through the stoma. The most effective method for achieving a proper seal involves using a smaller mask that conforms to the neck. In cases of a partial laryngectomy, two rescuers are required: one to occlude the mouth and nose, while the other applies the mask and administers ventilation.

Question 13

Identify which of the following is not recognized as an early indicator of respiratory distress in a 7-year-old female.

☐ **Bluish discoloration of the lips**

Explanation: Except for cyanosis, all the provided options are EARLY indicators of respiratory issues in children. Cyanosis is considered a LATE sign.

Question 14

The evaluation of respiratory parameters in anaphylactic patients reveals ____________ and ____________.

☐ **severe respiratory distress and wheezing to diminished lung sounds**

Explanation: The evaluation of respiratory parameters in patients undergoing anaphylaxis reveals severe respiratory distress alongside wheezing or diminished lung sounds. This occurs due to bronchoconstriction and angioedema secondary to anaphylaxis, which can precipitate profound respiratory difficulties. The auditory characteristics of the lungs can range from wheezes, indicating bronchial constriction, to markedly reduced or absent sounds, reflecting severe obstruction.

Question 15

Cyanosis is frequently indicative of ____________.

☐ **The presence of hypoxia**

Explanation: Cyanosis, characterized by a bluish discoloration of the skin, typically occurs in regions of the body that are experiencing low oxygen levels or hypoxia.

Question 16

What is the proportion of oxygen present in the air we inhale?

☐ **21%**

Explanation: The atmospheric air that humans inhale consists of roughly 21% oxygen. Upon exhalation, the oxygen content decreases to approximately 16%.

Question 17

A 61-year-old male patient presents with shortness of breath, without any evidence or history of trauma. Which diagnostic history and physical examination approach would you select for this patient, and what is the most probable diagnosis of his condition?

☐ **Focused:Focused / The patient has an inflammation of the lower airway**

Explanation: Considering the patient's primary complaint of respiratory distress and the absence of trauma, the primary focus should be on the history related to his breathing issues and a targeted physical examination of the respiratory system, including the lungs and airways. While multiple answers offer potential explanations for his condition, only one combines the correct history and physical examination approach.

Question 18

Upon arrival at the scene, you encounter a 78-year-old male positioned in a chair, staring blankly. His respiration is labored, accompanied by audible wet lung sounds. He does not respond when you call his name or instruct him to move his toes. However, he exhibits a slight wince and withdraws when you apply pressure to his chest. What is his Glasgow Coma Scale (GCS) score?

☐ **9**

Explanation: The absence of a verbal response scores a 1, withdrawal from painful stimuli scores a 4, and spontaneous eye opening scores a 4, yielding a total score of 9.

Question 19

Identify the condition that does not lead to respiratory arrest in pediatric patients.

☐ **Hilscot syndrome**

Explanation: Hilscot syndrome is a fictitious term and thus cannot result in respiratory failure.

Question 20

During a conversation with a group of children at a daycare center, you observe that one child appears to be struggling to breathe. Which of the following observations led you to this conclusion?

☐ **Head bobbing**

Explanation: When evaluating a child's respiratory effort, look for indicators of increased respiratory workload such as: the use of accessory muscles, retractions, head bobbing, nasal flaring, or an increased rate of respiration (tachypnea).

Question 21

When utilizing a bag-valve mask (BVM) for ventilation, one should administer air ________________.

☐ **With only the necessary volume to achieve proper chest elevation**

Explanation: Administer just sufficient air to ensure visible chest rise, without expending the full capacity of the BVM.

Question 22

A 75-year-old male patient under your care is suspected of having experienced a cerebrovascular accident. He remains unresponsive, exhibiting snoring respirations. After administering the head tilt-chin lift technique, the snoring persists. What is your optimal next step?

☐ **Utilize a nasopharyngeal airway, ensuring it is measured from the nostril to the earlobe**

Explanation: The likely cause of the snoring is the tongue obstructing the pharyngeal passage. Using a correctly sized nasopharyngeal airway device, measured from the nostril to the earlobe, may alleviate the snoring. Given that the head tilt method proved ineffective, it is improbable that the jaw thrust would be more successful. Snoring respirations are generally not attributed to oropharyngeal secretions.

Question 23

Emergency services have contacted your team following a distress call from an individual by a nearby lake. The caller reported that a boat had crashed onto the shore, propelling several individuals into a forested area. Upon arrival, you and your colleague Zeek discover three individuals with minor abrasions performing CPR on a woman in her 30s. They inform you that the patient was thrown into the trees when the boat struck land. Zeek quickly checks for a pulse and finds none at the carotid artery. Both of you initiate CPR. As you prepare to transport the patient to the ambulance, you should provide approximately ____________ per minute using a BVM. During the 30-minute journey, an oral airway adjunct is placed, and a subsequent pulse check indicates the woman now has a strong palpable pulse. What is the appropriate ventilation rate for this patient now? ____________

☐ **6 breaths / 10 to 12 breaths per minute**

Explanation: In accordance with the American Heart Association's CPR and rescue breathing guidelines, CPR on the woman should involve a 30:2 compression to ventilation ratio, resulting in approximately 6 breaths per minute. Once a pulse is detected, the ventilation rate should transition to the rescue breathing rate of 10 to 12 breaths per minute.

Question 24

You are attending to a 6-year-old girl suffering from an asthma exacerbation. She is having difficulty breathing, and you provide her with oxygen through a non-rebreather mask. Which of the following statements is incorrect in the context of pediatric asthma exacerbations?

☐ **Pediatric asthma episodes typically resolve without intervention**

Explanation: Pediatric asthma exacerbations necessitate the use of bronchodilators, oxygen therapy, and vigilant monitoring for signs of worsening. These events rarely resolve spontaneously and can pose a serious risk.

Question 25

During expiration, what condition is commonly suggested by the abnormal, contradictory excursion of the thoracic cage?

☐ **Flail chest**

Explanation: The phenomenon of paradoxical chest movement typically arises from a 'flail chest,' where a segment of ribs detached from the rest exhibits aberrant behavior due to compromised structural integrity, allowing the lung to bulge through the resultant opening.

Question 26

Crackles in the lungs are indicative of:

☐ **An indication of lower respiratory tract obstruction**

Explanation: Crackles are respiratory sounds produced when air passes through fluids within the lung tissue. This condition is typically associated with lower respiratory issues and is more commonly linked to left-sided congestive heart failure (CHF) than to right-sided CHF.

Question 27

You and your colleague, with whom you have been collaborating for two years, respond to a residence where a female patient reports experiencing chest discomfort and difficulty breathing. She presents with diaphoresis, a heart rate of 110 beats per minute, a respiratory rate of 22 breaths per minute, and a blood pressure of 140/80 mmHg. She denies any prior cardiac or pulmonary conditions. What is the most appropriate course of action?

☐ **Conduct an assessment, administer oxygen at a rate of 15 lpm, and proceed with transportation**

Explanation: The optimal approach entails administering oxygen and expeditiously transporting her to a medical facility.

Question 28

The left atrium and ventricle of the cardiac system are responsible for ______________ and ______________.

☐ **receives pulmonary circulation, drives systemic circulation**

Explanation: The left atrium and ventricle are pivotal in accepting blood from the pulmonary veins and propelling it through the systemic circulation.

Question 29

Identify the elements that constitute components of the lower respiratory tract from the options provided:

☐ **Trachea - bronchial tree - alveoli**

Explanation: The anatomical structures comprising the lower respiratory tract include the trachea, the bronchial tree, and the alveoli. In contrast, the upper respiratory tract encompasses all structures located above the trachea.

Question 30

After your colleague Gina has used a French tip catheter to clear a patient's airway of vomit, what is the appropriate subsequent action?

☐ **Ready the catheter for future use by rinsing it with sterile water**

Explanation: Proper protocol calls for preparing for potential further suctioning by rinsing the catheter with sterile water.

Question 31

Identify three pathological states frequently associated with an accelerated respiratory rate (tachypnea).

☐ **Hypoxia, CHF, and shock**

Explanation: Hypoxia, heart failure with fluid overload (congestive heart failure, CHF), and circulatory collapse (shock) are appropriate answers for the following reasons. Hypoxia refers to insufficient oxygenation of bodily tissues, leading to acid-base imbalance (acidosis). Tachypnea can ensue as the body attempts to enhance oxygen intake by increasing respiratory rate. Congestive heart failure arises when the ventricular myocardium suffers damage, impairing its ability to manage blood return from the atria. This leads to pulmonary congestion, where fluid accumulation in the lungs impairs oxygen exchange within the capillaries (pulmonary edema). The body's response often includes tachypnea to optimize oxygenation. In the case of shock, the cardiovascular system fails to maintain adequate circulation for tissue function, leading to early onset of metabolic acidosis. Tachypnea occurs as a compensatory mechanism to counteract the acidosis and maintain homeostasis.

Question 32

In pediatric care, certain interventions are necessary to ensure the airway remains unobstructed. Which of the following techniques is deemed appropriate?

☐ **Employ an oral or nasal airway adjunct**

Explanation: The sole recommended practice is the use of an oral or nasal airway adjunct. Alternatively, a rolled-up towel approximately one inch in height should be positioned beneath the shoulders, not the neck. Utilizing the Trendelenburg position accompanied by high flow oxygen will not facilitate airway maintenance. Furthermore, employing Magill forceps to reposition the tongue is not advisable.

Question 33

A report has indicated that a male individual is found unconscious behind a grocery store and is not exhibiting signs of respiration. Upon arrival, you encounter a male sitting solo against a wall with his eyes shut, unresponsive to verbal stimuli. His respiratory rate is 8 irregular breaths per minute, interspersed with episodes of apnea. Adjacent to him lies a small plastic bag containing a white substance. Upon administering a sternal rub, he clutches his chest but remains silent. How would you assess his Glasgow Coma Scale (GCS) score, and what is the most appropriate intervention?

☐ **GCS score of 7 / Facilitate ventilation using a Bag-Valve Mask (BVM)**

Explanation: Intervention to support breathing is essential due to his low respiratory rate and intermittent apnea, indicating inadequate oxygenation. His lack of ocular response to any stimulus scores 1 point. His absence of verbal response also scores 1 point. However, his response to pain by localizing it to his chest earns 5 points, resulting in a total GCS score of 7.

Question 34

Upon arrival at the scene where a man is experiencing unexplained respiratory distress, what can you ascertain?

☐ **It might involve the trachea, epiglottis, or alveoli**

Explanation: Given only the information about the man's respiratory distress, the only certainty is that the problem must be related to the respiratory system. Determining the need for Advanced Life Support or whether the patient has sustained a head injury cannot be concluded from the present information.

Question 35

Faced with a respiratory failure case, you and your colleague must determine the main objective of providing ventilatory support. What is the primary rationale for this intervention?

☐ **Providing ventilatory support enhances both oxygenation and ventilation**

Explanation: The primary rationale for offering ventilatory support during episodes of respiratory distress or failure is to enhance both oxygenation and ventilation processes.

Question 36

What causes gastric distention in patients undergoing cardiopulmonary resuscitation (CPR)?

☐ **Excessive air volume during ventilatory support**

Explanation: Excessive air volume and a blocked or partially blocked airway can lead to the abdomen becoming distended.

Question 37

During a pulmonary examination of a healthy 23-year-old woman, what type of respiratory sounds would you anticipate detecting?

☐ **Vesicular breath sounds**

Explanation: Vesicular breath sounds are typical over the lung fields in a healthy individual. In contrast, bronchial breath sounds are expected near the trachea and larger airways, not over the peripheral lung tissue.

Question 38

The initiation of resuscitative efforts should be withheld in cases where unequivocal indications of death are evident. Which of the following is not considered one of these signs?

☐ **Lack of cardiac activity**

Explanation: Definitive signs of death encompass: rigor mortis, dependent lividity, putrefaction or advanced decomposition, and injuries incompatible with life.

Question 39

What is the primary therapeutic intervention for a patient exposed to noxious gases?

☐ **Assisted Ventilation**

Explanation: While administering oxygen is essential, addressing the primary cause is crucial. Irritant gases compromise the lungs' capacity to ventilate, thus prioritizing the necessity for assisted ventilation.

Question 40

A young male, aged 20, has sustained a back injury at a nearby swimming location. Upon arrival, you and your colleague, Missy, find him groaning and partly submerged in water near a rock formation. Bystanders report that he fell approximately 30 feet from a tree he was climbing over the swimming area, landing on the rocks. His breathing rate is 12 breaths per minute, characterized by very shallow breaths with intermittent pauses of apnea. His heart rate is 72 beats per minute, and his skin appears slightly moist and pale. Following the provision of cervical spine stabilization, what should be the next immediate step in managing his condition?

☐ **Provide assisted ventilation and elevate his legs**

Explanation: This individual requires ventilatory assistance due to inadequate respiratory rate and depth. Management should include slight elevation of the legs to address potential shock, along with using blankets or heat packs to maintain body warmth.

Question 41

Individuals with tracheal stomas require distinct methods of ventilation compared to those without such openings. Which of the following statements regarding these ventilation methods is accurate?

☐ **An effective assisted ventilation technique involves sealing the patient's mouth and nose when ventilating through a stoma, and then unsealing them during passive exhalation.**

Explanation: A tracheostomy constitutes a permanent aperture at the midline or base of the trachea. During ventilation via a stoma, maneuvers like head tilt or jaw thrust are ineffectual as they only lift the tongue away from the pharynx, positioned above the tracheostomy opening. There is no unique adapter for tracheostomies; the typical adapter included with a bag-valve mask (BVM) is utilized. The adapter cannot attach directly to the stoma; a child or infant mask should be used to create a seal in the absence of a tube. Employing an oropharyngeal airway (OPA) provides minimal benefit to patients ventilated through a tracheostomy and should be removed if the patient vomits, with suctioning limited to the base of the tongue.

Question 42

What is a clinical reason for employing a tracheostomy mask?

☐ **The patient has a tracheal stoma**

Explanation: A tracheostomy mask facilitates the administration of oxygen directly into a patient's tracheal stoma. This device is designed to cover the stoma while being secured around the patient's neck.

Question 43

How is the term 'golden hour' best defined?

☐ **The interval from the moment an injury occurs to when surgery is performed**

Explanation: The 'golden hour' refers to the critical time period from the occurrence of an injury until surgical intervention.

Question 44

Identify the procedure that should be avoided in a 9-year-old with a cranial fracture resulting from a horseback riding incident.

☐ **Nasopharyngeal airway**

Explanation: Utilization of a nasopharyngeal airway is not advisable for individuals with potential basilar skull fractures, as the device risks penetrating the brain through the fracture site.

Question 45

An 84-year-old male patient presents with auditory crepitations during lung auscultation, along with reports of chest discomfort and pulmonary congestion. These clinical manifestations may be indicative of which condition?

☐ **Left ventricular failure**

Explanation: These clinical signs are suggestive of potential left ventricular dysfunction. The heart's pumping efficiency is compromised, leading to fluid accumulation in the lungs.

Question 46

What is a clinical sign that necessitates the suctioning of the upper respiratory tract?

☐ **A gurgling noise noted during a patient's respiration.**

Explanation: A gurgling noise perceived during respiration indicates the need for suctioning.

Question 47

What is a key benefit of using supplemental oxygen therapy?

☐ **Increasing the concentration of oxygen can enhance cellular respiration and replace some inert gases**

Explanation: Increasing the proportion of oxygen in the gas mixture during supplemental oxygen therapy can enhance cellular respiration by providing a higher concentration of available oxygen, thereby substituting some of the inert gases.

Question 48

After attending to a call concerning an unidentified ailment or injury alongside your colleague Aaron, you arrive at an apartment complex and notice a woman lying supine with her eyes closed in the parking lot. Following an assessment ensuring the safety of the environment, what would be the most effective method for obtaining pertinent information about her condition?

☐ **Assess her pulse manually while placing your ear near her mouth and watching the sternum for signs of chest movement**

Explanation: It is essential to evaluate her consciousness level, check her pulse, and confirm whether she is breathing. The second option is optimal for achieving this.

Question 49

Calculate the respiratory minute volume for an individual with a respiratory rate of 20 breaths per minute and a tidal volume of 300 milliliters.

☐ **6000 mL/min**

Explanation: The respiratory minute volume is determined by multiplying the tidal volume by the frequency of breaths per minute. In this case, 20 breaths multiplied by 300 mL results in 6000 mL/min.

Question 50

You are summoned to a childcare center where a 3-year-old boy has lost consciousness after choking on a plastic toy. Upon arrival, you observe the child in a supine position on the floor while the caregiver is unsuccessfully attempting to administer artificial respirations. 'I am unable to get any air into him!' she exclaims. Upon a swift examination of the oral cavity, a partially visible object deeply embedded near the glottis can be seen. What is the appropriate immediate action to take?

☐ **Start chest compressions to dislodge the obstruction and periodically check the airway.**

Explanation: For a patient who has lost consciousness due to a foreign body airway obstruction

(FBAO), initiating chest compressions is recommended upon confirming airway blockage. Chest compressions can generate intrathoracic pressure equivalent to or greater than that of abdominal thrusts, thereby enhancing the likelihood of dislodging the object in an unconscious patient. During compressions, regularly inspect the mouth to see if the object has been dislodged and attempt ventilations if feasible.

MEDICAL / OBSTETRICS / GYNECOLOGY

Question 1

When a patient experiencing chest pain inquires about the number of chambers in the human heart, how do you respond?

☐ **There are 4 chambers: the right and left atria, and the right and left ventricles.**

Explanation: The human heart consists of 4 chambers: the right and left atria, along with the right and left ventricles.

Question 2

Encountering an individual lying on their stomach is best described as which position?

☐ **Prone**

Explanation: A supine position refers to lying on one's back, a prone position pertains to lying on the abdomen, a lateral position involves lying on the side, and the Fowler's position is characterized by sitting up.

Question 3

A male motorcyclist involved in a collision with a car displays multiple injuries, including head trauma and several lacerations on his knees and feet. Despite efforts, such as verbal requests and a sternal rub, he does not open his eyes. He mumbles unintelligibly, and his arms and hands are drawn tightly to his chest. He does not respond to instructions to raise his arm. What is his Glasgow Coma Scale (GCS) score?

☐ **6**

Explanation: The patient's failure to open his eyes scores a 1. His production of incomprehensible sounds scores a 2. The abnormal flexion of his arms and hands scores a 3, leading to a cumulative GCS score of 6.

Question 4

In which anatomical structure within the maternal body does embryonic and fetal development occur?

☐ **Uterus**

Explanation: Embryonic and fetal development takes place within the uterus. The cervix, on the other hand, serves as the passage situated at the lower part of the uterus.

Question 5

Upon evaluating a stroke patient, you observe the presence of dysarthria. This condition is defined by which of the following symptoms?

☐ **Slurred speech**

Explanation: Dysarthria is characterized by slurred speech resulting from neurological damage.

Question 6

Which of the following accurately characterizes the role of plasma within the human body?

☐ **It carries cells to different parts of the body**

Explanation: Plasma serves as the liquid medium that carries cells across various parts of the body. It constitutes approximately 55% of the entire blood volume.

Question 7

Among the following physiological responses, which is regulated by the sympathetic division of the autonomic nervous system?

☐ **Narrowing of blood vessels**

Explanation: The activation of the sympathetic nervous system typically results in the constriction of blood vessels, leading to elevated blood pressure. Conversely, the deceleration of heart rate is associated with the activity of the parasympathetic nervous system.

Question 8

At which phase of labor is the rupture of the amniotic sac most commonly observed?

☐ **Initial stage**

Explanation: The initial stage comprises contractions and cervical dilation. The second stage encompasses the period from the baby's descent into the birth canal until delivery. The third stage involves the expulsion of the placenta.

Question 9

Which of the following is not a role of the pancreas?

☐ **Controls the level of iron in the bloodstream**

Explanation: The pancreas is involved in the breakdown of fats, starches, and proteins, and it also secretes insulin to control blood sugar levels.

Question 10

Given the rising threat of nerve agent exposure, emergency medical service (EMS) teams must be equipped with appropriate antidote kits. Which of the following options correctly identifies these antidote kits?

☐ **Mark 1 kits or NAAK**

Explanation: The antidote kits specifically designed for nerve agent exposure are referred to as Mark 1 kits or Nerve Agent Antidote Kits (NAAK). These kits typically contain two auto-injectors: one filled with atropine and the other with pralidoxime chloride (2-PAM chloride). Alternative names for these kits include Duo-Dotes or Chempaks. The implementation and usage of these kits vary based on regional guidelines.

Question 11

Upon arriving at a senior care facility, you and your colleague Rodrigo discover that both staff and residents are experiencing vomiting and dizziness. What is the most likely cause?

☐ **The presence of a harmful chemical or substance**

Explanation: When multiple individuals exhibit similar symptoms simultaneously, it often indicates an environmental hazard that must be thoroughly investigated to prevent further exposure.

Question 12

What is an alternative medical term used to describe inadequate blood flow to tissues?

☐ **Shock**

Explanation: A state in which the body's tissues receive insufficient oxygen due to reduced blood flow is referred to as shock.

Question 13

Upon arrival at a multi-casualty incident with your colleague Lola, which of the following patients should be deemed the highest priority for immediate medical intervention?

☐ **A 45-year-old woman with a blood pressure of 169/92**

Explanation: A patient presenting with a blood pressure reading of 169/92 necessitates prioritized attention. Compared to this, patients with 12-minute interval contractions, a minor fracture, or wasp stings are secondary.

Question 14

A severe winter storm has left numerous individuals stranded on a highway for several days. You have been called to assist with the National Guard to provide aid to those suffering from cold exposure. As you gather your supplies, what items should you prioritize and why?

☐ **Drinking water; Dehydration is a highly probable issue**

Explanation: While both external warming techniques and glucose are beneficial, the availability of drinking water is paramount. This is because cold environments diminish the body's thirst response, resulting in reduced fluid intake. However, a significant amount of moisture is lost through breathing in cold air, and this combined with the lack of thirst leads to rapid dehydration. Thus, it is essential to ensure that those impacted by exposure are encouraged to consume fluids, whether hot or cold.

Question 15

Which clinical manifestations would signify that a patient's condition has escalated from a mild allergic response to anaphylaxis?

☐ **Circulatory shock or severe respiratory distress**

Explanation: An individual presenting with severe respiratory compromise and signs of circulatory shock is diagnosed with anaphylactic shock or anaphylaxis.

Question 16

What is denoted by the abbreviation 'mmHg'?

☐ **Millimeters of mercury**

Explanation: The abbreviation 'mmHg' represents millimeters of mercury.

Question 17

What is the term for an infant born with the buttocks presenting first?

☐ **Breech**

Explanation: Infants delivered with the buttocks or feet first are termed 'breech.' The name 'Ryan' can still be used for such babies, but it does not describe the presentation type at birth.

Question 18

Syncope can arise from various emergency situations. Which term is commonly used to refer to Syncope?

☐ **Fainting**

Explanation: The term Syncope is commonly known as fainting.

Question 19

What are the primary etiologies of shock?

☐ **Inadequate cardiac output, fluid depletion, and excessive vessel dilation**

Explanation: Shock fundamentally arises due to inadequate cardiac function, depletion of blood or bodily fluids, and excessive dilation of blood vessels.

Question 20

What does the term 'Hemiparesis' signify?

☐ **Unilateral body weakness**

Explanation: Hemiparesis refers to a condition characterized by reduced muscular strength or partial paralysis affecting one lateral side of the human body, commonly observed during cerebrovascular incidents such as strokes.

Question 21

Upon arriving at the location of an unidentified medical incident with your colleague Abner, what should be your primary focus as you assess the scene?

☐ **Potential hazards that could compromise scene safety**

Explanation: Ensuring the safety of the scene is paramount, following your Body Substance Isolation (BSI) protocol. This is crucial even if the environment appears serene and well-controlled at first glance.

Question 22

Regarding the prevalence of seizures in the United States, it is noted to be _______. Emergency Medical Services (EMS) report that approximately _______ of their emergency 911 calls are related to seizures.

☐ **high, 30%**

Explanation: The prevalence of seizures in the United States is HIGH. EMS systems report that approximately 30% of their 911 calls are related to seizures.

Question 23

Identify the perineum from the following options.

☐ **Region between the anus and vaginal opening**

Explanation: The perineum refers to the region located between the anus and the vaginal opening.

Question 24

Determine the equivalent weight of 150 pounds in kilograms.

☐ **67.5 kilograms**

Explanation: One efficient method for converting pounds to kilograms is to calculate 50% of the pound value, then compute 10% of this result and deduct that from your initial 50%. For instance, 50% of 150 pounds is 75 pounds, and 10% of 75 pounds is 7.5 pounds. Subtracting 7.5 pounds from 75 pounds yields 67.5 kilograms. Alternatively, one can approximate the conversion by dividing the pound value by a factor of 2.2.

Question 25

In the context of the mnemonic OPQRST, what does the letter 'T' represent?

☐ **Time**

Explanation: The term 'Time' refers to the duration and pattern of the symptoms. Specifically, it addresses whether the symptoms are intermittent or continuous.

Question 26

In the context of a detailed ocular examination, upon which of the following should attention not be concentrated?

☐ **Pigmentation of the pupils**

Explanation: A thorough ocular assessment should prioritize evaluating: the size of the pupils; their symmetry and reaction to light; as well as the presence of pink, moist conjunctiva. The pigmentation of the pupils is typically irrelevant as it consistently appears dark in the majority of individuals.

Question 27

In conducting a detailed history of a patient's presenting symptoms, healthcare professionals utilize the acronym OPQRST. What inquiry does the letter 'O' denote?

☐ **When did it start?**

Explanation: Onset, referring to the initiation of symptoms. Did they begin suddenly or gradually?

Question 28

In the course of conducting a secondary evaluation of the abdominal region, which of the following should not be closely examined:

☐ **Retractions**

Explanation: When performing a secondary evaluation of the abdomen, focus should be given to pain, rigidity, distention, scars, and the presence of medical devices.

Question 29

Which of the subsequent factors can induce hypoglycemia?

☐ **All of the mentioned factors**

Explanation: Each listed factor has the ability to decrease glucose levels in the bloodstream.

Question 30

Which of the following symptoms is not characteristic of alcohol withdrawal?

☐ **Pinpoint pupils**

Explanation: Symptoms of alcohol withdrawal typically encompass: tremors, sweating, weakness, hallucinations, and seizures.

Question 31

The temporal characteristics of the immune system's response to an allergenic stimulus can be classified as ________________ and _____________.

☐ **slow (more than 30 minutes) and rapid (within 30 minutes)**

Explanation: The temporal characteristics of the immune system's response to an allergenic stimulus are categorized as slow (exceeding 30 minutes) and rapid (within 30 minutes). According to the National Emergency Medical Service Education Standards, the distinction is made at the 30-minute mark.

Question 32

The most frequent site of an aneurysm is the __________ and typically presents as ________________.

☐ **abdominal region / symptomless**

Explanation: An aneurysm is characterized by an abnormal dilation of a blood vessel. Predominantly, these occur in the abdominal region and generally do not exhibit symptoms, though they can sometimes cause intense discomfort. The likelihood of rupture escalates as the arterial wall thins.

Question 33

The ___________ stage of a seizure, which involves convulsive movements, is the third in sequence.

☐ **Clonic phase**

Explanation: Seizures initiate with the aura stage, where the individual responds to sensory stimuli. This is followed by the tonic stage, characterized by muscle rigidity and an arched back posture. The third stage is the clonic phase, marked by convulsive movements. The final stage is the postictal phase, during which the patient gradually regains awareness.

Question 34

How do the primary structural differences between pediatric and adult airways manifest?

☐ **In pediatric airways, the Cricoid ring is the most constricted section, and the tongue occupies a larger proportion of the oral cavity.**

Explanation: The anatomical proportions of a pediatric airway differ, with a larger tongue relative to the mouth's size. Moreover, in children, the Cricoid cartilage represents the most constricted segment of the airway.

Question 35

What classification do bacteria and viruses share?

☐ **Pathogens**

Explanation: Both entities are considered pathogens capable of being transmitted between individuals via multiple mechanisms.

Question 36

Which of the following is not an instance of toxic substances that can be absorbed?

☐ **Chlorine**

Explanation: Toxic substances known to be absorbed include: acids, alkalis, petroleum derivatives, poison ivy, and poison oak.

Question 37

Upon arriving at the residence of a 32-year-old male experiencing epistaxis, he is conscious, and no other medical issues are present. Interventions to arrest the hemorrhage include all of the following, except:

☐ **Instruct the patient to sit up and lean back**

Explanation: Effective measures to control nasal bleeding in an alert individual include: instructing the patient to sit upright and lean forward, applying firm pressure by pinching the nostrils together, and advising the patient to refrain from sniffing or blowing their nose. Leaning the patient backward can result in blood flowing down the throat and into the stomach, potentially inducing nausea and vomiting.

Question 38

Which category of shock is likely to be observed in a patient exhibiting symptoms of vomiting, increased urination, and diarrhea?

☐ **Hypovolemic shock**

Explanation: The condition known as hypovolemic shock can occur due to the excessive loss of body fluids through vomiting, urination, and diarrhea. Such fluid depletion disrupts the body's ability to maintain proper balance, potentially necessitating intervention to stabilize metabolic functions.

Question 39

All of the following are classifications of seizures except:

☐ **Postictal**

Explanation: Seizure types encompass: Generalized tonic-clonic seizures, partial seizures, and status epilepticus. General seizures originate from multiple regions within the brain, typically characterized by a loss of consciousness coupled with full-body convulsions. Partial seizures originate from a single area in the brain and may or may not include loss of consciousness. Status epilepticus is defined as prolonged or continuous seizure activity lasting more than five minutes or recurrent seizures without regaining consciousness. The postictal phase follows the seizure, during which the patient experiences a reduced level of consciousness, generally serving as a recovery period for both the body and brain after the seizure.

Question 40

A 46-year-old female, while trekking in the forest close to her residence, inadvertently disturbed a hornet's nest and sustained numerous stings. She managed to call 911 from her mobile device and will meet you at her address. Upon arriving, you discover her prone on her front lawn. Following the completion of your initial scene assessment, which treatment protocol would be considered most appropriate according to the NREMT Patient Assessment/Management - Medical Skill Sheet?

☐ **Evaluate consciousness level - Identify immediate threats - Evaluate airway, breathing, and circulation**

Explanation: In the first option, without a complete assessment, administering epinephrine is premature. The second option recommends oxygen therapy but neglects the initial steps of primary survey and takes vital signs before conducting a SAMPLE history. The fourth option also overlooks the initial steps of the primary survey and incorrectly prioritizes a secondary assessment and transport decision. Administering epinephrine would be warranted during ABCs if she was experiencing anaphylaxis.

Question 41

On a warm afternoon in August, you receive an emergency call to attend to a 78-year-old male who has frequently been a patient in your ambulance. The dispatch indicates that his caregiver discovered him lying in an empty bathtub, unable to exit on his own. Upon your arrival, the patient recognizes you and expresses regret for the 911 call, stating that he merely needs assistance to get out of the tub. Observations reveal that his respiratory rate is 20 breaths per minute with normal depth, his skin is slightly flushed, his pulse rate is 118 beats per minute, and his blood pressure reads 138/78. He denies experiencing any pain. What could be the probable cause of his condition and what is the recommended course of action?

☐ **He is experiencing hypothermia. Cover him with a blanket and help him out of the bathtub. Apply heat packs to his underarms and groin area, provide high-flow oxygen, and transport him to the nearest hospital for further evaluation.**

Explanation: The most plausible cause for this patient's condition is mild hypothermia. Despite the warm weather, the bathtub facilitates thermal conduction away from his body. Additionally, the body loses heat through radiation, and air circulation exacerbates heat loss via convection. Any remaining water in the tub could further lower body temperature through evaporation. Early indicators of hypothermia include an elevated pulse rate, rapid breathing, and flushed skin. Elderly individuals, due to a less efficient thermoregulatory system, are particularly vulnerable to urban hypothermia.

Question 42

You are attending to a 46-year-old male individual diagnosed with Type 1 diabetes mellitus. Emergency services were contacted by his partner, who discovered him in a fetal position on the bathroom floor, with a towel positioned beneath his head upon her return home from work. There are no apparent signs of physical injury. The patient is non-responsive, but his respiratory rate is stable at 16 breaths per minute, with adequate depth. His partner reports having a phone conversation with him earlier in the day, during which he appeared to be in good health. What is the most plausible reason for this individual's altered level of consciousness?

☐ **He administered his insulin dose but did not consume food, resulting in hypoglycemia.**

Explanation: It is most probable that the patient is experiencing hypoglycemia due to skipping meals. Option 2 is unlikely as hyperglycemia develops slowly, and his partner had only recently conversed with him, noting no issues. Moreover, his regular breathing negates hyperventilation, which would be typical in hyperglycemia if the body were expelling excess carbon dioxide. Option 3 is incorrect because omitting insulin leads to hyperglycemia, not hypoglycemia. Option 4 is also incorrect, as in Type 1 diabetes the pancreas is incapable of producing sufficient insulin. Excessive insulin causes hypoglycemia (insulin shock), not hyperglycemia (diabetic coma).

Question 43

Upon responding with your colleague Wanda to a multi-vehicle collision, you are the second ambulance to reach the site. Your primary assessment reveals seven individuals involved across two vehicles, and extrication is unnecessary for any. In the first vehicle, you find a 42-year-old pregnant woman at 28 weeks gestation who is unconscious, a distressed 14-year-old girl reporting back pain, and a 7-year-old boy with a facial laceration but otherwise uninjured. The second vehicle contains an 86-year-old male driver slumped over the steering wheel and three teenagers in the back seat. The two teens on the impact side exhibit nausea and altered consciousness levels. The third teenager, a girl in the back seat, mentions she experienced seizures and vomiting earlier and her grandfather was driving her to the hospital; she shows no signs of injury and was wearing a seatbelt. Whom should your medical team prioritize for immediate attention?

☐ **The 86-year-old male and the pregnant woman**

Explanation: The unconscious 86-year-old male and the unconscious pregnant woman require urgent medical intervention due to their severely diminished responsiveness.

Question 44

You are summoned to the Shadypines elder care facility to attend to an octogenarian male exhibiting altered consciousness and tachycardia. Upon arrival, a nurse is measuring his blood pressure, which registers at 98/62 mmHg. The patient is diaphoretic, tremulous, and febrile. The nurse informs you that he has diabetes mellitus and was recently discharged from the hospital following a surgery for diverticulitis two days prior. Despite multiple attempts to rouse him by calling his name, he fails to open his eyes. The only verbal response he provides when questioned is the repetition of the name "Katherine." He is unresponsive to commands to move his extremities but withdraws his hand to his chest and moans when subjected to a sternal rub. What is this patient's Glasgow Coma Scale (GCS) score, and what is the most probable diagnosis for his condition?

☐ **GCS of 9/ He is in septic shock**

Explanation: This patient receives a score of 1 for the eye-opening category due to no response. His verbal response of repetitively uttering "Katherine" is deemed inappropriate, earning him 3 points verbally. He localizes pain when sternal rub is performed, awarding him 5 points for motor response, culminating in a total GCS score of 9. The clinical indicators such as hypotension, diaphoresis, and recent surgical history are indicative of septic shock.

Question 45

Given no additional context, assess the condition of the following pediatric patient: A 12-month-old male presenting with a heart rate of 110 bpm, a respiratory rate of 30 per minute, and a systolic blood pressure of 90 mmHg.

☐ **Healthy**

Explanation: All vital signs fall within the expected range for a child of this age group. A 12-month-old child can be categorized at the intersection of infancy and toddlerhood, wherein both sets of vital parameters are applicable. Evaluate the patient based on his physical condition and the parents' description of normal versus abnormal behavior.

Question 46

How is 'behavior' most accurately characterized?

☐ **Observable responses by an individual to their environment, including their actions.**

Explanation: 'Behavior' is optimally characterized as: 'Observable responses by an individual to their environment, including their actions.'

Question 47

The phenomenon where a blood clot dislodges and migrates to another part of the circulatory system is known as ______________.

☐ **Embolism**

Explanation: Such a clot can obstruct smaller blood vessels, depriving downstream tissues of oxygen and leading to potential damage.

Question 48

All of the following are recognized long-term consequences of chronic alcohol consumption, except:

☐ **Seizures**

Explanation: Chronic alcoholism can result in numerous long-term health issues: liver damage, hepatitis, cirrhosis, pancreatitis, erosive gastritis, elevated risk for breast and colorectal cancers, cerebral atrophy, impotence, and infertility.

Question 49

In the context of a diabetic crisis, the preference for administering glucose over sucrose is due to what reason?

☐ **Glucose, being a monosaccharide, is metabolized more rapidly**

Explanation: The body's ability to quickly utilize glucose stems from its classification as a monosaccharide, whereas sucrose is a disaccharide requiring additional metabolic steps before use.

Question 50

Define the term Hyperglycemia.

☐ **A medical condition characterized by elevated blood glucose levels beyond the normal range.**

Explanation: Hyperglycemia refers to a medical condition characterized by elevated blood glucose levels beyond the normal range. This condition arises due to an excessive amount of glucose circulating in the bloodstream.

Dear Reader,

We understand that preparing for the NREMT exam can feel like a challenging task, and that's why we want to provide you with additional tools to support your journey toward success.

As a valued customer, you have exclusive access to our advanced e-learning platform, "Learnik," designed to enhance your study experience and offer targeted resources to help you excel in the NREMT exam. By scanning the QR code below, you'll unlock a wealth of supplementary learning resources directly related to the topics covered in this book.

On Learnik, you'll find a variety of interactive features to optimize your preparation:

> **Scenario-Based Quizzes:** The platform generates personalized quizzes based on real-life scenarios and the content of the book you've purchased. These quizzes are designed to reinforce your understanding of key concepts and skills essential for the NREMT exam and help you track your progress.

But there's more! Learnik also offers a wide range of bonus content to enrich your learning experience:

> **Audiobooks:** Study on the go with our professionally narrated audiobooks, allowing you to learn during your commute or downtime.
>
> **Flashcards:** An effective tool for quickly memorizing essential medical terminology, procedures, and guidelines. Our flashcards are structured to present critical facts in a clear and concise format.

These resources are designed to complement your study routine, making your preparation more comprehensive and efficient. They are available exclusively to our valued customers like you, helping to maximize your chances of success in the NREMT exam.

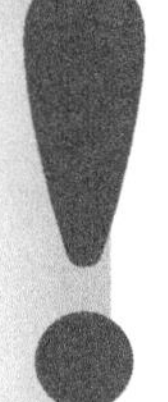

So why wait? Scan the QR code below and embark on your learning journey with Learnik. It's the perfect way to elevate your NREMT exam preparation. We're here to support you every step of the way as you work toward your goals.

Thank you for choosing our educational materials, and we wish you all the best in your NREMT exam preparation!

For any issues, feel free to contact us at ***info@learnik.com***

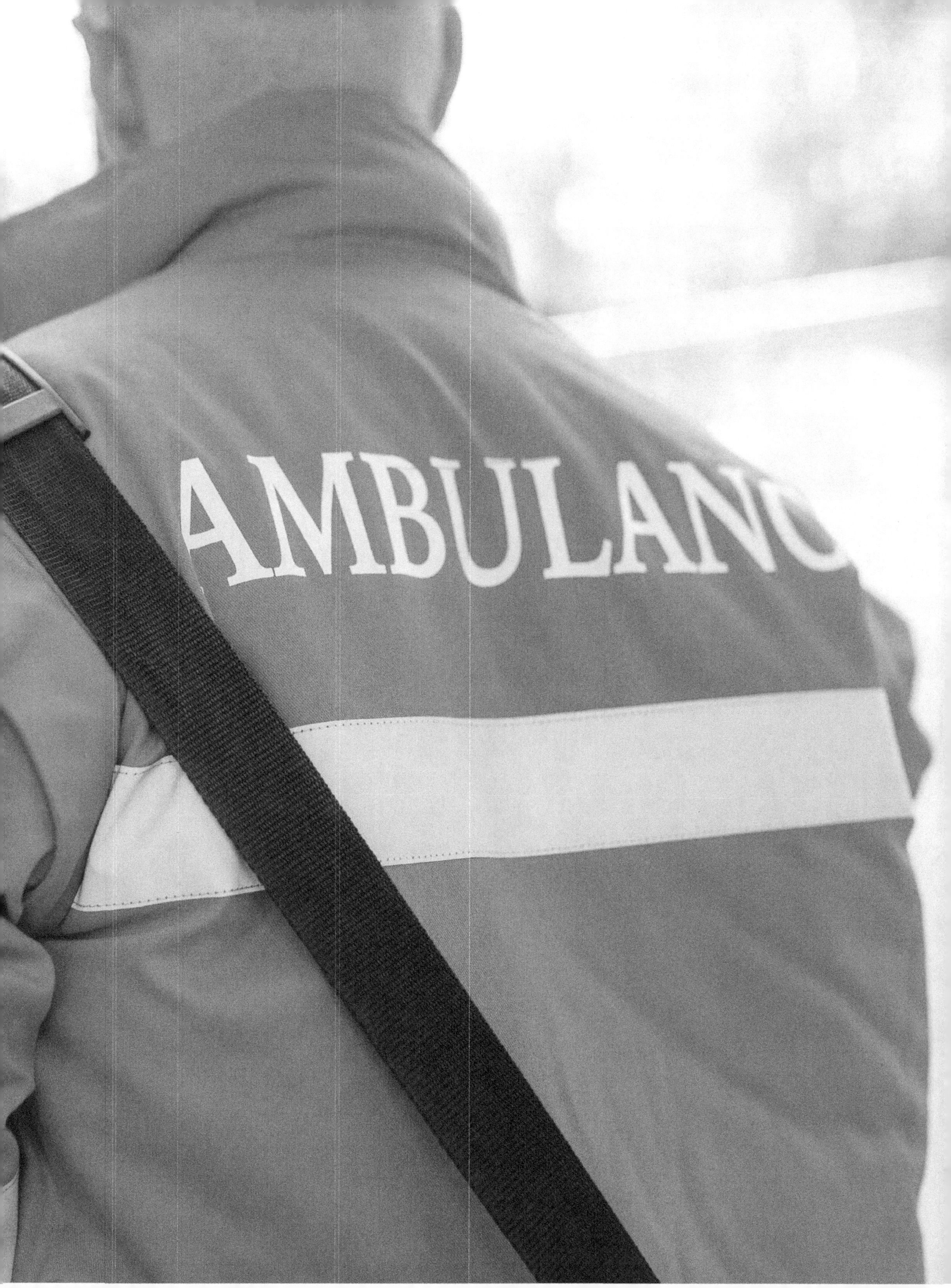

AMBULANC

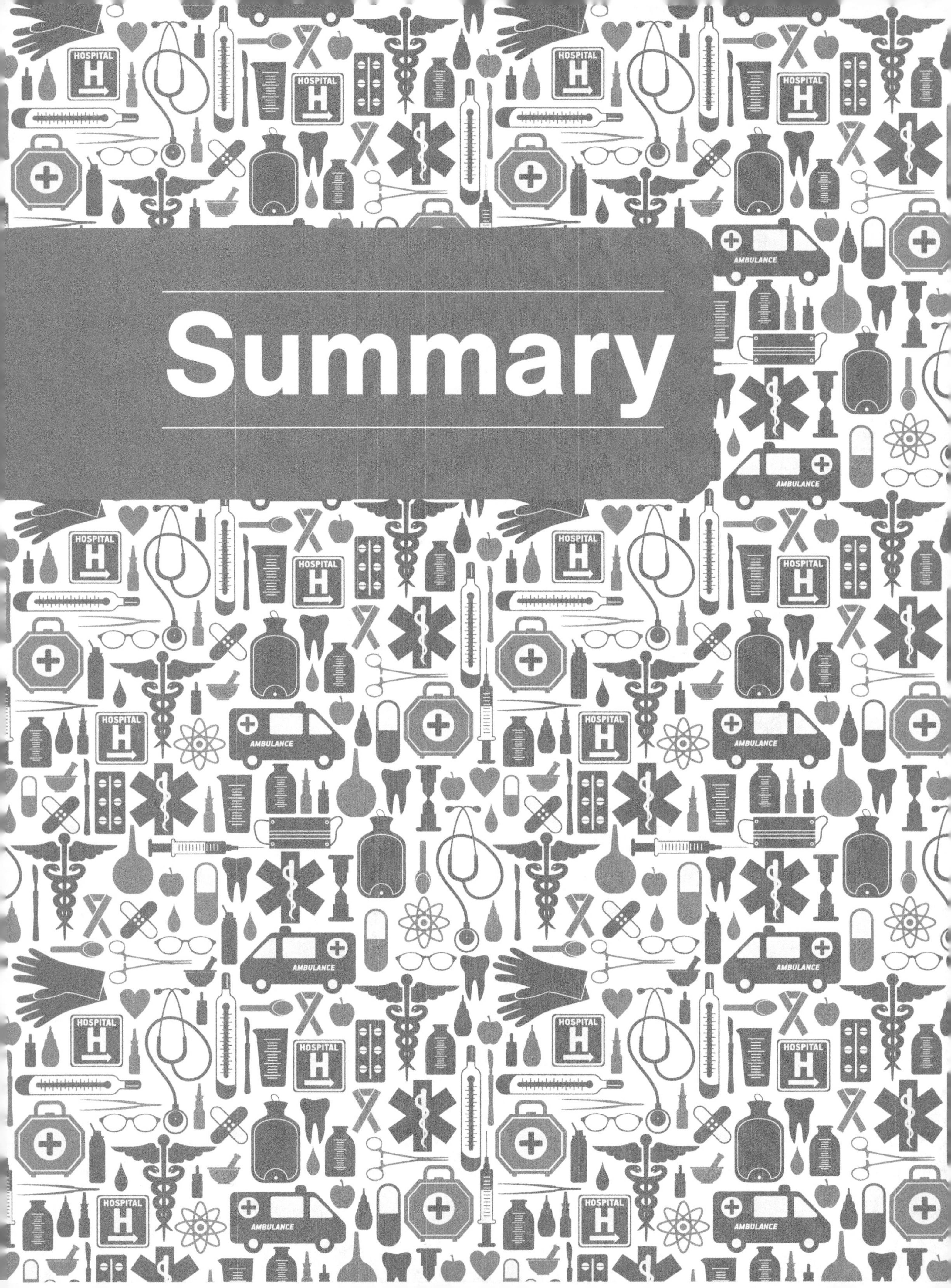
Summary

HOSPITAL
H
AMBULANCE

Made in the USA
Las Vegas, NV
27 February 2025

18798987R00136